PART 1

The Devil Is Diabetes

Praise for

DIABESITY

"A compelling combination of medical insight, practical treatment strategies, and Fran Kaufman's special passion for ways to prevent this devastating epidemic."

—James R. Gavin III, M.D., Ph.D., President, Morehouse School of Medicine; Chair, National Diabetes Education Program

"Parents today are unwittingly leading their children into a dietary danger zone. Dr. Kaufman's wise book lays out a clear path guiding families back to safety."

—Harvey Karp, M.D., author of *The Happiest Baby on the Block* and *The Happiest Toddler on the Block*

"A dramatic personal account of the modern obesity epidemic."

—Greg Critser, author of *Fat Land*

"Francine Kaufman is a warrior. Her enemies are type 2 diabetes and obesity, preventable conditions that menace our nation's health. In this inspiring book, she leads us toward solutions."

—Miriam Nelson, Ph.D., author of *Strong Women Stay Young* and *Strong Women Stay Slim*

"Francine Kaufman writes with clarity and compassion, blending cutting-edge science with the stories of those affected. She makes a compelling case for change as individuals and as a society."

—David S. Ludwig, M.D., Ph.D., Director, Obesity Program, Children's Hospital, Boston

"A gem . . . coupling insightful analysis with creative recommendations for what might be done."

—Kelly D. Brownell, Ph.D., author of *Food Fight;* Director, Yale Center for Eating and Weight Disorders

"Francine Kaufman is a passionate crusader in the battle to turn the tide of one of the largest epidemics in the history of man."

—Paul Zimmet, M.D., Ph.D., Director of the International Diabetes Institute, Melbourne, Australia

DIABESITY

A Doctor and Her Patients

on the Front Lines of the

Obesity-Diabetes Epidemic

FRANCINE RATNER KAUFMAN, M.D.

Professor of Pediatrics
The Keck School of Medicine
of the University of Southern California

Head, Center for Diabetes,
Endocrinology and Metabolism, Childrens Hospital Los Angeles

Past President of the American Diabetes Association

BANTAM BOOKS

New York   Toronto   London   Sydney   Auckland

DIABESITY

A Bantam Book

PUBLISHING HISTORY

Bantam hardcover edition published March 2005
Bantam trade paperback edition / February 2006

Published by
Bantam Dell
A Division of Random House, Inc.
New York, New York

Book design by Patrice Sheridan

Library of Congress Catalog Card Number: 2004054189

ISBN-10: 0-553-38379-5
ISBN-13: 978-0-553-38379-9

Printed in the United States of America
Published simultaneously in Canada

www.bantamdell.com

BVG   10   9   8   7   6   5   4   3   2

To Neal

In memory of my parents and Grandma Sadie

Contents

Part 3: Engines of Change

DIABESITY

A Tale of Two Children

The blaring telephone woke me from the already fitful sleep of a night on call. I struggled desperately to lift my mind from semi-consciousness. The year was 1981; the time was 1:30 a.m. At that hour, a ringing phone meant a critically ill child.

I'm a pediatric endocrinologist. Since 1978 I have cared for youngsters with diabetes. I've also worked with adults with this dread disease, as a researcher, teacher, and advocate. In 2002, I was elected president of the American Diabetes Association.

Many people today think of diabetes as a slow-moving chronic disease. But it can be swift and merciless, particularly when it attacks young children. An abnormally high blood sugar level, the hallmark of diabetes, is always a medical emergency. In my early years as a doctor, first as an intern and then as a resident, I spent every third night on call, ready to go into battle against diabetes. The telephone call on that night in 1981 came from the emergency department resident. He told me that a nine-month-old baby named Cameron had been rushed to Childrens Hospital Los Angeles in a coma. Cameron's blood sugar was ten times higher than normal. No one in the emergency department had ever seen such a high number. By the time the resident finished his terse description, I was on my feet, fully awake.

I had recently completed my fellowship in pediatric endocrinology, the specialized training that follows residency, and I'd joined
the staff at Childrens Hospital, where I now head the Center for Diabetes, Endocrinology and Metabolism. My husband, Neal, who
was also establishing a medical career, was out of town at a professional meeting. We had two young children: Adam, age three, and
Jonah, who was almost one. Our babysitter had quit that afternoon,
and I'd spent most of the evening patching together child care
arrangements for the coming week. I'd fallen into bed at midnight,
even more exhausted than usual.

A close friend had promised to babysit if I needed to go to the
hospital in the middle of the night, but time was too short. Cameron
was already unconscious. If his blood sugar wasn't brought down to
a normal level in just the right way, he might not survive the night. I
ran to the kitchen with a tote bag and grabbed a plastic bottle of
juice for Jonah and other supplies. Then I carried both boys to the
car and fastened them into their car seats, trying not to awaken
them. I drove with dread anticipation to the hospital.

Cameron was my first concern, but I also had to find some secure spot for my children. Carrying one sleeping child in each arm,
I entered ER Room 2. This is the room nearest to the ambulance
bay. It's larger than the other ER rooms, with special equipment and
extra space so more people can fit. You're brought to Room 2 when
you're in real trouble. The resident brushed past me; he was rushing
a blood sample to the lab. Cameron lay on the bed, naked, his tiny
body pale and motionless. Hovering over him were two of the ER
interns, a respiratory nurse, and Esther, the ER's senior nurse.
Around them, machines beeped and monitors flashed. An IV
dripped fluid into Cameron's limp body.

Cameron was so thin I could count every rib. His lips were dry;
his eyes were sunken in his head and tearless—all obvious signs of
dehydration. Despite the lack of fluid in his body, the sheet under
him was soaked, indicating he was urinating copiously because of his
diabetes. His breathing was deep and labored. I could smell a fruity
odor on his breath, another sign of his disease.

Even though his appearance was what I had expected, I was still
shocked to see such a gravely ill infant. His mother—slender,

young, and alone—sat in a corner of Room 2. She looked over-whelmed by the commotion surrounding her child. Holding my own two children in my arms, I ran to Cameron's mother and intro-duced myself as Dr. Kaufman, the diabetes specialist. Then I mo-tioned to Esther to step into the hall. "I'm going to need some help with my boys," I told her.

Esther shook her head. "We're already short of staff," she said. "I can't spare anyone for babysitting. Put them on those arm-chairs"—she pointed to two chairs in the hallway—"so you can keep an eye on them." Esther slid the chairs to face each other, forming a makeshift crib.

Adam curled up on his chair without awakening. But when I put Jonah on the chair facing Adam, he began to whimper. I dug the plastic bottle out of the tote bag. Jonah grabbed it and flung it across the hall. Juice sprayed out like a fountain. Now he was crying incon-solably. I knew that if he awakened Adam I'd be sunk. So I lifted him up and held him against my shoulder. As soon as he quieted, I hur-ried back into Room 2 and began to examine Cameron.

Carrying my own son with my left arm, I poked Cameron's ab-domen with the fingers of my right hand. He didn't flinch, which told me he was deeply unconscious. When I removed my fingertips, little white circles remained on his skin, indicating extremely poor circulation. Cameron's mother stared, no doubt startled by the sight of a doctor at work while holding her own baby.

SUGAR TURNS TOXIC

Diabetes can devastate nearly every system of the body, but it all starts with the metabolism of glucose, a type of sugar. Glucose is what fuels our every move and our every thought. The glucose we need comes from the food we eat. But our body can't use it without insulin, a hormone produced by the pancreas. As I'll explain shortly, diabetes comes in different forms. In all of them, insulin is unable to play its proper role.

Because Cameron had lost the ability to process sugar, his cells were starving. That's why he was so thin. Meanwhile, sugar had accumulated to toxic levels in his blood—a condition called hyper-glycemia. His body was drawing water from his tissues, trying to flush out the excess sugar in his urine. That's why he was urinating excessively. And because so much water was leaving his body, he had become severely dehydrated. Desperate for calories, he had begun burning stored fat. The fruity aroma of his breath came from ke-tones, a by-product of his abnormal metabolism. The ketones were making Cameron's blood dangerously acidic. Despite his body's at-tempt to blow these acids out with his breath, he could not exhale them fast enough. This condition, called diabetic ketoacidosis, can lead to coma and even death.

To bring Cameron back to life, he would need infusions of in-sulin, as well as salts and fluids to counter the effects of dehydration and ketoacidosis. Balancing these inputs is crucial and never easy. But it's especially tricky with a tiny infant. Intravenous fluid was es-sential, but fluid with the wrong salt concentration or excess fluid—or in some cases even the right amount of fluid—could cause fatal swelling of the brain.

The resident burst in from the lab with the test results. "The first blood sugar was 1,050 milligrams per deciliter; the repeat is down to 953," he told me. A normal sugar level for an infant is no higher than 110 milligrams per deciliter (mg/dl). Back then, in 1981, we could measure blood sugar in the ER with a drop of blood and a glucose strip. But the strips in the ER didn't register if the level was that high, so Cameron's blood had been checked in the hospital laboratory. "I didn't think someone could be alive with blood sugar at that level," the resident whispered, not wanting Cameron's mother to hear.

I told Esther what fluids Cameron needed and at what rate they had to be given. Jonah lifted his head from my shoulder and began to whimper. I ordered more blood tests to assess Cameron's body chemistry. Jonah was crying now. I rocked back and forth, trying to soothe him as I struggled to calculate how much insulin to put into Cameron's intravenous infusion. By the time I gave Esther the or-der, Jonah was screaming.

Cameron's mother was watching all this, visibly nervous. Finally she approached and said to me, "Dr. Kaufman—that's your name, right?"

"Yes," I responded. My child was crying hysterically, but I spoke as calmly as I could, trying to look as if I had the situation under control. Cameron's mother knew her son's life was in danger. She was terrified and exhausted and I wanted desperately to reassure her. But Jonah was inconsolable. I felt frustrated and embarrassed.

"I'll tell you what," she said. "I'll hold your child if you'll save mine."

We were two mothers. Our eyes met, and a look of understanding instantly passed between us. I transferred my baby to her, just as she had given hers to me. She took my son and held him tight. He quieted down. She rocked him, ran his blanket gently across his cheek, and hummed to him. Tears streamed down her face. Within minutes, my son was asleep in her arms.

Shortly after 6:00 a.m., Cameron's eyes opened. He took in the unfamiliar surroundings and the hovering strangers in white coats. Then he opened his mouth and screamed—the first sound he'd made through this terrifying night, other than his labored breathing. Cameron's mother lifted her head. We smiled at each other. Even Esther, whose face had been set in a worried frown, grinned with delight. Cameron had made it back from the abyss; he had recovered from diabetic ketoacidosis. Now he faced the rest of his life with diabetes. But as I told his mother, with scrupulously careful management of his disease, that life could be a long and healthy one.

TYPE 1 VERSUS TYPE 2

Diabetes takes two forms. Cameron suffered from type 1. His immune system had destroyed the beta cells in his pancreas, the cells that produce insulin, so he was unable to make this essential hormone. Type 1 diabetes typically appears in childhood and progresses rapidly. Fortunately, type 1 is relatively rare. Ninety percent of people with diabetes have the other kind, which is known as type 2. In type 2 diabetes, the key problem is not that insulin is lacking; rather, the body's cells don't respond normally to it. As with type 1, the cells go hungry while, paradoxically, glucose accumulates in the blood.

When I was in medical school in the 1970s, we were taught that type 2 diabetes was a disease of aging. It usually comes on gradually, typically making its appearance after age fifty. Over time, cells throughout the body become less sensitive to insulin, and the pancreas compensates by producing more. After a while, the pancreas is no longer able to manufacture this excessive amount of insulin, and the blood sugar level rises.

No one could ignore for long the dramatic symptoms of type 1 diabetes. Until insulin treatment became available in 1922, people with this disease typically died within months of diagnosis. But the signs of type 2 diabetes can be hard to spot: fatigue, frequent urination, slower healing of sores. In fact, the symptoms are so subtle that almost a third of those with this form of diabetes have no idea they have the disease. If they're lucky, they'll discover it during a routine physical examination. But some people first learn they have diabetes when they develop complications: suddenly their vision is blurred, or they're felled by a heart attack or stroke.

There's another important difference between the two forms of diabetes. Though we can treat type 1, we can't cure it and we don't yet know how to prevent it. But type 2 is different, because it's strongly associated with excess weight. Simply by maintaining a healthy weight, people can significantly cut their risk of developing this terrible disease. What's more, they can even cure it at its early stages if they achieve and maintain a normal weight.

Though the vast majority of adult diabetes cases are type 2, the reverse is true in children. In fact, during my first fifteen years as a pediatric endocrinologist, I never saw a young patient with type 2 diabetes. But then everything changed.

"I CAN'T FIGURE OUT WHY SHE STILL LOOKS SO GOOD"

In the middle of a spring day in 1995, I received a call from an emergency department doctor, asking if I could see a thirteen-year-old patient named Tanesha and her family right away. Tanesha's blood sugar level was 427 mg/dl, at least four times higher than normal for a young teen.

I was in my office at the hospital, and my appointment schedule was solidly booked. The waiting room and all the examining rooms were filled with patients and parents. But that didn't matter. I had to see Tanesha immediately because of her alarmingly high blood sugar. Hearing the number, I pictured a typical type 1 patient referred from the emergency department: thin and severely weakened by dehydration, nausea, and fatigue—maybe even comatose, like Cameron. But I soon learned that Tanesha didn't fit that picture.

"Tanesha has been hyperglycemic for at least two weeks," the ER doctor told me. "I can't figure out why she still looks so good. And you won't believe how big this girl is. She's the fattest kid with diabetes I've ever seen." Despite her elevated blood sugar, Tanesha was barely symptomatic. She didn't feel weak or exhausted; she hadn't vomited. Instead, she was hungry. While Tanesha waited in the ER, she'd eaten a bag of fries and downed a can of soda. "By the way," the doctor added, "Tanesha is African American." This too was puzzling. Type 1 diabetes is rarer in non-white children.

Even though I'd been told that Tanesha was overweight, and even though she was not sick after a long bout of hyperglycemia, it didn't dawn on me that she might have type 2 diabetes. Not in 1995. Only when I walked into the examining room did it become apparent that my thinking was all wrong. Tanesha was there with her mother and her grandmother, who was in a wheelchair. Each of them weighed at least 250 pounds. I realized that I might be walking into a whole new world. I felt scared and shocked.

Two weeks earlier, during a routine health evaluation at a pediatric clinic in Los Angeles, Tanesha's urine test had revealed a high level of sugar. Despite the fact that large amounts of sugar in the urine require immediate attention, Tanesha was not called back for a confirmatory blood test for ten days. When she returned, her blood sugar level was 443 mg/dl. Though this pointed to a potentially dangerous situation, it was another two days before Tanesha arrived at the Childrens Hospital's emergency department.

I had visited that underfunded and understaffed pediatric clinic in downtown Los Angeles. The doctors who worked there were dedicated. But they were overwhelmed by enormous caseloads and the catastrophic health problems that poverty brings. It was easy to understand why no one had considered Tanesha's situation urgent— after all, she didn't seem sick. But I was pained by the knowledge that if she had been an affluent suburban child, it most likely wouldn't have taken nearly two weeks for her to receive appropriate medical attention.

I introduced myself to Tanesha, her mother, and her grand-mother. Tanesha shook my hand, smiled, and looked me straight in the eye. I was impressed by her poise. A glance at her chart told me that her height—5 feet 3 inches—was normal for a girl of thirteen. But she weighed 267 pounds. As I examined her, I was struck by something I had rarely seen in children: extensive darkening of the skin around her neck. I'd seen this condition, called *acanthosis nigricans*, in adults with type 2 diabetes. Could this thirteen-year-old girl have type 2 diabetes? That would explain why she wasn't acutely ill; unlike a child with type 1 diabetes, she was still producing insulin.

I began to question Tanesha about her symptoms. Her answers confirmed the possibility.

"Are you thirsty?" I asked.

She told me she'd been drinking a lot of juice and soda. "My mama told me to stop drinking so much, but I told her I was just thirsty all the time, day and night," she informed me. I appreciated her candor.

"How about urination?" I asked. "Do you have to pee at night?"

"Yeah, but that's only 'cause I get up to drink," she explained. "If I didn't need to drink so much, I mightn't need to pee so much."

Tanesha was intelligent, and she'd clearly thought about her symptoms. But she actually had it backward. Her body was trying to rid itself of excess sugar by urinating. And because she was losing so much water, she was constantly thirsty.

I asked, "How long have you been waking up at night to urinate?" This would tell me how long her blood sugar had been elevated.

She thought and then answered, "At least for this whole year."

Her response crystallized my thinking: Tanesha had type 2 diabetes. How could that be? And then I looked over at her grandmother and thought: "Just like her grandma."

I didn't need to see blood test results to guess that Tanesha's grandmother had type 2 diabetes. She was obese and sat in a wheelchair. Her face drooped on one side, suggesting that she'd had a stroke. People with diabetes have an elevated risk for strokes and heart attacks.

I asked the grandmother about her medical history, half expecting her daughter, Tanesha's mother, to reply on her behalf. But the older woman's physical problems had not diminished the force of her personality. Her daughter and granddaughter sat silently as she answered my questions.

"They told me I had the sugar in 1966," she said. "They took my foot in 1987. Gangrene." I looked at the footrest of her wheelchair and recognized the special orthopedic shoe. Her right foot had been amputated, probably a result of the nerve and blood circulation problems that can develop from diabetes. In 1990 Tanesha's grandmother had suffered a mild heart attack, followed by a stroke in 1993. The stroke had left her left leg spastic and her left arm paralyzed. "I been going to therapy for two years pretty regular. Still can't open my hand," she said.

"What medications do you take?" I asked.

"Them doctors tried to get me to take insulin. But insulin makes you sick," she said defiantly.

Tanesha's mother rolled her eyes at this. She pulled a sheet of paper from her purse and handed it to me. Tanesha's grandmother was supposed to take three medications to control her blood sugar, two more to lower her blood pressure, aspirin to prevent heart attacks and strokes, and a cholesterol-lowering drug. I wondered how many of those pills she actually took.

"Tanesha will be okay, Doc," the elderly woman continued. "Everybody has a little bit of the sugar in our family, 'cept my daughter here. We don't need to pay it no mind. And we don't need to think 'bout putting her on no insulin shots. Don't you worry, Tanesha," she said, turning to her granddaughter. "You don't need none of those shots, and we don't need to pay the doctor no mind, either."

I was shocked. This woman needed handfuls of medicines; she'd been through a heart attack, a stroke, and an amputation—all because of diabetes. If that was only a "little bit of the sugar," what would be a lot?

Tanesha would require insulin injections, at least at the beginning of her treatment. After that, I hoped, her blood sugar levels would stabilize and she'd be able to take pills for her diabetes. I hadn't expected her grandmother to attempt to thwart me. I turned my attention to Tanesha's mother. I needed to convince her that her daughter's condition was serious and to win her over to my side. Tanesha also needed to be persuaded. But I didn't want to frighten either of them too much.

"The blood tests show that Tanesha has diabetes," I explained. "There's no doubt about it. Any sugar test above 200 indicates diabetes—and hers is over 400." I quickly turned to Tanesha and added, "We'll do some more tests to find out what kind of diabetes you have. That will help determine how to treat you." Tanesha nodded, her expression somber. Her mother blinked back tears.

"Almost all children with diabetes have what we call type 1 diabetes. But Tanesha may actually have type 2, just like her grandmother," I explained. I didn't want to get too technical—not after the shocking news I'd just delivered. "If Tanesha has type 2 diabetes, we may be able to treat her with pills eventually. But her blood sugar is too high now for the pills to work. The first step is to get her blood sugar levels normal, to stop all that drinking and urinating." Then I added, "We must get her well again, so that she doesn't ever have to face what her grandma has faced because of her diabetes."

I looked at Tanesha's mother to see if I'd made an impression. She remained expressionless for what seemed like a lifetime. Finally she responded in a quiet but very firm voice: "We will do what you say, Dr. Kaufman. My whole life, I've watched diabetes eat my mother to pieces, because she doesn't take care of herself. No way will I let that happen to Tanesha." As she spoke, Tanesha's grandmother glared at her but remained silent.

I sighed with relief. The first battle was won; I would be allowed to treat Tanesha with the medications she required. But that was just the beginning. Tanesha was only thirteen years old. She would need to control her blood sugar for the rest of her life. Would she be able to meet this challenge? If not, I feared the diabetes complications that might affect her. Problems that typically take two or three decades to develop could strike Tanesha by age forty. I also worried about her mother, who was as overweight as her daughter. Had she been checked for diabetes? Would this disease overtake the entire family?

One thing was clear: we would have to do everything possible to encourage Tanesha to modify her eating habits and become more active. She desperately needed to lose weight. I hoped her mother would do the same for her own sake. It seemed unlikely that her grandmother would change, but maybe I could persuade her not to stand in Tanesha's way. Then there would be the constant battle with the rest of the world. Everywhere Tanesha turned she'd be surrounded by the junk food, soft drinks, and candy that threatened her health.

In that clinic room in 1995, I knew that a world of battles would have to be fought for Tanesha. What I didn't know was that this skirmish was the harbinger of a much larger war to come.

THE EMERGENCE OF DIABESITY

In 1990, 4.9 percent of the American adult population had diabetes. The prevalence was up to 6.5 percent in 1998—and by 2002, it had soared to 8.7 percent in adults. Ninety percent of them have type 2. In just over a decade, diabetes nearly doubled. Unless current trends can be stopped, experts predict that within a few years over 10 percent of adults in the United States will have diabetes.

Why this dramatic change? The answer is simple. The increase in diabetes mirrors the increased incidence of obesity, which has reached epidemic proportions in our nation and around the world. Currently, there are 45 million obese adults in the United States. That is almost 30 percent of the adult population—and they're all at elevated risk for diabetes. As experts became alarmed by the closely linked epidemics of obesity and type 2 diabetes, some began referring to the two as a single problem. They called this dual epidemic *diabesity*. Shape Up America, an organization founded in 1994 by former United States Surgeon General C. Everett Koop to raise awareness of the adverse health effects of obesity, trademarked the term diabesity as part of his effort to promote a healthy lifestyle.

At first, these disturbing trends didn't seem directly relevant to my pediatric practice. But families like Tanesha's are common now: a massively obese child and that youngster's equally heavy relatives, some of whom—even men and women in their twenties, thirties, or forties—already show the terrible long-term effects of diabetes. Once the province of the elderly, type 2 diabetes has become a disease of middle age and even young adulthood. Now type 2 is attacking children, too.

Before the mid-1990s, it was so rare for pediatric centers to diagnose children with type 2 diabetes that doctors sometimes wrote up these cases for medical journals. In fact, the most common term for type 2 used to be "adult-onset diabetes." By 1996, reports in the medical literature from across the country confirmed that type 2 diabetes was occurring in greater numbers of children and youth. In 1997, an international committee sponsored by the American Diabetes Association recommended that the term "adult-onset diabetes" be dropped. Obviously, type 2 was no longer limited to adults.

The reason we're seeing type 2 diabetes in children, and the reason it's appearing in adults at earlier ages than ever before, is that obesity is escalating in our youth. In the early 1970s, 4 percent of children and 6 percent of adolescents were obese. Over the past three decades, both of these numbers have climbed to nearly 16 percent—and they will continue to increase unless we act. Think of youngsters with type 2 diabetes as the proverbial canaries in the coal mine: they signal that something is very wrong and endangers us all.

An estimated 18.2 million Americans have diabetes. This number is an estimate because we know that about a third of people with type 2, by far the most common form, are not yet diagnosed. Even more ominous: more than twice as many people—41 million Americans—have blood sugar in a higher-than-normal range, a condition we call pre-diabetes. They don't have diabetes yet, but they're on the path and have begun marching in that direction. My colleagues and I are racing after them, trying to head them off. If we can pull them back from pre-diabetes, they may never develop type 2 or its dire complications.

Diabetes is the sixth leading cause of death in the United States. The disease was directly responsible for 71,000 deaths in the United States in 2002, but a total of more than 186,000 people died from reasons linked to diabetes, such as cardiovascular disease. Diabetes increases the risk for heart disease sixfold and multiplies the risk of stroke by four.

This supreme medical villain damages organs, destroys cells, and shortens lives. Every year in the United States, 24,000 people go blind because of diabetes. Twenty-eight thousand people end up in kidney failure from diabetes. To survive, they must either undergo frequent dialysis to have their blood cleansed by a kidney machine or obtain a kidney transplant. Eighty-two thousand people with diabetes will have an amputation this year, losing a toe, a foot, or even a leg. A recent study by scientists at the Centers for Disease Control and Prevention (CDC) estimated that men diagnosed with diabetes by age forty will lose more than eleven years of life and women will lose more than fourteen years. The CDC investigators also looked at what medical researchers call "quality-adjusted life years"—life expectancy adjusted for ill health or disability. After all, an extra year of vibrant good health is more meaningful than an extra year in which illness greatly limits normal activity. These findings were even more horrifying. Men diagnosed at age forty lost nearly nineteen years of quality life to diabetes; for women, the loss was twenty-two years.

Although this disease can strike anyone, the danger is even greater among certain racial and ethnic groups. African Americans are 1.6 times more likely to develop diabetes than whites of a similar age. On average, the risk is 1.5 times higher for Hispanic Americans—but it's 2.0 times higher for Mexican Americans. Native Americans also have 2.0 times the risk of diabetes compared to whites. These differences are in part due to genetics and in part due to lifestyle.

In my day-to-day life as a doctor, I see the human toll of diabetes. I see children suffering with this unrelenting illness, pregnant women burdened, adults ravaged, and the elderly put in their graves. Watching this suffering compels me to push forward to find better answers, more effective treatments, and a more equitable environment. When I attend meetings of the American Diabetes Association, work on my grants from the National Institutes of Health, and read the medical journals, the shocking economic costs come to light.

Many of my patients struggle to pay for the treatments they need to be well. But all of us—even if we're in perfect health—pick up the bill for the devastation caused by diabetes. This disease ranks number one in direct costs, consuming one healthcare dollar of every seven. In the U.S. in 2002, the tab for diabetes-related doctor visits, medications, and hospitalizations was a staggering $92 billion. The bottom line comes to $137.7 billion if you add the indirect costs for lost wages and lost work productivity due to diabetes. And unless the diabesity epidemic is reversed, these numbers will rise even more.

If we could prevent obesity, type 2 diabetes would become rare. On one level, the solution is simple. Obesity, as we all know, results from consuming more calories than are burned in physical activity. In theory, all it should take to prevent the problem is for people to eat less and move more—in other words, to become personally responsible for maintaining a healthy lifestyle. But obesity and diabetes are much more complex than that. The genes hidden inside each of our cells predetermine if diabetes can happen or not. And the genes related to diabetes likely make someone want to eat more and end up weighing more. In addition, a person's environment is critically important. The children and teens who develop type 2 diabetes typically live in families, go to schools, and inhabit neighborhoods where it's difficult to find nutritious, affordable food and safe places for physical activity.

We can't simply blame diabesity on gluttony and laziness. Nor can we assume that the sole solution is individual change. Listening to my young patients talk about their lives, I become angry at a society that doesn't seem to care, at an economic structure that makes it cheaper to eat fries than fruit, and at the food industry and the mass media luring children to consume what should not be consumed. As

I walk by the nursery in Childrens Hospital, I shudder to realize how many of these babies will develop diabetes sometime during their lives unless our society can make drastic changes: more than one in three whites, about two in five blacks, and one in two Hispanics.

The diabetes and obesity epidemics are not confined to the borders of the United States. We are witnessing an epidemic that is the scourge of the twenty-first century. In 2002 I attended a conference in Hong Kong on type 2 diabetes. Countries from across the globe were represented, and it became obvious that most developed nations and many developing ones were facing the same problem. In fact, some of the world's nations were experiencing worse epidemics than ours.

A CALL TO ACTION

In 2002 I was honored to be chosen president of the American Diabetes Association, which is the nation's leading nonprofit health organization providing diabetes research, information, and advocacy. A year later, as is customary, I gave my presidential address. My speech was a call to action. In the audience were healthcare providers, educators, researchers, and people touched by diabetes. Diabesity requires action from every one of them—in fact, from everyone. To solve this problem will require drastic changes in our society. That's why I decided to write this book. I want to share my experiences as a diabetes doctor, researcher, and advocate. I want you to see what diabetes and obesity have done to the many patients and people I know and care for, so you will understand why we must restructure the way we live.

The first section of my book explains the impact of diabetes on children, adults, and families. You'll learn more about the two kinds of diabetes, how they are diagnosed, how they affect the body, and how they're treated. I'll take you to the bedside as a young wife clings to her dying husband, to the emergency room as we rush to bring children back from the brink, and to the clinic at Childrens Hospital Los Angeles where families learn the daunting routine of daily diabetes care. You will walk with me into their lives, open their medicine cabinets, see their fingers stuck with needles and their cells damaged by disease. I'll show you that diabetes leaves emotional as well as physical scars—yet patients and their families learn to triumph over adversity.

In the second section of the book, I'll present the history of diabetes and obesity, describing how they have emerged as human disorders. We humans evolved over 2.5 million years and many thousands of generations. But our basic DNA has changed surprisingly little over the past 40,000 years. In other words, our genes were designed for living in caves, eating the plants we gathered and the animals we killed, communicating via smoke signals, and running around pretty much stark naked. Meanwhile, our lifestyle has altered dramatically. Only in the past few decades have our genes needed to figure out how to metabolize a bacon cheeseburger, soda, and fries. Our ancient genes and our modern environment have collided. Unless our environment changes, the diabesity epidemic imperils human existence as we now know it.

The last section of my book offers solutions for individuals, families, workplaces, schools, and the healthcare sector. These changes will require resolve, bold leadership, and a set of comprehensive strategies that cross the breadth and depth of our lives.

The course of our ancestors over thousands of years has been to transform the world so that we may eat and thrive. Nothing illustrates this better than America, the land of plenty, where there's a chicken in every pot and a car in every garage. My relatives came to her shores dreaming of such miracles, but they discovered that even miracles can be tainted with disaster and disease.

Americans have defined progress in terms of the quantity rather than the quality of our food. We've also defined progress as the elimination of any requirement for physical activity in our jobs and for transportation, ignoring its importance for our health. And thanks to this brand of "progress," we've managed to devise a world designed to kill us.

But we don't have to be the creators of our own demise. We don't have to watch 300 million people worldwide develop diabetes by 2020, as is presently projected. We have the opportunity to demand of our leaders, of our healthcare system, of our communities, and of ourselves that the world become a place in which it is possible to live not just a long life but a healthy one—a world in which we can have normal blood sugar, normal blood pressure, normal blood fats, normal weight, healthy meals, and a safe walk through the park. I hope you will join me to set a new course, redefine and redirect progress, and stop the diabesity epidemic.

Diabetes Descends on My Grandma Sadie

Ilearned to hate diabetes in 1960, when I was nine years old. One morning I woke up and my grandmother Sadie, whose room was right next to mine, wasn't there. My mother told me, "Grandma Sadie got sick in the middle of the night, and your father had to take her to the hospital. When she comes back, nothing will be the same."

My mother spent the day cleaning out our entire kitchen and pantry. The cookies and cakes disappeared. The candy box that she kept in the freezer was brought over to my aunt's house. I was mystified—and frightened.

In the evening, my mother sat down with my two brothers and me. She explained that our grandmother had diabetes. She would take shots every day. And she would need to eat special food to be healthy—no candies or cookies or cake. "All of us will follow Grandma's diet," my mother announced. "So there will be no more treats in the house. This diet will be healthy for all of us."

I didn't think this diet sounded healthy at all. I thought it sounded unfair. Just because my grandmother had this thing called diabetes, why did I have to give up treats? In that instant, I hated diabetes. I hated diabetes because it made my grandmother sick and I was worried she would die. I hated diabetes because it took away all my favorite foods. I didn't know exactly what this disease was, but I vowed to get back at diabetes some day.

My father brought my grandmother home from the hospital a few days later. He carried three large shopping bags into the kitchen. I watched him make room in the pantry for packages of medicine and the needles and syringes for my grandmother's insulin injections. My grandmother sat at the kitchen table, waiting for her first shot. Even though my brothers were older, they were scared and didn't want to watch. But I was fascinated. My father was a physician, and I was already determined to be one, too. As my father put the needle into her arm, my grandmother screamed. I ran to her side. "Does it hurt, Grandma?"

"Not so much," she answered in her thick Russian accent. "I'm just a little scared. Even grandmas get a little scared."

I looked at her arm, expecting to see blood. But there was none. "Can I touch it?" I asked.

"Vhy not?" (My grandmother's *W*'s always came out as *V*'s.) Gently, I touched her arm where my father had given her the insulin injection. It didn't feel any different.

I asked her why she'd gotten diabetes. She shrugged. "The doctor at the hospital told me my veight not good. Such a young man— from vhat does he know? He said I got diabetes 'cause I eat too many sweets. Maybe I eat a piece of that chocolate cake your mother makes, and sometimes, when no one looks, I sneak maybe some candy. Vhy not?"

My mother's chocolate cake was rich and incredibly delicious. Wow, I thought, Grandma got diabetes because of my mother's chocolate cake. If such a thing could happen, then there was little that was safe anywhere at all.

LEARNING ABOUT MEDICINE— AND DIABETES

I grew up in a suburb of Chicago, Illinois, in the 1950s and 1960s. One day my father removed my doll collection from a shelf in my room and replaced it with his old medical books. "I want you to become a doctor," he told me, and I agreed. I was four years old.

My desire never wavered. In sixth grade my teacher assigned an essay topic: What You Want to Be When You Grow Up. I wrote what was in my heart: "I want to become a doctor so I can do good, help other people, and diminish suffering." This treatise earned me an F. I was a conscientious student and had never before received a failing grade in anything. I ran home with tears streaming down my face. Sobbing, I called my father at his office. He left work immediately and went straight to my school. The teacher explained to him that she'd given me an F because girls weren't supposed to be doctors. I don't know exactly how my father responded, but the next day my teacher told me that my grade had been changed from an F to an A.

In college, I was a pre-med major from the start. On the first day of freshman biology the professor said, "Look to the left and look to the right. Half or more of you will be gone soon, and it's likely to be those wearing dresses." I was wearing jeans that day, not a dress, and I had no intention of leaving. The course was tough. By the end of the semester, close to 75 percent of the students, including most of the women, had dropped out. Today, about half of medical students are female. But when I entered medical school, only about 10 percent were women.

The first two years of medical school were spent in classrooms and labs. At that point, I hadn't yet decided what kind of doctor I wanted to become. During the third and fourth years, we were sent out of the classroom and into hospitals to learn first-hand how to care for patients. In a series of rotations, each lasting eight to twelve weeks, we were divided into small groups and exposed to all the specialties—internal medicine, emergency medicine, obstetrics and gynecology, neurology, surgery, psychiatry, and pediatrics. Five to ten medical students would trail an experienced specialist as he or (rarely) she examined and treated patients. Under supervision, we began to perform examinations, order tests and medications, and perform procedures. After two or three months, we'd rotate to a new specialty.

One day during our internal medicine rotation, we were called to the emergency room. A heavy middle-aged man had been brought in by ambulance with severe chest pain. He was clutching his chest and barely able to catch his breath. His wife, torn between anger at her husband and terror that he might die, told us that he had been given medication by his doctor but refused to take it. The ER staff quickly made the diagnosis—an acute heart attack—and leaped into action. My fellow students were thrilled by the medical heroics: defibrillation paddles clapped to the patient's chest, the continuous electrocardiogram (EKG) tracing spilling its paper onto the floor, the intravenous drip of lifesaving medications. But I felt frustrated that we hadn't been able to prevent this disaster. On that day I knew that I didn't want to deal with disease only after it reached a crisis point, when it might be too late to help.

Pediatrics appealed to me because it was different. It offered the opportunity to work with children and adolescents to teach them how to stay healthy, physically and psychologically. I'd be able to prevent disease, to catch it early. I wanted to make a difference at the beginning of life—not just to intervene at its end.

During my internship in pediatrics, I decided to train in a sub-specialty. I wanted to learn one field in depth. The subject that appealed to me most was endocrinology, the study of glands, hormones, and the body's regulatory systems. I liked the logic of this field—the explanations of how things worked and how they went awry. Endocrinology captured the body's cadences and rhythms. Hormones were secreted in different concentrations throughout the day. Some ebbed and flowed like the tide; others rose and fell continuously, like the swells of waves. Some gushed like torrents; others trickled. I found poetry in the study of glands and decided I wanted to spend my life understanding them more.

I know that my decision to become an endocrinologist was also linked to memories of my grandmother. Diabetes is the most common endocrine disease, and its rhythms fascinated me. As insulin falls to a trickle, sugar swells to a storm. That storm overtook my Grandma Sadie. From the memorable day when the chocolate cake disappeared, until her death almost two decades later, diabetes was my grandmother's nemesis and it was part of our family life.

After Grandma's diagnosis, I pestered my father with questions

about the disease. My father was an internist, and he loved to teach
me about medicine. He told me that diabetes was first described in
antiquity, in 1535 BC. He read to me the quotation that had been
found on an Egyptian papyrus:

> Diabetes is a terrible affliction, not very frequent among men,
> being a melting down of the flesh and limbs into urine. The pa-
> tient never stops making water and the flow is incessant, like
> that of an aqueduct.

The word *diabetes* comes from the Greek word meaning
"siphon"—a pipe that's used to transfer liquid—because when you
have untreated diabetes, you can't stop urinating.

"The symptoms of diabetes are polyuria, polydipsia, and
polyphagia. They're called the three polys," my father told me.
Then he waited for me to ask what the words meant. *Poly*, I learned,
comes from the Greek word *polus*, meaning "many." The three
polys, translated into English, meant too much urination, too much
thirst, and too much eating.

My grandmother was always sipping a cup of tea, and she went
to the bathroom more often than anyone else in the family. But I'd
thought all elderly women were like that. During the months before
she was diagnosed with diabetes, it seemed like she was going to the
bathroom all the time. But only my grandmother and I knew about
this, because we shared a bathroom. Until my father explained it all
to me, I didn't realize she was showing warning signs of diabetes. I
also knew that my grandmother was heavy and that she loved to eat.
She often told us how she'd gone hungry during her childhood in
Russia. One of her brothers had starved to death. To her, the abundant food in America—being able to eat whatever and whenever she
wanted—was a miracle. My grandmother had once owned a candy
shop. She always carried candies in her pocket so she could eat them
and give them to everyone else. I wondered if she'd offered candies
to the doctors and nurses at the hospital even as they were telling
her she could have no more.

Though diabetes was known in ancient times, its cause was not discovered until many centuries later. In 1869 Paul Langerhans—a German doctor who studied anatomy—identified special cells arranged in peculiar islands in the pancreas. The islands were later named the *islets of Langerhans*. At the time of his discovery, Langerhans had no idea what purpose the pancreas or the islet cells served in the body. Because the pancreas is a gland located just behind the stomach, most scientists of that period assumed it played some role in digestion. They knew that the pancreas was damaged in some people who died from diabetes. But no one was sure whether this was cause or effect. Perhaps the damage was one of the many changes produced by the disease.

The mystery of the pancreas and diabetes was solved in 1889 by Oskar Minkowski and Joseph von Mering, two physiologists working at the University of Strasbourg, which was then in Germany and is now in France. They removed the pancreas of a healthy dog—and within days, the animal developed diabetes. This verified that the pancreas was responsible for maintaining normal sugar metabolism. Later experiments pinpointed the specific area of the pancreas: the islets of Langerhans. More than a century later, in September 2003, I lectured in Oskar Minkowski's hometown, Kaunas (now part of Lithuania), at the Third Oskar Minkowski Memorial Course of the European Association for the Study of Diabetes. Minkowski's picture hung above the podium. I have a photograph taken during my talk that I cherish, because it looks as though he is standing next to me.

In the decades after Minkowski and von Mering's discovery, scientists tried to isolate the essential component—the key to sugar metabolism—from the islets of Langerhans. Finally, in 1921, Frederick Banting, a Canadian surgeon, and associates at the University of Toronto succeeded after months of experimentation. They extracted material from the islets and injected it into dogs whose pancreases had been removed to induce diabetes. The preparation, which they called "isletin" at first, lowered the dogs' abnormally high blood sugar.

Shortly after this triumph, in December 1921, a fourteen-year-old boy named Leonard Thompson, near death from diabetes, was admitted to Toronto General Hospital. Because his body couldn't utilize glucose, Leonard weighed only 65 pounds and was as emaciated as a famine victim. The boy was listless, and his mind was dulled by his disease. He spent most of the day in bed. His skin was pale and his hair was falling out. Despite the efforts of his doctors, he continued to deteriorate. In January, Leonard's desperate father allowed Banting's team to inject his son with an improved version of their extract—and the child recovered dramatically. His abnormally high blood sugar quickly dropped, his energy returned, and his mind became sharp again. When the researchers reported their stunning news in a medical journal, they called the extract "insulin," from the Latin word for island.

Insulin, one of the great miracles of modern medicine, soon became widely available. In 1923, Frederick Banting and one of his associates shared a Nobel prize. Leonard Thompson—who had not been expected to live for more than a few months—survived another thirteen years. Insulin allows people with diabetes to manage their disease; it's not a cure. But it has saved millions of lives over the past eight decades.

THE DELICATE SUGAR BALANCE

Every time we eat, we set off the amazingly complicated series of events that make up our metabolic processes: all the chemical reactions that enable us to use food. We use food for energy; we use it for repairing old cells and for making new ones. Thanks to our metabolism, a tuna salad sandwich can fuel a walk in the park or find its way to a double chin. In healthy people, metabolic processes function automatically, without our thinking about them. But if you have diabetes, you need to understand how the food you eat affects your blood sugar levels. People diagnosed with diabetes should be immediately referred to a nutritionist to learn the basics, so they can manage their disease.

Everything we eat must be broken down into components that can circulate in the bloodstream. That's the job of the digestive system. The three major types of nutrients in food are fat, protein, and carbohydrates.

When fat is metabolized, it's turned into fatty acids and lipids that are released into the blood. If you're concerned about excess weight, you might not realize that fat is actually essential to good health—but it is. We need dietary fat to manufacture cells and some of the chemicals our body requires, including certain hormones and digestive acids.

The protein in our food is made up of long chains of amino acids. As food is metabolized, the chains are broken apart. These "links" of amino acids are sometimes called the building blocks of life. Our bodies reassemble them into new proteins, which are made into muscles, hormones, and other chemicals required for our functioning.

Carbohydrates—sugars and starches—are essential, too. To enter the bloodstream, starches and sugars must be broken down to glucose, a simple form of sugar. Our body extracts glucose not only from sweets such as candy and cake, but also from starchy foods such as grains and beans. Glucose is the body's main fuel. Without glucose, we couldn't move and we couldn't think. Our cells, particularly our brain cells, require a constant supply simply to maintain life.

Glucose can reach certain cells directly—the cells of the nervous system (including the brain), the red blood cells, and the cells that line our blood vessels. But most of our cells can't use glucose without insulin. In a healthy person, insulin and glucose match their moves like graceful dancers. As soon as we eat, the glucose level rises in our bloodstream. Sensors in the pancreas detect the change, and the pancreas releases a corresponding amount of insulin from special cells, called beta cells, in the islets of Langerhans. The insulin goes to receptors on cells throughout the body. Receptors are like docking stations: when insulin docks in its receptors, responses are triggered inside the cells that allow glucose to enter them. As glucose moves into our cells, the glucose level in our bloodstream drops. The pancreas senses the change and stops releasing insulin.

These mechanisms keep blood sugar levels remarkably steady. That's vitally important, because our body can't function properly if blood sugar is too low or too high. In the morning, after an overnight fast in which we've consumed no food at all, our blood sugar level normally doesn't fall below 70 milligrams per deciliter (mg/dl)—enough to ensure a steady supply of fuel to our brain and essential organs. And even after a large meal, our blood sugar concentration normally doesn't exceed 140 mg/dl, so we're protected against the harmful effects of excess sugar in the blood.

Our bodies are designed to maintain stability—or, as we say in medicine, homeostasis. Another important mechanism for this is our reserve fuel supplies. Thanks to these stores, we don't have to worry about running out of glucose if we skip a meal on a busy day or exercise for an hour or two. Indeed, most of us could survive for weeks or even months without food. The body's short-term storehouse—which might be tapped if we miss lunch or join a volleyball game and need extra energy—is the liver. The liver stockpiles glucose in the form of glycogen, which is made up of glucose molecules strung together. When our blood sugar level becomes low, the pancreas releases a hormone called glucagon, which signals the liver to discharge some of its glycogen stores. Glucagon is made in the islets of Langerhans of the pancreas, in the cells right next to the beta cells, which manufacture insulin. These cells communicate with one another, helping our blood sugar levels to remain stable. As insulin production rises—which happens when there's abundant glucose in the blood—glucagon production falls, because there's no need to tap the liver's glycogen stores.

We have another great fuel reserve: our body fat. When a person consumes more calories than his or her body can burn, insulin helps trigger metabolic processes that turn the excess food into fat. The average man or woman of normal weight has enough body fat to serve as fuel for a month or so. Of course, many people accumulate much more because they chronically eat more than their body requires. Stored fat is consumed as fuel when caloric intake is insufficient for our needs—for example, when we go on a diet or become ill and can't eat. In a dire situation, including starvation or following an unhealthy diet, the body can also use muscle tissue for fuel. But under normal circumstances, the glycogen reserves in our liver, along with our body fat, can provide all the backup energy we need.

METABOLISM DISRUPTED

The delicate balance of sugar metabolism is completely disrupted by diabetes. In type 1 diabetes, the insulin-producing cells—the beta cells in the islets of Langerhans—are destroyed by the body's own immune system. That's the type of diabetes that struck Cameron, the baby you met in Chapter 1. The immune system's normal job is to destroy outside invaders, such as germs, viruses, bacteria, and the abnormal cells that can cause cancer. The immune system is not supposed to attack the body itself. But in type 1 diabetes and other autoimmune disorders, it does. This happens when someone whose immune system has certain genetic alterations is exposed to a series of triggers—infections, toxins, and other environmental factors that are ubiquitous in our world. We haven't yet identified all of the type 1 diabetes genes or the exact triggers. But we do know that in order for the disease to occur, there must be interplay between genes and the environment.

In type 2 diabetes—the type my grandmother and Tanesha had—the story is very different. The problem starts when the cells become insulin-resistant: they can't use insulin properly, even though the pancreas is producing it. Insulin circulates in the blood, as it normally does; it attaches to receptors on the cells. But the cells don't respond properly. It's as if someone is knocking on the door, trying to deliver a package, but no one is answering. At first the body makes more insulin to compensate. This may work for a while. But at some point the pancreas falters and diabetes develops.

Type 2 diabetes is almost always associated with obesity. It's not an autoimmune disorder like type 1, but this form of diabetes has genetic components, too. Genes make some individuals more susceptible to both obesity and diabetes. That's why both conditions tend to run together in families. As I'll explain in Chapter 8, our Paleolithic ancestors evolved with genes that enabled them to survive in a world where food was often scarce and vigorous physical activity was a required part of everyday life. Back then, the ability to store body fat was an advantage. Though times have changed, we're all linked genetically to our primitive forebears. However, some people carry more of these Paleolithic genes. If those individuals happen to live in an environment that makes it easy to eat too much and exercise too little, their risk of diabetes is greatly elevated. For example, Grandma Sadie—whose genes made her susceptible—gained weight on my mother's chocolate cake. But my mother, her daughter-in-law, who had a different genetic heritage, was slender all her life.

Diabetes treatment is tailored to the individual. Depending on the type of diabetes and how far it has progressed, a doctor might prescribe insulin or other medications to regulate sugar metabolism. Daily blood sugar testing is necessary to monitor the condition. Diet and physical activity are key parts of the metabolic equation. People with type 2 diabetes can sometimes control their disease simply by losing weight and making healthy lifestyle changes. Years ago, a diabetes diagnosis meant severe dietary restrictions, but that's no longer true. Grandma Sadie, who loved sweets, was ordered to give them up. Guidelines are much more permissive these days. Treats containing sugar are now allowed in limited quantities, as part of an overall dietary plan.

Women and men are equally likely to develop type 2 diabetes. But women face an additional risk: gestational diabetes—a condition in which type 2 diabetes appears temporarily during pregnancy. The problem occurs because pregnancy-related hormonal changes can create insulin resistance. A pregnant woman needs up to three times the normal amount of insulin. If her body can't make enough, glucose builds up in her blood. Approximately 4 percent of pregnancies—about 135,000 per year—are complicated by gestational diabetes, according to the American Diabetes Association. The problem usually emerges late in pregnancy. Expectant mothers who are overweight are at elevated risk. Gestational diabetes, like other forms of the disease, requires careful attention to diet and physical activity. Treatment also may involve multiple insulin injections each day, as well as daily blood tests.

Finding and treating gestational diabetes is important for both baby and mother. If there's extra glucose in the mother's blood, excess levels reach the developing child via the placenta. In effect, she's overfeeding her baby while it's still in the womb. If a baby is born atypically large, that could be a sign of gestational diabetes. Childbirth may be more difficult if a baby is very big. And a baby who starts life with excess weight is at greater risk for obesity and type 2 diabetes later on.

Usually, gestational diabetes goes away after the baby is born. But a mother who's had the problem once faces a two-in-three chance that it will return in subsequent pregnancies. Also, many women who experience gestational diabetes go on to develop type 2 diabetes.

Years ago, when I first told my fellow pediatric interns that I'd decided to specialize in endocrinology, they were baffled. To them, endocrinology meant rare disorders of metabolism and uncommon problems with hormones gone awry. Several close friends tried to change my mind. "You'll spend your life dealing with the arcane and obscure," they said. The worldwide epidemic of diabesity proved them wrong.

More than forty years after Grandma Sadie's diagnosis and my father's lectures in the kitchen, I still hate diabetes—and it still fascinates me. I've learned a great deal about this terrible disease from books and lectures, from research, and from my patients and their families. But there is much yet to discover—and more to do with the knowledge we already have—if we are to hold back the tide of the diabetes epidemic before it engulfs us all.

THREE

The March to Type 2 Diabetes

Type 2 diabetes sneaks up on people. At first, there are no symptoms, no signs that anything is wrong. But hidden changes begin and the damage slowly mounts. Diabetes snuck up on my friend Elizabeth. I first met her in college, when we lived in the same dorm. Everyone liked Elizabeth because she was so cheerful and generous. If you were up late studying and felt lonely or hungry, you could go to her room for upbeat conversation and something to eat. She had a distinctive laugh—high-pitched and loud enough to hear from down the hall.

Elizabeth was petite, about 5 feet 2 inches, and enviably curvy. Her weight was normal when she first arrived at college. But by the end of our first year, she'd put on the "freshman twenty": 20 excess pounds from not getting enough exercise plus eating starchy cafeteria food, snacking on candy and chips, and drinking soda and beer. Through the remaining years of college, Elizabeth tried this diet and that. Her friends cheered her on. But each time she lost weight, she gained more back. By graduation, there was no polite way to put it: Elizabeth was obese.

"I can't believe how much weight I've gained at school," she told me one night. "Forty-eight pounds!" It was our last semester in college. We were sitting on one of the ratty sofas in the dorm lounge, taking a break from studying for midterms. Elizabeth, as usual, had brought a box of doughnuts to share with anyone who happened to be there. She continued, "I went to Student Health the other day, and the nurse put me on the scale. She told me I had to lose weight, and I said, 'I've been losing—and gaining—all year.'" Elizabeth laughed her high-pitched laugh.

I liked her too much to hurt her feelings, so I didn't say anything. But it was obvious why she'd gained weight. Except for brief periods when she went on an unrealistically strict diet, she ate constantly. And she was completely sedentary. The rest of us often went for walks in the evening or played Frisbee on the grass in back of the dorm. But Elizabeth refused to join us. Taped to her door was a quote from the famous educator Robert Maynard Hutchins: "Whenever I feel the urge to exercise, I lie down until it passes." If she needed a study break, she'd watch TV. When we had a class across campus, I'd try to persuade her to walk with me, but she always took her car.

After we graduated, Elizabeth and I lost touch, though I heard about her from mutual friends. I knew that she taught fifth grade, that she'd married late and had three children, one when she was forty. The next time we met was at our thirtieth reunion. We hadn't seen each other for three decades, but I recognized her laugh, which I heard from across the room.

Many of my classmates were thicker around the middle than they'd been in college. But Elizabeth was one of the heaviest. Looking at her, I guessed she weighed close to 200 pounds. When we greeted each other, my arms couldn't fit around her for a proper hug. "Elizabeth!" I cried. "How are you!"

"Terrible," she said. This was not the upbeat Elizabeth I remembered.

"Really?" I responded, puzzled. "Why?" The doctor in me was talking at that point, not the college friend.

"I just found out I have borderline diabetes," she said. "This came totally out of the blue. I mean, I get a checkup every single year, and my blood sugar has always been normal." Elizabeth was surprised, but I wasn't. I knew that her excess weight put her at very high risk.

FAT DOESN'T JUST JIGGLE

Physicians and scientists are starting to unfold the complex story of how obesity causes diabetes. We know that the leading player is the fat cell, the cell known as the adipocyte. When I was in medical school, fat tissue was billed as relatively inactive. I used to think of the fat cell as Jell-O: it just sat there and jiggled. These days, I picture adipocytes as those greedy little creatures in a Pac-Man video game, gobbling fuel and storing it as fat molecules until they're ready to burst.

After we eat, any extra glucose, fatty acids, and amino acids in the bloodstream are picked up by our adipocytes, the fat cells, and converted into fat. That's how we build our reserve fuel supply. Once we're past childhood, our body doesn't make many more fat cells. Rather, the new fat molecules are crowded into existing fat cells, making them larger.

Insulin plays a role in fat storage. One of its contributions is to help liberate fatty acids from food. Because more fatty acids are available, there's more for fat cells to store. In addition, insulin inhibits the release of stored fat by adipocytes. These effects mean that people who are insulin-resistant—and who therefore have excess insulin circulating in their bloodstream—have an increased tendency to store fat and gain weight.

Body fat isn't merely a warehouse. We now know that fat—especially the fat around our midsection—is incredibly active metabolically. It responds to hormones, including insulin; it also manufactures and secretes hormones and other chemical signals. For example, fat cells contribute to production of estrogen, the female hormone. Women need some body fat for normal hormonal cycling: if a pre-menopausal woman becomes too thin—whether because of famine, illness, extreme physical training, or an eating disorder—she stops menstruating. But an excess of fat can mean an excess of estrogens. That's why obesity is linked to breast cancer. And it also explains why obese men may develop breast tissue. Obesity can also decrease production of male hormones (androgens), a change that can reduce libido.

When fat cells are overstuffed, our body chemistry can go awry, leading to diabetes and other serious problems. We don't yet completely understand all the mechanisms that link obesity and type 2 diabetes, but hormones and other chemicals released by the adipocytes undoubtedly are involved. For instance, one important factor could be resistin, a hormone made in fat cells that promotes insulin resistance. Scientists recently discovered that when they inhibited the production of resistin in mice with elevated blood sugar, their response to insulin improved and their blood sugar levels dropped. The next question is whether inhibiting resistin might be a viable strategy to prevent or treat type 2 diabetes in people.

Chemical regulators made by our fat cells affect our weight. One example is a hormone called leptin, which is released by fat cells when fat molecules build up. In people of normal weight, leptin signals the brain that it's time to stop eating. But for reasons that we don't yet understand, leptin doesn't have the same effect in people who are obese. Some regulators released by fat cells influence the digestive tract, affecting whether or not nutrients will be absorbed; others switch fat deposition on and off.

As fat cells expand, their chemical output changes in ways that actually increase fat accumulation. Adipocytes thereby guarantee their own existence at the peril of the whole organism. One mechanism involves adiponectin, a hormone secreted by the adipocyte. Adiponectin helps muscle cells burn glucose, which contributes to weight control. It also makes the cells more sensitive to insulin, which lowers the risk of type 2 diabetes. But the more fat your body stores, the lower your level of adiponectin. Researchers are investigating adiponectin for its potential in treating obesity, and we're all waiting to see if this approach will have clinical significance.

APPLES AND PEARS

If you've ever prepared a whole chicken for cooking, you know that fat is deposited in two ways: there's a thin layer just under the skin and also larger lumps deeper inside. The same is true for us. We have a layer of fat under our skin, called subcutaneous fat, and invisible fat, called visceral fat, in our abdominal cavity.

Subcutaneous fat acts as insulation and serves as a cushion upon which we can sit. The bumpy fat on our thighs and rear ends—the fat that's sometimes referred to as cellulite—is subcutaneous fat. Though some women agonize about cellulite, it actually has little significance for health. According to a study published in the *New England Journal of Medicine* in 2004, obese women showed no improvement in risk factors for cardiovascular disease after liposuction—despite the fact that an average of more than 20 pounds of subcutaneous fat was removed from their abdomens.

Visceral fat is more metabolically active than subcutaneous fat—and more dangerous. It churns out more of the potent chemicals produced by adipocytes, and its location in the trunk of the body adds to the risk. If the fat cells are so overstuffed that they would burst if more was added, fat molecules actually spill into nearby organs, including the pancreas and liver. Fat molecules can also enter our muscles.

We've recently learned that when fat gets inside muscle cells, they can't respond properly to insulin, so the muscle doesn't take up sugar normally or metabolize it as efficiently as it should. Fat inside the pancreas appears to shorten the lives of beta cells, which can lead to insufficient insulin production and type 2 diabetes. And if fat enters the liver, it alters the liver's response to insulin. Normally, the liver refrains from releasing its stored glucose when there's insulin in the blood, since the presence of insulin indicates an ample supply of sugar. But when there's fat inside, the liver is resistant to insulin and releases glucose into the bloodstream unnecessarily. So blood glucose rises to abnormal levels. A liver with excess fat also makes more cholesterol, which elevates cholesterol in the blood and contributes to cardiovascular disease.

Because of the problems associated with visceral fat, doctors are beginning to look not only at height and weight but also at body shape when they assess the risks of overweight patients. People with an "apple" shape—those with excess weight concentrated in their midsection—are especially likely to have invisible visceral fat inside the abdominal cavity and around the liver and other organs. As a result, individuals with this body type are at much greater risk for diabetes and other serious health problems. In contrast, those with a "pear" shape—excess weight carried on their thighs and buttocks— have fewer health risks. A simple way to assess shape is to measure the waistline: a waist larger than 40 inches in a man or above 35 inches in a woman is a sign of elevated risk.

As we learn more about the adipocyte—its complex connections with other systems of the body, as well as the substances it releases and their unique effects—we may be able to develop new therapies for diabetes and for obesity. In the meantime, this much is all too clear: nearly everyone diagnosed with type 2 diabetes has weighed too much for many years.

THE SILENT FIRST STAGE

Though neither of us knew it back then, Elizabeth had probably begun the long march to type 2 diabetes when she was in college. The first steps in this unfortunate journey are silent. There are no symptoms, not even ones that can be recognized in retrospect. Routine glucose tests can't detect the problem. But as Elizabeth began to gain weight in college, her body chemistry changed and her cells became increasingly insulin-resistant.

When someone is insulin-resistant, the beta cells in their pancreas produce plenty of insulin—but the cells throughout their body don't respond normally to it. To maintain homeostasis, the pancreas makes more and more insulin. This works temporarily: the extra insulin compensates for the cells' insensitivity, so blood sugar remains normal. That's why the condition is silent.

Over time, the beta cells become exhausted and can no longer sustain their abnormally high insulin production rate. Why this happens is still not completely understood, but we assume that multiple factors are at work. Some of these factors are linked to obe-sity: the beta cells may be damaged by excess fat deposited within them; other hormones released by visceral fat may interfere with the function or even the survival of beta cells. In addition, a person's ge-netic heritage and early life probably play a role, since these factors help determine how the beta cells develop and how robust they will be later on.

Ironically, Elizabeth had always been conscientious about med-ical checkups, even as a college student. Her blood sugar was checked at each annual physical and even more frequently during her three pregnancies. The test results were always normal—but that was because her pancreas was working overtime. An abnormal process had begun without her realizing it. After many years, her beta cells began to falter. Her insulin production dropped, and her blood sugar levels began to rise.

PRE-DIABETES

Blood sugar fluctuates throughout the day. Overnight, when no food is consumed, blood sugar drops to its lowest point—about 70 to 100 milligrams per deciliter (mg/dl). After a meal, blood sugar rises, normally reaching no higher than 140 mg/dl; as the meal is di-gested, it falls again.

Because of these fluctuations, it's best to perform routine blood glucose tests—the kind used to screen apparently healthy people—after an overnight fast. Fasting blood sugar under 100 mg/dl is con-sidered normal; 126 mg/dl or higher means diabetes. Sometimes blood is checked over the next one to three hours after a person drinks a liquid that contains a fixed dose of glucose. This is called an oral glucose tolerance test. If blood is tested this way—or if it's sim-ply checked at a random time during the day, rather than after an overnight fast—a level of 200 mg/dl or greater indicates diabetes.

Pre-diabetes is diagnosed when fasting blood sugar is elevated but not high enough to be considered diabetic: between 100 and 125 mg/dl after an overnight fast, or between 140 and 199 mg/dl at the two-hour point during an oral glucose tolerance test. Though many of them don't know it, more than 41 million Americans have pre-diabetes. Sometimes doctors refer to this as borderline diabetes, or they call it "glucose intolerance" when it's diagnosed via an oral glucose tolerance test or "impaired fasting glucose" if a fasting glucose test was used. By any name, the diagnosis should serve as a loud warning signal. Studies have shown that each year about 10 percent of people with pre-diabetes will develop diabetes.

Elizabeth, who had just passed age fifty, had been given notice. "My dad died of diabetes," she told me. "I'm petrified that I'll get it, too. Fran, I shouldn't burden you with all this at a party, but I literally found out two days ago, and this is your field. Do you know what my odds are?"

I hated to tell her, in the middle of our college reunion, that if she didn't lose weight, she would almost inevitably get diabetes within the next ten years. So I simply said, "Most people with what you have will go on, over years, to get diabetes." As soon as I said that, I felt I had doomed Elizabeth. I needed to soften the blow, so I touched her arm and added, "But it's possible to prevent that by losing weight."

We know that lifestyle changes can prevent type 2 diabetes, even in people who have already begun the march. We know this because of the Diabetes Prevention Program (DPP) study, which was chaired by Dr. David Nathan of Harvard University, one of the most gifted clinical researchers in the field of diabetes. This investigation, which began in the mid-1990s, was the single most important study ever conducted in diabetes prevention.

Twenty-seven medical centers across the United States participated. They put out the call for volunteers at high risk for diabetes. More than 3,000 participants were selected. They ranged in age from twenty-five to eighty-five, and they represented a wide range of racial and cultural backgrounds. But every single one of them was overweight. And they all had pre-diabetes.

The volunteers were assigned at random to one of three groups. The first group received metformin, a medication that makes cells more sensitive to the insulin the pancreas produces naturally. If insulin sensitivity could be improved in people with pre-diabetes, the investigators reasoned, perhaps diabetes could be prevented. The second group was given a placebo, a pill that contained no active in-gredients. This part of the study was blinded, which means that nei-ther the participants nor the investigators knew who received the real medication. Members of both groups also were given printed information on diet and exercise.

The third group, with more than 1,000 high-risk participants, received no pills at all. Instead, they underwent extensive training with lifestyle coaches, who taught them how to alter their lives to lose weight and to become more physically active. The coaches counseled them about diet and exercise. They learned how to set goals and keep track of their success. Group members were ex-pected to eat less fat and fewer calories overall, and to exercise for a total of at least two and a half hours per week. The coaches led problem-solving discussions to help participants deal with lapses. Members of the lifestyle change group also attended classes on healthy eating, physical activity, and behavioral topics. In addition to all this, they participated in special events, such as group walks or competitions. Meanwhile, those in the other two groups simply took their pills and went about their usual lives.

At the end of the three-year study period, investigators com-bined the data from all twenty-seven centers. Then they tallied medical test results from all three groups. Everyone had entered the study with pre-diabetes: how were they doing three years later?

Twenty-nine percent of the participants who received only a placebo now had diabetes. Those who took the medication fared better—just 22 percent of that group had developed diabetes. But the people in the lifestyle change group enjoyed the most success of all: only 14 percent developed diabetes during the three years of the study. What's more, they lost an average of 12.3 pounds. In contrast, those taking the placebo dropped only a fraction of a pound, and those taking medication lost just 4.6 pounds, on average. In 2001, as president-elect of the American Diabetes Association, I was part of a press conference to announce these findings, along with U.S. Health and Human Services Secretary Tommy G. Thompson. It was thrilling to learn conclusively that each of us has it within our power to reverse diabesity.

I told Elizabeth about the study. She listened. But when I finished, she said firmly, "That's enough about me. Let's talk about you." Reluctantly I let her change the subject. As a doctor, and as a friend, I wanted to help. But I know that the motivation for weight loss ultimately must come from within and not from anyone else. So I didn't press her. I felt deeply concerned—and frustrated. If Elizabeth hadn't gained all that weight during college and in the years afterward, she might never have become insulin-resistant. If she lost weight now, her beta cells probably could recover. She didn't have to get diabetes, but I feared she would.

METABOLIC SYNDROME: A CLUSTER OF RISKS

A year after our college reunion, I attended a meeting in the city where Elizabeth lived. I called her and we arranged to get together for an early breakfast. To my dismay, she was even heavier than she'd been the year before. As soon as we sat down she told me, "You were right. I knew you would be, but it still hurts. I have diabetes now—plus metabolic syndrome."

Approximately one-third of obese adults, and perhaps as many overweight teenagers, have metabolic syndrome, which is also called syndrome X or insulin resistance syndrome. Metabolic syndrome is defined as a cluster of risk factors for diabetes and cardiovascular disease: high blood sugar, high waist circumference, high blood pressure, high levels of triglycerides, and low levels of high-density lipoprotein (the good cholesterol).

Metabolic syndrome is in large part caused by visceral fat. A key mechanism involves chemical signals from our fat cells that trigger inflammation. We've all experienced inflammation—swollen nasal passages when a cold strikes, or swelling, heat, and tissue sensitivity near an infected cut. This kind of acute inflammation reflects a cascade of responses by our immune system. Normally, inflammation helps us recover from illness and injury, then it disappears when healing is complete. But when we have too much fat, we also have a chronic overabundance of the inflammation-triggering chemical signals. And that can mean chronic inflammation—not inflammation we can see, but invisible inflammation throughout our bodies, including inside our blood vessels.

We're beginning to understand that systemic inflammation plays a significant role in cardiovascular disease. Inflamed blood vessels become narrower. If there are cholesterol deposits in the blood vessel walls, the wall becomes distorted and the cells may even rupture. This can cause formation of small blood clots, which may block the already narrowed blood vessels, cutting off the flow of blood to the heart (a heart attack) or brain (a stroke). The link between fat cells and inflammation helps explain the connection between obesity and cardiovascular disease.

Doctors have begun to identify people at elevated risk for heart attacks and strokes by testing their blood for an inflammation marker called C-reactive protein (CRP). In 2002 a landmark study in the *New England Journal of Medicine* reported that CRP level predicted cardiovascular events—including heart attacks, strokes, and deaths from cardiovascular causes—even more accurately than blood cholesterol level. Investigators had tracked nearly 28,000 women, all over age forty-five and apparently healthy at the start, for an average of eight years. Those whose CRP level showed systemic inflammation were the most likely to have had cardiovascular problems.

Most people with metabolic syndrome—and this was true of Elizabeth—have the characteristic apple shape, with their excess weight concentrated in their midsection: men wear their pendulant potbellies over their belts, and women look as if they're halfway through a pregnancy. The heavier they are, the greater their risk for type 2 diabetes and cardiovascular disease.

Elizabeth told me that her blood pressure was elevated and that her lipid profile—her triglyceride and cholesterol numbers—was unfavorable. I asked about her treatment. Her doctor had prescribed several medications to lower her blood pressure, improve her lipids, and make her cells more sensitive to the insulin her body produced. "The doctor told me that if I exercise and eat right, I might not need all the pills. My diabetes might even go away," she said.

If Elizabeth could only lose weight and become fit—a Herculean task for someone like her, with a decades-long history of obesity—she might be able to bring her blood sugar to normal or near-normal levels. It was still possible that her beta cells could recover and that her diabetes could be cured. But even if it was too late for that, exercise and a healthier diet could improve her diabetes management, reducing the chances of complications. "He's right," I told her. "Lifestyle changes really make a difference."

Elizabeth rolled her eyes. "Let me tell you about my lifestyle. My mother broke her hip last year, and now she's in a nursing home. By the time I finish work and visit her, I'm wiped out. No way am I going to take an hour to shop and cook dinner. I can't ask my husband to do it—his schedule is even crazier than mine. So most nights we eat take-out. And forget exercise. After dinner there's the kids and the dishes and the laundry and the mail and the answering machine. When I'm finally done, I just collapse in front of the TV." She looked defiant.

I nodded sympathetically. This was a familiar story. "You teach, you take care of your children and your husband, you take care of your mother. You have time to take care of everyone—everyone except Elizabeth," I observed. She seemed surprised by my words; I think she was expecting me to criticize her. I continued: "But Elizabeth, you must take care of yourself, for your family's sake as well as yours. Diabetes is relentless, and the complications are terrible. I don't want to scare you, but I've just seen too much. I'm talking about blindness, heart attacks, strokes, kidney failure, amputations."

I reached across the table and took her hands. "It's likely not too late to fix this whole thing," I said. "And it doesn't take as much as you think—thirty minutes of physical activity a day. You could walk with your husband or your kids. It would be good for them, too. Some decent food, nothing fancy." Elizabeth listened. But when I finished, she changed the subject and I reluctantly followed her lead.

All through my meetings later that day, my mind kept returning to Elizabeth and our conversation. I agonized. Should I have been more forceful? Did she really understand what diabetes could do to her body? That evening I sent her an e-mail. I repeated the warnings—and the encouragement. I urged her to call me if there was anything I could do to help.

She didn't reply, and I felt awful. I'd probably said too much; maybe she was angry with me for being intrusive. Then two months later I had an answer. Her message was short: *10 lbs gone, off some of my meds. Forget walking 30 minutes a day—I don't stop before 60. Thanks, Fran!*

FOUR

The Blood Sugar Balancing Act

Diabetes sucks!" That's what one of my teenage patients, Gordon, told me after he'd had diabetes for two years. I was surprised. Gordon had seemed to adjust well. He'd been faithful about his daily blood tests and insulin shots. I've pricked my finger and stuck myself with those needles to see how they feel, so I know that they're a little unpleasant but don't really hurt. Gordon had never complained before. "Why?" I asked, wanting to understand his pain. "Why is it so bad?"

"It's that it's every day. No matter what," Gordon said simply. "Wherever I go, I've got diabetes." Gordon was right. He had diabetes, and he had it 24/7. He had it come rain or come shine, day or night, weekdays and weekends, now and for the rest of his life.

DIAGNOSING THE DISEASE

Type 1 diabetes usually begins abruptly. Suddenly a person is much hungrier and thirstier than usual. Despite eating and drinking more, he or she loses weight. Urination is copious. Excess urination, excess drinking, and excess eating are the three "polys" my father told

me about: polyuria, polydipsia, and polyphagia. People who experience these changes may seek medical care. But if they don't, serious
symptoms are likely to follow in a month or two as insulin defi-
ciency becomes more profound: significant malaise, vomiting, and
even loss of consciousness. If the diabetes hasn't yet been discovered, surely it will be at that point.

The course of type 2 diabetes is different. It begins with silent
changes that may continue for years, as was the case with my friend
Elizabeth, whom you met in Chapter 3. Since the disease itself usually progresses slowly, the diagnosis is often made by routine tests
during a medical checkup, before symptoms become severe enough
to prompt a special visit to the doctor.

Blood sugar testing should be part of regular medical checkups
for everyone who is over age forty-five—and for everyone over age
ten who has two or more risk factors for diabetes. Risk factors include being overweight; having a family history of diabetes; showing
signs of insulin resistance, such as high blood pressure, high cholesterol, or other abnormal blood fats; or being a member of an ethnic
or racial minority known to have above-average risk (for example,
African Americans, Hispanics and Latin Americans, American Indians, Asian Americans, and Pacific Islanders).

The best way to perform the test is to draw blood from a vein after an overnight fast and send it to a laboratory for analysis. If
blood sugar is at or above 126 mg/dl, that indicates diabetes. Sometimes blood is drawn on the spot during a checkup and simply
checked with a glucose meter. A level of 200 mg/dl or greater suggests diabetes. But these findings are less reliable—for example,
blood sugar may be elevated temporarily because the person has
eaten recently—so additional tests are needed to confirm the diagnosis.

After a blood test reveals elevated blood sugar, many patients
realize they've experienced symptoms that had seemed too minor
to mention, such as increased thirst and hunger, more frequent
urination, unexplained weight loss, sores that are slow to heal, or occasional blurry vision. A diagnosis of diabetes can be made immediately if high blood sugar is accompanied by symptoms. But if the
person is asymptomatic, it's important to repeat the blood test to

make sure blood sugar is consistently high. Sometimes an oral glucose tolerance test, which I described in Chapter 3, is given at this point.

Once elevated blood sugar is detected, it's essential to determine which kind of diabetes a person has. That's because types 1 and 2 require different treatments. Some doctors assume that any child with high blood glucose has type 1 and that any newly diagnosed adult has type 2. While these assumptions are usually correct, they could be wrong. More children and teenagers are developing type 2. And about 10 percent of adults diagnosed with diabetes have type 1. We can't even assume that an obese child with diabetes has type 2, because childhood obesity has become so common.

One way to differentiate types 1 and 2 is to look for specific antibodies in the blood. Type 1 diabetes is an autoimmune disease, in which the body's own immune system attacks the beta cells in the islets of Langerhans that make insulin. The blood of a person with type 1 diabetes will have islet cell antibodies; the blood of someone with type 2 will not. Another approach is to measure insulin secretion, since people with type 2 diabetes—unlike those with type 1—don't completely lose the ability to make insulin. Insulin secretion is measured with a test for C-peptide, a substance released by the pancreas along with insulin.

George, the brother of one of my type 1 patients, developed diabetes while he was away at college. He went to the student health service and described his symptoms: he hadn't been feeling well and he was urinating a lot. Because his sister had been diagnosed with type 1 diabetes when she was four, George knew what his problems might mean. The doctor checked his blood sugar. Sure enough, it was elevated. Simply because George was twenty years old, the doctor assumed he had type 2 diabetes. He prescribed a pill that makes the cells more sensitive to insulin. But that couldn't help anyone with type 1 diabetes, whose pancreas was no longer producing insulin.

George's symptoms continued, and his mother called me. I suggested that he come home from college immediately so we could take care of him. When he arrived, his blood sugar was 513 mg/dl. We checked his blood for islet cell antibodies and confirmed that he had type 1 diabetes. Once he began taking insulin, his blood sugar dropped and his symptoms subsided.

DIABETES REVEALS ITSELF

My grandmother's diabetes wasn't diagnosed until she developed a lung infection serious enough to require a middle-of-the-night emergency room visit. Like many women of her generation, she refused to talk about her health or any aspect of her body's function. Every morning my mother would ask Grandma Sadie how she was, and every morning she'd reply, "I'm fine. Vhy shouldn't I be?" My parents didn't know that for a few months before her diagnosis, Grandma was awakening multiple times each night to urinate. They could tell she was losing weight, but they had no idea she was still sneaking candies and cookies. When my mother commented that she looked a little thinner, Sadie said, "Vhy not? You told me I should try to lose veight, so now maybe I do." I knew the truth, but I didn't know what any of it meant.

Diabetes may be discovered on a medical visit prompted by some other problem connected with diabetes, such as fatigue, sores that don't heal, blurry vision, recurrent infections, and tingling, numbness, or burning pain in the hands and feet. In women, recurrent yeast infections can be caused by diabetes. That's because yeast, which is normally present in the vagina, thrives on sugar that escapes in the urine and clings to the vaginal walls. In men, erectile dysfunction—impotence—may be an early signal of diabetes. What's the connection? Excess sugar in the bloodstream can damage nerves and blood vessels in the penis.

Type 2 diabetes can cause so many diverse medical problems that even a healthcare provider may not recognize it. That happened with Jaime, who came to my office because a school nurse referred him—but not for diabetes. Her consultation request said: *Please evaluate this twelve-year-old boy. He is obese and has severe body odor. I think he has some kind of hormone problem. By the way, he is filthy.*

My secretary was appalled. "How insensitive can this woman

be?" she asked. "What does being 'filthy' have to do with his medical problems?"

I answered, "Looking filthy has a lot to do with it. I'll bet you that this school nurse is talking about acanthosis nigricans, though she has no idea what it is." Acanthosis nigricans is a darkening of the skin that often affects the neck, armpits, or groin. It's a sign of insulin resistance—the body's cells not responding properly to insulin—and can appear in someone with diabetes or obesity.

Five days later, Jaime came to my clinic with his mother and father. A technician weighed and measured him and took a blood sample, which was sent to the hospital's laboratory. An hour later, the lab results tentatively confirmed my guess: Jaime's blood sugar was 212 mg/dl, which meant that he probably had diabetes.

I entered the examining room to speak with the family. At age twelve, Jaime weighed 220 pounds; he was 5 feet 6 inches tall. Though he was not yet into his teens, he was nearly finished with puberty and looked like a man. It's not unusual for heavy children to go through puberty early. His father was about 6 feet tall and appeared to weigh close to 300 pounds. But his mother was tiny. When I looked at her, then looked at her husband and son, it was difficult to imagine they were all part of the same family.

Jaime's mother immediately said, "He has diabetes, doesn't he? I knew he would get it! My husband has diabetes, his father has diabetes—all the men in their family have it. I kept telling his doctor he would get it, but the doctor kept saying, 'Not at his age.'"

"You're right—a preliminary test suggests that he has diabetes. Because of his weight and family history, it's almost certainly type 2. But to be sure, we'll need to check his blood again tomorrow morning, before he has breakfast," I told her. Then I turned to Jaime and quickly added, "The good news is, we caught it early. Your blood sugar level is not so high that we must give you medicine right away. We'll see how you do with some changes in your diet and exercise every day. Maybe you won't need medication."

Jaime's father interrupted, "Listen, Doc, I know I need to lose weight, but I take good care of myself. My sugars are good; I'm healthy. We'll work with Jaime, that I can assure you."

I discussed the importance of lifestyle changes, speaking directly to Jaime. "Jaime, you could actually reverse the diabetes process and get rid of your diabetes forever. But you'll have to eat differently," I said. Jaime and his parents nodded in agreement. "You'll also need to exercise," I added.

Suddenly they all looked uncomfortable. Jaime lowered his head, and I thought he was going to cry. His mother fidgeted and finally spoke. "He sweats really bad. When he exercises, his BO smells terrible. We've tried everything, but his armpits are dark and dirty all the time. I've taken a Brillo pad to his armpits and his neck, but it just doesn't come out."

"That's not dirt," I told them. "Jaime has a skin condition we call acanthosis nigricans. It happens because his body can't respond normally to insulin. Brillo isn't going to help. But the acanthosis nigricans may fade if he loses weight and gets his diabetes under control."

Jaime looked up, his face suddenly brighter. His parents stared at me. With that information, I had lifted a weight from the entire family. They were exonerated. Jaime wasn't dirty. His darkened skin was part of a medical condition. Now they understood its cause and knew how to resolve it. I continued: "Jaime, body odor is a common problem in heavy youngsters as they go through puberty, because they sweat a lot. And it's worse for some people than others. But I promise, we can show you how to control it." The whole family was smiling now, and I smiled, too.

HERALDED BY COMPLICATIONS

In some cases, the first sign of type 2 diabetes is the appearance of one of its severe complications. Vision is suddenly lost: a person wakes up in the morning to find everything dark and blurry. Or the kidneys fail, causing severe headaches, weakness, and water retention. When the body retains water—a condition called edema—a person can gain weight rapidly; legs and ankles swell uncomfortably, and the face looks puffy. Diabetes can also cause gastrointestinal symptoms, including severe abdominal bloating, constipation, or explosive diarrhea. And people as young as forty may be brought to the emergency room with a heart attack or a stroke. They arrive on a stretcher clutching their chest, to learn that not only is a blockage killing their cardiac muscle as they lie there, but they also have out-of-control diabetes.

Gordon—the teenager who told me, "Diabetes sucks"—was diagnosed in the emergency room of Childrens Hospital Los Angeles. He arrived by ambulance, unconscious, and was rushed into Room 2. That's the room I mentioned in Chapter 1, the ER room for our most desperately ill or severely injured patients. No one knew why Gordon was unconscious. Doctors were called over their beepers in anticipation of his arrival. Specialists streamed into Room 2 and waited to see if they were needed. A neurosurgeon and a general surgeon arrived just in case.

The senior emergency room physician ordered a host of blood tests immediately, trying to determine what was wrong. Anyone who arrives unconscious receives a blood glucose test in the ER, since the cause might be extremely high or low blood sugar. Within one minute the answer was known: Gordon's blood sugar was above 600 mg/dl, the highest level the emergency room glucose meter could register. I was paged. I raced to the ER from my clinic, nearly crashing into one of the surgeons as she left.

Gordon lay on the gurney in Room 2. One glance told me that he was obese. That meant he probably had type 2 diabetes. His condition was just as life-threatening as the diabetic coma of someone with type 1. When the report came back from the laboratory, we learned that Gordon's blood sugar was 984 mg/dl. Quickly I reviewed his medical records. The boy was thirteen years old. Though his mother realized in retrospect that he'd been urinating excessively for about four months, he had been noticeably sick for only the past week, with flu-like symptoms that included abdominal pain and three days of vomiting. Now he was unconscious.

Intravenous lines were placed so we could pump desperately needed fluids and medicine into Gordon's body; a urinary catheter was inserted through his penis into his bladder, so we could measure his fluid output. I began my least favorite balancing act: racing to bring a child back to normalcy without killing him in the process. I needed to get his blood sugar level down by giving him more intra-venous fluid, but I couldn't give too much at once for fear of causing brain swelling. Gordon's mother, Denita, stood in the corner of Room 2, tears pooled in her eyes. Once the insulin and fluid drips were established, I approached her and introduced myself. "I will tell you everything as we go along," I promised. "He's really sick now, but most of the children do okay in the long run."

"Do okay with what?" she asked. Apparently, no one had ex-plained why her son was unconscious.

"He has diabetes," I said. Denita gasped, covered her face, and began to sob. A social worker appeared. She wrapped her arms around Denita and led her out of Room 2. For a moment I felt envi-ous. I needed a hug, too; I needed support and confirmation and en-couragement. I needed all that because I was the one who had been sent out to battle the giant. I returned to Gordon's side to examine him. Although his blood sugar was extremely high, that didn't ex-plain why he had become so gravely ill so quickly. Usually a teenager with type 2 diabetes would not reach such a point until after months of severe symptoms that only a negligent parent would fail to no-tice—for example, an unexplained 40-pound weight loss. But Denita was clearly a devoted mother.

Was anything complicating Gordon's diabetes, I wondered. I put my stethoscope over his chest and listened. An extra heart sound would indicate heart failure; crackling sounds as he breathed would suggest a lung infection. I moved the stethoscope to his abdomen. If he had a ruptured appendix, bacteria in his blood might account for his condition. In that case, I'd be unable to hear the sounds that his bowels would normally make as food and fluids coursed through them. But I could hear faint rushing bowel sounds, so a ruptured ap-pendix was unlikely.

I lifted Gordon's eyelids and looked into his eyes with the oph-thalmoscope. If the optic discs at the backs of his eyes were blurry, that would suggest swelling of his brain or a possible infection in his spinal fluid. But the edges of the discs were sharp. I touched his skin and pressed the tips of his fingers to determine how well his vessels were circulating his blood. When you press on the skin, you force all the blood out of the capillaries and the skin turns white. Then you let go. If circulation is normal, the capillary blood comes back instantly and skin color returns. But if blood return is sluggish, the skin stays white for several seconds. Poor circulation is one sign of dehydration. Gordon's circulation was sluggish, indicating he was dehydrated, but even dehydration didn't explain why he was so profoundly ill.

I tapped his knees and ankles to check his reflexes. If there had been a difference in the responses of his left and right foot, that could have meant he'd had a stroke. But Gordon's reflexes, though slow, were not abnormal. I palpated his abdomen with my fingers. His belly rose like a mountain and seemed very tender, especially around the middle and upper sections. Gordon hadn't responded to other stimuli—the bright light of the ophthalmoscope, the sound of his mother calling his name, my touch on his legs, chest, and face. But when I probed his belly, he involuntarily winced. This type of abdominal sensitivity suggested the possibility of pancreatitis, an inflammation of the pancreas. It could explain why he was so sick. Pancreatitis is uncommon in children but not unheard of with type 2 diabetes. After I'd ordered the blood tests and the X-rays that could confirm the diagnosis, I threaded a tube through Gordon's nose into his stomach to drain its contents. A full stomach is a danger to an unconscious person. If Gordon had vomited, undigested food and stomach acid could spill into his lungs and cause inflammation severe enough to kill him.

Gordon was wheeled from the ER to the intensive care unit. Denita joined us, clinging to his limp hand. Every drop that went into his body was measured, as was every drop that came out. I calculated and manipulated, continuing to adjust his IV drip. Four hours later Gordon stirred. "Gordon!" I called, trying to penetrate his hazy consciousness. He opened his eyes for the first time. I felt relieved and exhausted. Denita wept.

Tests confirmed my hunch that Gordon had pancreatitis and type 2 diabetes. One of the causes of pancreatitis is a high level of triglyceride—fat—in the blood. Normally the blood triglyceride level is less than 125 mg/dl. But Gordon's was 845 mg/dl. This elevation was caused by his genes, plus obesity, terrible eating habits, and uncontrolled diabetes. I told Denita that we would teach them all they needed to know for Gordon to stay healthy and well. Much later, Denita told me that she'd made a promise to God in Room 2: if He would bring Gordon back, she would do whatever she could to make sure he never got sick again. She has kept that promise.

TAKING CONTROL

The key to staying well with diabetes—both type 1 and type 2—is simple: control blood sugar. Until a decade ago, we weren't certain what caused the long-term complications of diabetes. Many specialists had hypothesized that elevated glucose was responsible for the devastating problems of blindness, kidney failure, and nerve damage. But some disagreed. Maybe, they argued, the problems could be explained by genetic defects associated with diabetes; perhaps insulin treatment caused the complications that were blamed on the disease. A study was designed—the Diabetes Control and Complications Trial (DCCT)—to settle the matter once and for all. Twenty-nine medical centers in the United States and Canada participated, led by a team of distinguished doctors and scientists.

Between 1983 and 1989 nearly 1,500 men, women, and teenagers enrolled in DCCT. All had type 1 diabetes, but at the time they volunteered to participate, none had any serious complications. The original plan was to follow everyone until 1994, checking them regularly to see if the rate and severity of complications could be decreased by strict control. Such control requires considerable effort. But perhaps it could make a real difference in the lives of people with diabetes.

Half of the volunteers were assigned at random to receive the then-standard therapy: they took insulin injections once or twice a day; they checked their blood glucose once daily. As long as they felt well, they did not adjust their insulin dose. Every three months they were examined by a doctor.

The remaining DCCT participants were put on an intensive regimen designed to control their blood sugar strictly, keeping it as close to normal as possible. They took insulin injections at least three times a day; or they used an insulin pump—a device that's attached to a small tube inserted just under the skin, which automatically delivers a continuous trickle of insulin throughout the day. In addition, the patient can use the pump's manual controls to send an extra dose just before a meal or at any time when blood sugar is too high.

Participants in the strict control group tested their blood glucose at least four times a day, and once a week they were required to measure their blood sugar in the middle of the night. Rather than focusing on how they felt, they were given strict numerical goals for their blood sugar levels. Using test results, as well as information about their food intake and exercise, they adjusted their insulin doses or reprogrammed their pumps frequently. Instead of visiting the doctor every three months, they had monthly checkups plus even more frequent telephone conferences to review and adjust their regimens.

At periodic intervals throughout the study, members of both groups underwent tests to determine if they'd developed complications of diabetes. Their retinas were photographed every six months, and the pictures were evaluated by eye specialists for evidence of damage. To guard against bias, the study was blinded: the specialists who examined the photographs did not know the participant's group. Other tests looked for damage to the kidneys and nerves. Meanwhile, an independent monitoring committee tallied the findings.

As the study went on, evidence mounted that strict sugar control reduced the risk of diabetes complications. In 1993, one year before the study was supposed to end, the difference between the two groups had become so large that the monitoring committee ordered a halt to the trial. Strict control had reduced the risk of retinal disease by 76 percent. The risk of kidney disease was cut by 50 percent, and there was a 60 percent decrease in nerve complications resulting from diabetes. Those in the standard care group were urged to change their regimens immediately. These dramatic results were announced to the public. Strict sugar control became the new standard of care not only for people with type 1 but for those with type 2 diabetes as well.

The DCCT study also showed the value of an ingenious blood

test that has come to be known as the diabetes report card: the gly-cohemoglobin test, now called the hemoglobin A1c test, or just A1c, after the specific part of hemoglobin that's measured. This test can determine how well a patient has controlled blood sugar levels over the previous few months. Here's how it works: glucose in the blood-stream becomes attached to some molecules of hemoglobin, the part of the red blood cells that carries oxygen. These hemoglobin molecules are now said to be "glycated." The more sugar in the blood when a blood cell is being made, the higher its proportion of glycated hemoglobin molecules. Red blood cells have a life span of about four months. When they die, new ones replace them. So the blood circulating in our bodies contains red blood cells of different ages—some as old as four months, some brand-new. The number of glycated hemoglobin molecules is directly proportional to the amount of sugar that has been in our bloodstream over the past sev-eral months.

The A1c test has become a vital part of diabetes management. A normal A1c level is 3 to 6 percent, indicating that 3 to 6 percent of red blood cells have glucose attached. In diabetes, the level can climb to 14 percent, which is the highest that can be measured by most A1c tests. In the DCCT study, the average A1c was 9.2 percent for the standard care group. But the strict control group—whose rate of diabetes complications was much lower—had an average A1c of 7.5 percent. Since DCCT, our goal at Childrens Hospital Los Angeles has been to get the children we treat into the 7.0 to 7.9 per-cent range. For older teens and young adults, we aim for the 6.0 to 6.9 percent range. Over the last few years, more than half of our patients have met those goals, and another 30 percent are not far behind.

"YOU MUST BECOME YOUR OWN PANCREAS"

The first step in sugar control is education. Every new patient in my clinic at Childrens Hospital Los Angeles spends a lot of time in the teaching room. They sit down with family members, a doctor, a nutritionist, and a nurse, and they learn about their illness. We explain what diabetes is, and tell them about types 1 and 2. We answer questions like "How did I get it?" Mostly, though, we provide the detailed instructions they need to keep glucose levels under control.

Insulin production normally varies throughout the day, as the pancreas responds to our needs. But in diabetes, the pancreas doesn't work properly. Instead, people with diabetes need to figure out how to balance physical activity, food, insulin, and other medications. As I tell patients, "You must become your own pancreas."

We tell patients to test their blood at least four times a day—before each meal and before bedtime, and occasionally at other times as well. Extra blood checks after meals make sure that medication keeps a lid on the post-meal sugar peak. It's also important to perform a test if symptoms of abnormal blood sugar are noticed. Excess thirst or urination suggests the possibility that blood sugar is too high; irritability or shakiness might indicate low blood sugar. In addition, we recommend that people taking insulin test their blood sugar in the middle of the night, at least occasionally; for those who experience episodes of low blood sugar, it's a prudent nightly routine.

They prick their finger to extract a drop of blood, put the drop on a special strip of paper, and insert it into a glucose meter. Depending on the reading, they might need to adjust their medication, food intake, or both. We urge them to keep a detailed diary of their blood sugar readings, their medication doses, their food intake, and their exercise. At each medical appointment, we review the diary and their laboratory tests to assess how well they are controlling their disease. If necessary, we adjust their prescriptions or suggest lifestyle modifications.

With type 1 diabetes, the body makes no insulin. So this essential hormone must be injected or delivered through the catheter of an insulin pump. Unfortunately, we don't yet have any way to deliver insulin in a pill or other oral form. That's because insulin is made of amino acids, just like protein. If it entered the stomach, it would be digested as if it were a piece of meat. But pharmaceutical companies are trying to develop insulin pills that will resist digestion, as well as forms of insulin that can be inhaled or taken via skin patches.

About a fifth of people with type 2 diabetes require insulin injections just like those with type 1, because their beta cells have lost the ability to make insulin. In addition, doctors sometimes prescribe insulin temporarily when a patient's blood sugar is extremely high, to help bring it down to normal levels. But if the beta cells are still functioning and blood sugar is not extremely high, other medications—all taken in the form of pills—are used.

Prescribing medicine for type 2 diabetes is an imperfect science that often involves trial and error. Usually treatment begins with one of the sulfonylureas, a class of drugs that increase insulin secretion, or with metformin, which makes the cells more sensitive to insulin and also inhibits the release of stored glucose from the liver. A sulfonylurea and metformin are often used together: the combination of increased insulin and improved insulin sensitivity usually brings blood sugar down, especially if the patient also makes dietary improvements and becomes more active. Sometimes, a combination of different sulfonylureas is used. Or a class of drugs like the sulfonylureas, the meglitinides, can be given because they enhance insulin secretion with less risk of lowering blood sugar too much.

If blood sugar is on target and there are no side effects, the medication regimen is a success. But if the outcome is unsatisfactory, we try a different type of drug or a new combination. There is a category of drugs called thiazolidinediones that markedly enhance insulin sensitivity. When I see that metformin, which also improves sensitivity to insulin, is helpful but not sufficiently so, I might prescribe a thiazolidinedione. Since the thiazolidinediones also seem to lower blood lipids a bit, I tend to use them for patients who have metabolic syndrome, with elevated cholesterol and triglycerides.

The alpha-glucosidase inhibitors, a class of drugs that interfere with carbohydrate absorption, are useful when I'm trying to help a patient who is obese and struggling to lose weight. Many patients find weight loss easier when they're taking an alpha-glucosidase inhibitor.

New medications—and new types of medications—are promising. For example, a new class of drugs, called glucagon-like peptides, still in clinical trials, appears promising when added to other medications. Glucagon-like peptides slow the emptying of the stomach, increase insulin secretion, and inhibit the release of glucagon, the hormone that tells the liver to send its glycogen stores into the blood. More exciting is that these drugs appear to help the beta cells regenerate. If this preliminary finding proves correct, glucagon-like peptides might help people make more insulin on their own.

When I evaluate medication for an individual patient, I also take side effects into account. For example, the alpha-glucosidase inhibitors, which interfere with carbohydrate absorption, can cause gas and abdominal discomfort. Metformin sometimes produces diarrhea and abdominal pain; the thiazolidinediones may cause water retention and weight gain; the sulfonylureas increase the risk of abnormally low blood sugar.

If a patient has side effects, I might switch to a different kind of medication, reduce the dose, or suggest a different timing for the dose. For example, people who experience gastrointestinal problems if they take two metformin tablets twice a day might have no difficulty if they reduce the dose to one pill twice a day. That might be sufficient to keep blood sugar under control.

With Gordon—the teenager with type 2 diabetes I first met when he was brought unconscious to the emergency room—I began treatment with insulin. A couple of weeks later, I reduced his insulin dose and added metformin. It was not yet clear if his beta cells would recover from the dual assault of pancreatitis and type 2 diabetes, and his blood sugar was still high enough to require supplemental insulin. We monitored his condition closely. After a month, his pancreatitis had been resolved and his natural production of insulin increased. As a result, he was experiencing frequent, though mild, hypoglycemia—a sign of excess insulin. We reduced his insulin dose, then a month later discontinued it altogether. He continued to take metformin before breakfast and dinner.

Medication alone can't maintain strict sugar control. It's critical for people with either type of diabetes to follow a nutrition plan, to get regular physical exercise, and to maintain a healthy weight. In the past, a diabetes diagnosis meant a rigid diet. Sweets were forbidden; people were directed to weigh and measure their food and to eat the same amount at the same time every day. But starting in the early 1980s, when home glucose monitors became available, guidelines became more liberal. Clinical research showed that improved testing allowed patients to balance food, activity, and medication successfully without severe restrictions. These days people with diabetes can enjoy appropriate portions of sweets, and they need not weigh everything that goes into their mouths. Nevertheless, they must pay more attention to their diet than the rest of us, because it's harder for their bodies to adjust when meals are irregular or when food intake doesn't match their energy expenditure and medications.

Physical activity benefits us all, but it's especially important for people with diabetes. Exercise lowers blood glucose and increases the body's sensitivity to insulin, aiding sugar control. Furthermore, physical activity contributes to weight loss, which is an issue for most people with type 2 diabetes.

Jaime—the twelve-year-old patient I described earlier, who was referred by a school nurse who thought he was filthy—was diagnosed with diabetes in late December, during school vacation. Over the next week, the clinic nurses and nutritionists worked with him and his parents to establish new routines and new habits.

Since blood tests would tell us if he could control his diabetes adequately without medication, we told Jaime that he had to check his blood sugar four times a day for at least the next three months. At first he was reluctant to stick his finger, fearing that it would hurt. His mother offered to do it for him, but we pointed out that she couldn't be with Jaime during school and at all the other times when he needed to test his blood. We gave him a pen-like lancet device that performs the finger stick quickly and relatively painlessly. Jaime tried it, and—greatly relieved at how easy the procedure was—pronounced it "cool!"

His diet changed drastically. Because Jaime, like most people with type 2 diabetes, was overweight, he needed to cut back on calories. He began drinking water instead of juice and sweetened sodas; he stopped eating fried foods and candy.

A social worker arranged for Jaime to join the local YMCA, and he went to basketball clinic every afternoon. As I had promised, we helped him develop a routine to tame his body odor. He showered before exercising, using a strong antiseptic wash. Then he applied an antiperspirant combined with a deodorant. During the halftime break, he went to the locker room and refreshed his deodorant. After exercise he showered again if necessary.

When school resumed in January, Jaime brought his diabetes healthcare plan to the same school nurse who had referred him to me. The plan I'd written stated that Jaime needed to check his blood sugar before lunch, right after his math class. He'd keep an extra glucose meter and lancet pen in his math teacher's desk, along with a special container for used lancets and glucose strips. He would stick his finger, put the blood on a glucose strip, and wait for the glucose meter to tell him the results. Then he'd record the number in his glucose diary. All this would take only a minute or two, then he could go off to lunch.

Jaime's math teacher agreed to the plan. Since the testing equipment and container of used supplies would be locked in her desk, out of reach of the other children, there was no risk that anyone could get stuck or exposed to Jaime's blood. But the school nurse insisted that Jaime needed to test his blood in the health aide's office, on the other side of the school. Jaime either would have to leave math class fifteen minutes early to get there or else miss fifteen minutes of his lunch period, which was only twenty-two minutes long.

His father called me for advice. "Which would be better?" he asked. "This is his advanced math class, so it's important for him to be there. But I'm afraid that if he's so late for lunch, he won't have time for a healthy meal and he might just grab a candy bar."

I had fought this issue many times in the past. Each time, I was amazed and frustrated that a school would place insurmountable barriers before a child who was trying to maintain both health and academic success. "He shouldn't miss either!" I said to Jaime's father. "Your son has the right under the Americans with Disabilities

Act to take care of his diabetes in the least restrictive environment and with optimal access to educational opportunities, just like everyone else."

I sent Jaime's father to the Web page that the National Diabetes Education Program has set up for school nurses. The page—called "Helping the Student with Diabetes Succeed"—explains the rights of children with diabetes in the school. I told Jaime's father to show this to the school nurse, the principal, and anyone else in the school who was not aware of the law. I suggested he contact the American Diabetes Association if the problem was not resolved. If necessary, ADA would advise him, and might even assist with legal action to allow Jaime equal access to education and to take care of his health in school.

A few days later—after considerable back-and-forth among me, the school nurse, the principal, and Jaime's father—Jaime was checking his blood sugar levels after math class, so he missed none of his class and still had time to eat a healthy lunch. Three months after his diagnosis, Jaime had lost 15 pounds and his blood sugar was under excellent control. His acanthosis nigricans had faded considerably, and his body odor was acceptable. The school nurse never apologized. She simply told me, "I guess things are good. He isn't filthy anymore."

Some diseases are worse than diabetes. But none requires such a complex balancing act, where patients must do so much themselves. When you're diagnosed with diabetes, the disease infiltrates every moment and clouds the future. Gordon was right: diabetes sucks!

A Life-Altering Diagnosis

Every morning and every night after Grandma Sadie was diagnosed with type 2 diabetes, she would give my mother a urine specimen in a small cup. Urine tests are no longer used for routine diabetes care, because blood tests are much more precise. But until the beginning of the 1980s, the only way to assess day-to-day diabetes management at home was with a urine sugar test. I'd watch my mother dip a dropper into the cup, then place two drops of urine in a test tube with ten drops of water. To the mixture she would add a tablet containing a chemical that reacted with glucose. Then we would wait two minutes for the results. My mother seemed to hold her breath. My grandmother would busy herself in the kitchen, as if the test didn't matter. In fact, my grandmother acted as if her diabetes didn't matter. That frustrated my parents, and as I grew older it frustrated me.

After the two minutes were up, my mother and I would look at the test tube to see what color the mixture was; my grandmother showed no interest. If the liquid had turned blue, that was good, because it meant Sadie's urine had no sugar. But most of the time it was brown, and that was bad. Brown indicated a high sugar content. After the test, my mother would give my grandmother her insulin shot. Five extra units of insulin would be added to her usual dose if the urine test had been brown.

My grandmother's diabetes was not well controlled. After her brown tests and after her medical appointments, my parents would argue with her and with each other. My father would shout: "Mom, you've been sneaking candies again!" He would demand that she follow her nutrition plan. My mother would plead with her. And my grandmother would answer, "So it makes such a difference in the vorld if I have a piece of candy?"

When I was in high school, I frequently performed my grandmother's urine test and gave her the insulin injections. I often think back on those days now when I work with teenagers. My teenage patients—in fact, most of my preteen patients—take more responsibility for managing their diabetes than my grandmother ever did for hers.

By the time I started medical school, my grandmother had developed high blood pressure and early kidney disease as a result of her diabetes. Her legs were swollen, and she was always tired. The restrictions mounted. She could not eat pickles or add salt to her food; she could not get upset; she could not gain any more weight. But the more my grandmother was told what she could not do, the more she rebelled. My parents were exasperated.

As Sadie grew older, heavier, and sicker, it seemed cruel to deny her the pleasures she wanted. Yet my parents and I were baffled and frustrated that she couldn't curb her consumption of sweets, despite knowing how harmful they were. I realize now that after going to bed hungry for so many years when she was a child, feeling full must have made my grandmother feel more secure than following her diabetes regimen and controlling her blood glucose.

I visited Sadie as frequently as I could when I was in medical school. She'd introduce me to her friends when I picked her up: "You vant maybe to meet my granddaughter? She's almost a doctor."

As I helped her into my car for our excursion, I'd ask: "So, Grandma, how's your diabetes?"

"Diabetes, shmiabetes," she would answer. "From you too now I get diabetes? That's all I hear."

"Grandma," I would reply, "it's just that we are all worried about you. We want you to take better care of yourself."

"No, everyone just vants to tell me vhat to do. You know, I didn't have a mother to tell me vhat to do. The last time I saw my father vas vhen I vas sixteen, so he didn't have the chance to tell me vhat to do. Now that I'm an old lady, you and your parents don't need to start telling me vhat to do. And that young doctor," she continued—talking about her internist, who was at least fifty—"he don't need to tell me nothing."

After dinner I'd ask, "Grandma, how much insulin do you think you need tonight?" I was trying to get her involved in managing her disease.

"How should I know?" she would respond, annoyed.

"It's your body," I would reply.

"Then let me do vhat I vant."

I remember the day I told her I was thinking of becoming a diabetes specialist. "Such a big shot," she said. Then she thought for a while and asked, "So if you're a diabetes specialist, vill you be for or against diabetes?"

"Against diabetes," I answered. Then I quickly added, "But I'll be for all people with diabetes."

"You can only pick one," she retorted.

DEVASTATING NEWS

Diabetes is a chronic disease, one that can be fatal. The diagnosis is a shock and an immense challenge. Every time I must deliver this news, I'm filled with trepidation. I'm telling a child, an adult, or family members that diabetes has entered their lives, and I know I must pick each word with meticulous care.

Denial is a common reaction to bad news of any kind. Many newly diagnosed patients immediately say, "This can't be true." So my first task is to convince them that the diagnosis of diabetes is correct, that there is no doubt. Then I have to explain that diabetes requires them to alter their lives. Nothing will be as it was before. I need to figure out not only what treatments they need but also how to educate them, support them, and give them the skills to manage their own disease themselves—something my own grandmother could never do. As I speak, I worry that a slip of the tongue might confuse or upset them.

Diabetes requires radical lifestyle changes. Here's what a day looks like when a person has diabetes: wake up, prick finger and check blood sugar, take medication, eat breakfast, check blood sugar again before lunch, adjust medication, eat lunch, exercise and eat a snack if necessary to prevent blood sugar from becoming too low, check blood sugar before dinner, take medication, eat dinner, check blood sugar before bedtime, take medication, consider eating a bedtime snack to prevent low blood sugar overnight, and check blood sugar again in the middle of the night if anything out of the ordinary has occurred during the day. Plus, write everything in a detailed diary—the test results, the doses of medications, the meals and snacks, the physical activity.

In addition to the daily routine, there are frequent medical visits. Instead of an annual checkup, as recommended for healthy people, medical appointments come every three months—and are more stress provoking than ordinary checkups because of the specter of fearsome diabetes complications.

Understandably, people who are diagnosed with diabetes feel a loss of normalcy. Emotions run strong. Patients often experience depression, despair, and a sense of doom. They may become angry and refuse to accept the diagnosis. Or they may react with shame and embarrassment. Adults sometimes feel like failures because they've been unable to keep their own body healthy and strong. Children and teenagers often don't want anyone else to know—they feel like pariahs. For children who are too young to understand the concept of disease, diabetes means that their parents keep coming at them with needles. They may hide under their beds, terrified, and wonder why they're suddenly being punished.

Diabetes affects the entire family. Children whose parent gets diabetes worry that the parent may die and abandon them, just as I feared that my grandmother might die. Or they wonder if they're next to be diagnosed. They may be scared by the needles and other equipment, and wince as their mother or father pricks a finger for a blood test or injects insulin.

Spouses suffer enormously. They wake up in the middle of the night to make sure their partner is still breathing. If a loved one is late from work, they fear he or she is dead somewhere as a result of diabetes. Sometimes a partner will infantilize the person with diabetes, watching every morsel that goes into their mouth, telling them what to eat and what to do. Mutual resentment and anger can result.

Mothers and fathers of children who get diabetes often blame themselves. They wonder, "What did I do wrong to bring this disease upon my child?" Or they may blame each other. When I inform parents of the diagnosis, I sometimes hear, "Well, he didn't get it from *my* side of the family!"

Parents' lives become consumed with diabetes paraphernalia; their minds fill with diabetes-related fears and concerns. It's almost impossible not to become overprotective, not to hover. Siblings hate diabetes because it takes their parents' time and attention. They worry that something they did in anger might have caused their brother or sister to get sick, and they fear that they might get diabetes, too.

On top of everything else, there are costs in money and time. Diabetes treatment is expensive. People must buy multiple medications, syringes, a glucose meter, and supplies. Even those whose insurance covers these expenses may spend over $100 per month on co-payments. There are extra medical appointments, which means additional co-payments, transportation costs, and days off from work.

Diabetes management is time-consuming. Moreover, successful sugar control requires order in every aspect of a person's life. Those who love to live by the clock, and who are already bonded to routine, become fixated. They calculate their portions, their exercise, and their insulin doses over and over again, leaving them little time to think about anything else. Meanwhile, those who hate regimentation—who refuse to wear a watch, who are accustomed to eating at irregular hours, who like to stay out late and sleep until noon on weekends—chafe at the new need for order. For everyone, spur-of-the-moment is gone forever.

TAKING CHARGE

When I meet with people newly diagnosed with diabetes, I tell them: "Your doctor can't navigate for you. If you want to succeed with this disease, someone has to be in charge—and the best person is you." Of course, family members take full responsibility when the patient is an infant. But as soon as toddlers are able to speak, I begin to teach them that this is *their* diabetes. If I'm examining a two-year-old, I ask him to show me where he pricks his fingers and where he gets his shots; I'll say, "You're doing a good job with your diabetes," emphasizing that it's his. As children grow older, more of the questions and instructions are directed toward them during medical visits, and less toward their parents.

School-age children can participate in their own care. We teach them to recognize the signs of low blood sugar—feeling hungry, or shaky legs, or an aching tummy. We encourage youngsters to play a role in their blood tests: we ask them to pick which finger to use, to press the button on the device that pricks the finger, to put their blood on the testing strip. If they can't yet read numbers, we tell them if a result is high or low and explain if this means they'll need another shot before they can have something to eat. At this point, they need help with diabetes management from parents, teachers, and nurses or health aides. But by age eight or nine, many young patients can test their own blood sugar, make decisions about balancing insulin and food, and give themselves their own shots after an adult checks to be sure the dose is correct.

Teenagers take more and more responsibility for their own care. But they still need to check in with their parents and discuss their diabetes. It's important for parents to create an atmosphere in which adolescents can talk about their high and low blood sugar tests and be helped rather than judged or punished if their diabetes care isn't optimal. At medical appointments with teenagers, I try to make sure we talk alone for some of the time, but I also include parents for part of the discussion. I want to convey that although the teen has most of the responsibility for managing the diabetes, their parents and I are the support team.

When children leave home or turn eighteen, by law they are in charge of their own medical care. I must obtain their permission to talk to their parents, something I always encourage. Even at this age, parental involvement remains important, because most young adults need frequent validation to stay on track.

DIABETES CAMP

For almost twenty years I've run the teen session at Camp Chinnock, a camp in Southern California for children and teenagers with diabetes. There are similar camps around the country and throughout the world. For a few weeks in the summer, kids can be in a place where having diabetes is the norm. No one asks you what diabetes is or if it's contagious. No one says, "What are you doing?" when you check your blood sugar. Until 1996, only those taking insulin were allowed to come to the camp. But since the summer of 1997, in response to the rising tide of type 2 diabetes in youth, the camp has been open to all youngsters with diabetes, regardless of type or treatment.

Over a hundred campers—all kids age fourteen to sixteen with diabetes—attend the one-week session for teenagers. Another hundred counselors and staff participate. The counselors who oversee the teens range in age from eighteen to twenty-five, and they also have diabetes. I have a love/hate relationship with diabetes camp. It's a lot of work. On a typical day, I analyze 1,000 blood glucose levels and approve 600 doses of insulin; I must treat thirty to forty mild hypoglycemic reactions—incidents in which blood sugar dips too low and youngsters feel lightheaded or even confused. This happens because they're more physically active at camp and their bodies burn more glucose; also, they don't have continuous access to food. When I'm at camp, I miss the comforts of home. Though my cabin, the doctor's cabin, is Camp Chinnock's most luxurious, I must share it with the resident mice and bugs. I hate sleeping in a sleeping bag on a cot. Not that I get much sleep. Almost every night at camp, I'm awakened to attend to an emergency, such as an abnormally high or low blood sugar level.

Each summer at the end of camp, I vow never to return again. But I come back year after year. What draws me? It's watching the teenagers grow from the experience. Regardless of ethnicity, gender, race, or socioeconomic status, they face a common enemy together. They learn, find support, and have fun. They begin to understand that they can control their diabetes and that diabetes doesn't have to control them. Camp shows that there's no shame and no blame attached to diabetes.

These children come from the inner city, from affluent suburbs, and from rural areas I've never heard of. They come from poverty and privilege, from intact homes and broken ones, from hope and despair. They become friends and allies. I listen to them ask each other the questions they're afraid to ask me. They ask about their futures; they ask whether they can have normal sexual relations and normal babies. They ask how long they will live. They try to imagine what it must be like to not have diabetes. Later I talk with them about what I've overheard. We talk in the canoes as we paddle around the lake, in the mess hall while we're waiting for our food. I find them on the porch or at the pool. I try to give them the answers they need to hear, to dispel rumors and falsehoods. Whether the truth is harsher or better than what they had imagined, it's their right to know it and my responsibility to tell them.

In some way, the easiest part of being in a camp full of teens is managing blood sugar levels. Much more difficult is dealing with teenage rebellion—the need to break rules, the desire to buck authority. Fourteen-year-old girls emerge from their cabins wearing skimpy bathing suit tops and bottoms that are barely more than thongs. I tell them that they need to cover more of their body parts before they can be seen in public. I must remind some of the boys to keep their hands to themselves and to watch the words they use in conversation. But the real challenge is getting them to take control over their diabetes. For many of them, camp is the place where they first learn to manage their disease without their parents.

I have watched many of these children grow up at diabetes camp. I've watched my own children grow up there, too. When they were young, they stayed with me in my cabin. But later they were allowed to join the campers and even become counselors though they don't have diabetes. Doing all this has made them just a little more humble, a little more appreciative, a little more aware.

Diabetes camp has taught me more than I could have imagined about teens, about diabetes, and about how much I am willing to endure—insects, sleeping bags, and incredible fatigue. Helping people with diabetes is not just about science or state-of-the-art treatments. Help is about feeling and giving; it's about hugs. To help people with diabetes, you have to be state-of-the-art and state-of-the-heart.

In the early 1990s I also participated in family camps for children with diabetes. Not just kids but whole families would come to the wilderness for a weekend, to learn more about diabetes and to find support from those facing the same challenges. On the first morning, while the kids went off with the counselors, we would hold separate rap sessions for the mothers and for the fathers. These sessions were designed to break the ice and to get us on common ground.

The mothers would go first. We sat in a circle. Within minutes the mothers would start to cry. One by one they'd speak about how they never stop worrying, never stop checking: Did my son take his snack? Did my daughter test her blood? Did she remember to bring her lunch? Will he survive? The others would all nod, crying. All of them felt validated and relieved. Their concerns were the same. They were not crazy for feeling consumed by fears about their child's diabetes.

Next came the session for fathers. They would sit down quietly, defensively, with no tears. It was always a challenge to get them to speak and to open up. But one year—I will always remember this moment—a father started to talk even before we all sat down. I had never heard a father speak that way before. He said, "My son is five. Ben got diabetes when he was two years old. I couldn't believe it." Some of the other fathers looked uneasy, wondering how personal he would get.

Ben's father continued, "I didn't know right then what it meant to have diabetes, but I felt really bad. Like it was my fault, like I hadn't done my job to protect my kid. When Ben got that first shot, I just didn't know what to do. He was screaming and crying; the nurse was chasing him around the room. I grabbed him and told him, 'I have diabetes, too. We're going to take our shots together.'"

The other men were leaning forward now. He went on, "The nurse was a little miffed, but I convinced her to give me a shot of water. After that, Ben let her give him his shot. The problem was when we got home, I didn't know how to stop it. I didn't want to tell him I'd lied. And I didn't want to say that I was cured but he wasn't. So for the last three years I've been taking water shots every day." He sighed, obviously relieved by his confession, then said: "What I want to know is, how do I stop?"

Silence. I remembered my nurse telling me she had given this man a shot when Ben was diagnosed. The nurse felt bad about the subterfuge. But neither of us had known he was still doing it.

All eyes were on me. I was the doctor, the expert. I had brought everyone there to fix their problems. I felt a wave of nausea. Hey, I was an endocrinologist, not a psychiatrist and certainly not a magician. I gathered my thoughts and responded, "This is pretty tough. But I think you have to tell Ben the truth."

Some of the fathers nodded; others shook their heads in vehement disagreement. One father said, "No way you can tell him. He'd never trust you again. You just gotta keep it up."

"Trust is so important," I said. "What if you tell him why you did it—that you felt really bad for him and were just trying to help?" Even as I said it, I thought it was unrealistic to expect a five-year-old to comprehend such an explanation. Then I had an inspiration: "You could do it with a child psychiatrist with you," I added.

The fathers liked that: get some shrink to take the fall. There was a lively discussion about where to do it (not in the wilderness, everyone agreed); they talked about which shrink to bring. Everyone said I should be there, too. An army of experts would support Ben's dad.

When family camp was over, I talked to the head of psychiatry at Childrens Hospital. We came up with a simple strategy. Ben, his father, his mother, and the psychiatrist would meet in my office, which was familiar ground for Ben. His father would tell Ben he loved him. He would tell his son that when he'd learned that Ben had diabetes, he had become very sad. One of the reasons was that he knew Ben would feel bad because he was the only one in the family who had to take shots. So he wanted to make Ben feel he was not alone. But it wasn't true that his dad had diabetes. Now that Ben was a big boy, his dad wanted him to know the truth. Telling the truth is the most important thing to do, and sometimes even daddies make a mistake.

Three days later, everyone assembled in my office. Ben bounced into the room, followed by his parents. I was already seated next to the psychiatrist. I introduced Ben to her, and he plopped into his seat between his parents. "So, Ben," I began, "I asked your mom and dad to bring you here today because when we were all at family camp, your father told us something that we felt we needed to talk to you about." I hesitated, then blurted it out: "We felt we needed to talk to you about your father taking shots with you."

Ben squirmed in his chair. His father said, "I want to tell you the truth about my shots, Ben." He took a deep breath. "I want to tell you—" he began, but Ben interrupted.

"Daddy, why do you take shots? You don't have diabetes." Then he laughed and jumped up and hugged his father. That was it. Ben was five years old, but somehow he knew the truth. With that hug, he finally liberated his father.

DISCRIMINATION: SALT IN THE WOUND OF DIABETES

One issue that no one thinks about before they are diagnosed is discrimination. In Chapter 4, I described the discrimination that Jaime encountered in school. Other families in my practice have had similar problems. One of my young patients was told she couldn't go on her school trip to Washington, D.C., because of her diabetes. Another was excluded from the California Junior Lifeguard Program.

A young law school graduate was forbidden from sitting for the bar exam with her glucose meter and sugar tablets. All of these restrictions were successfully challenged, but not until my patients and their families were put through anguish and despair.

You might be surprised to learn that you're not allowed to enlist in the U.S. military if you have diabetes. Until a few years ago, you were immediately discharged if the condition developed while you were in the service. These days, the fate of people who are diagnosed with diabetes while in the military is decided on a case-by-case basis. The American Diabetes Association advocates a similar approach for those already diagnosed who would like to serve.

Workplace discrimination persists, despite state and federal laws designed to protect against it. Employers are not supposed to discriminate against people with any kind of disability who are qualified for a job and can carry out the work. What's more, employers are obliged to make reasonable accommodations to allow disabled individuals to perform their jobs. This means, for example, that an employer would have to adjust a worker's schedule to allow quick breaks for blood tests and insulin shots, provided that was feasible. Nevertheless, I've seen people get fired when they're diagnosed with diabetes. Promotions don't come; offers are withdrawn; doors close.

In 2003 a man named Jeff Kapche won an important victory over the city of San Antonio, Texas. The battle started in 1994 when he applied to become a police officer for the city. He'd worked hard, passed every hurdle, and aced every test. Yet when he went for his medical exam and disclosed that he had type 1 diabetes, he was taken out of the running. He was told that diabetes was an absolute exclusion to becoming a police officer in San Antonio—despite the fact he had well-controlled diabetes, with no blood sugar or health problems, and despite the fact that his application was otherwise totally acceptable.

Jeff Kapche had always wanted to be a police officer; he had never thought about being anything else. So he decided to fight back and sued the city of San Antonio. He did this because he was outraged and because he did not want anyone with diabetes to face the same kind of discrimination. Behind him was a stellar team: his family; a tough-minded attorney, John Griffin; two no-nonsense medical experts, Dr. Ralph DeFronzo and Dr. Edward Horton, former president of the American Diabetes Association (ADA); and the founder of the ADA's Legal Advocacy Network, Michael Greene.

The case worked its way up through the federal courts, with both sides refusing to give up. But finally, in 2002, the Fifth Circuit Court of Appeals issued a decision that vindicated Jeff Kapche and all people with diabetes: no one could be denied a job simply because of diabetes. Each person had to be evaluated as an individual, based on his or her own merits and frailties. In 2003 Jeff Kapche accepted a $325,000 settlement from the city of San Antonio. Ironically, he had been a police officer in a neighboring community since 1994—and was promoted to detective in 1999. He decided to remain there rather than reapplying to San Antonio.

Social discrimination takes an equally painful toll. But there's no appealing to the Fifth Circuit Court if a new boyfriend or girlfriend backs off when you reveal you have diabetes. Some people try to keep the disease a secret. If no one knows, they reason, no one will treat them differently or think they are less whole. I knew a man who checked his blood sugar in the bathroom stall at work before lunch every day. He would sit on the toilet seat and take his insulin injection. Then one day he dropped his syringe and it rolled onto the bathroom floor, in full sight of colleagues who were washing their hands. This man had to think for a minute: would he rather have people think he was a drug addict or that he had diabetes? He told me, "I told them the truth, but it was not an easy decision to make."

My grandmother died in her mid-eighties from cardiovascular disease, one consequence of her diabetes. She had struggled with diabetes and its many complications for almost two decades. Though lifestyle changes would have improved her health, she struggled against those, too. I learned from her experience that living successfully with diabetes requires people to assume responsibility for managing it.

Diabetes never takes a vacation and never gives anyone a break.

By the time one shot is finished or one pill is taken, it's time to prepare for the next. When one blood test is completed, the next one
must be anticipated. Each meal or snack requires thought. When
patients and families react to all this, I empathize. And I assure them
that they can adjust. Somehow, as time goes on and as diabetes
comes under control, the hurt and anger will diminish. They will
find inner strength and strength from the support of family and
friends, and they will learn how to get on with their lives.

S I X

Running on Empty

When people without diabetes talk about hypoglycemia, they're usually thinking of the slightly lightheaded or sluggish feeling they get when they're hungry. That's like a spring shower compared to the hurricane that can afflict someone with diabetes. Severe hypoglycemia can strike in an instant. One minute, you're standing; the next, you're in a coma, or you're on the floor having a convulsion, drooling, biting your tongue, and wetting your pants, with your arms and legs shaking with a rhythmic intensity that conjures up a medieval image of apocalyptic proportions. During this kind of hypoglycemic episode, you feel as if you've entered a black box and might not be able to find your way out again.

Hypoglycemia is not a complication of diabetes itself. Rather, it's a complication of the *treatment* of diabetes. It happens when there's an imbalance between diabetes medications—most often insulin—and food intake and physical activity. Diabetes medications are supposed to prevent high blood sugar. But if someone who is taking insulin or other diabetes drugs skips a meal, eats less, or is more active than usual, blood sugar can plummet.

Perhaps two or three times per week, someone with type 1 diabetes checks his or her blood sugar and finds that it's less than

60 mg/dl. Associated with this, he or she may experience symptoms: feeling shaky, sweaty, hungry, lightheaded, or even a little confused. The person may notice that his or her heart is racing. This is considered mild hypoglycemia. It's quickly and easily corrected by taking glucose in oral form—a glass of juice, glucose gel, or glucose tablets.

The problem occurs in only about a quarter of people with type 2 diabetes, usually those who are taking insulin or multiple diabetes pills, particularly the sulfonylureas, which increase insulin secretion. But it can also happen to type 2 patients who are beginning to lose weight from dieting and exercising and who haven't yet adjusted their medication. Similarly, kids with either form of diabetes may experience hypoglycemia during gym at school, and it's often a problem at diabetes camp or when people take an active vacation.

As a doctor, I share the frustration when someone with type 2 diabetes begins to exercise, eat right, and lose weight—and then, just as they're experiencing success, they develop hypoglycemia. They feel dizzy, confused, lightheaded. In addition to the anxiety caused by these symptoms, they're famished. So they eat more to compensate—and their weight comes right back on. Understandably, they become terribly discouraged. Fortunately, the situation can be corrected by decreasing some of the diabetes medications and by paying more attention to the timing of meals and snacks. For example, a small snack before exercise can prevent hypoglycemia without causing weight gain.

Mild hypoglycemia is a minor problem—unless it is not corrected. But if blood sugar plummets below 40 mg/dl and remains low, the condition is potentially life-threatening. When insufficient sugar is brought to the brain, the brain cells can't work properly. If the sugar level drops too low for too long, a person can become confused, have convulsions, and enter a coma. That's severe hypoglycemia, and it can be fatal.

Because severe hypoglycemia is so dangerous, our bodies have evolved many protective mechanisms to detect a falling blood sugar level and correct it. When blood sugar drops, adrenaline (also called epinephrine) is released by the adrenal glands. This causes us to feel anxious, hungry, and lightheaded. Our heart rate increases. These changes prompt us to search for food.

At the same time, the body sends signals to several glands, activating alternative fuel sources. The pituitary gland at the base of our brain releases growth hormone, which enables the body to make sugar from its fat stores. Another emergency fuel reserve is found in our muscles. When blood sugar falls too low, the adrenal glands release cortisol, which speeds up the normal turnover of muscle tissue. As muscle breaks down, its amino acids are released and used for energy. Cortisol also interferes with the action of insulin in our cells: if the cells can't absorb sugar, more remains in the blood. The brain doesn't need insulin to let sugar into its cells. Therefore, if there's more sugar in our blood, there's more for our brain to use. This preserves brain function. In addition, the pancreas releases glucagon from the alpha cells, which are right next to the beta cells that make insulin. Glucagon causes our liver to release its supply of stored glucose.

All these compensatory mechanisms usually bring blood sugar back to a healthy range, protecting us from severe hypoglycemia. But both types of diabetes can impair these crucial responses, as can the excess insulin in the bloodstream that's characteristic of type 2 diabetes in its early stages. Furthermore, the body's safeguards against low blood sugar are blunted by repeated episodes of hypoglycemia. As we explain to patients, hypoglycemia begets hypoglycemia. Over time, the autonomic nervous system—the part of the nervous system that controls our glands—becomes less responsive to falling blood sugar levels.

Most people with diabetes, whether type 1 or type 2, are alert to signs that their blood sugar level is becoming dangerously low. They realize that they're becoming overwhelmed by hunger or fatigue—especially if these feelings are associated with headache, lightheadedness, chills, shakiness, rapid heartbeat, or a sense of malaise. Quickly, they consume a ready source of sugar to push glucose into their bloodstream.

Hypoglycemia can turn deadly when the early signals are missed or aren't apparent. Sometimes blood sugar drops too quickly or the warning mechanisms are impaired by the disease itself. In other cases, drugs or alcohol interfere with judgment. If the person is lucky, someone else—a family member, friend, or colleague—will recognize the signs and intervene. Other people sometimes spot personality changes characteristic of hypoglycemia, such as irritability, impatience, or sadness; or they might notice confusion or odd behavior.

A particular danger time is during sleep. Though only a third of a person's time is spent asleep, over half of hypoglycemic episodes occur during sleep. That's because people aren't checking glucose levels or eating, and they're unaware of symptoms when they're asleep. I have never met someone with diabetes, whether type 1 or type 2, who doesn't worry about having hypoglycemia during the night. This fear is heightened once they learn about "dead in the bed"—death from severe night-time hypoglycemia. In this tragic situation, low blood sugar symptoms don't wake the person up. "Dead in the bed" occurs when there's no one nearby to hear them convulsing, no one to give them sugar or call for help.

THE ALBATROSS

Hypoglycemia is the albatross around my neck. It ties my hands as an endocrinologist, and it interferes with my patients' ability to reduce their overall glucose levels. As they get down to the range that's optimal for avoiding long-term complications of diabetes, they may experience more frequent hypoglycemia. It can happen at work, or at school, or on the street. If one of those episodes is severe, all hell breaks loose. After they recover, they don't care if their blood sugar soars way above the desired range. Anything is better than waking up and not knowing where you are, with a puddle of urine collected around your legs, and medics putting you in an ambulance.

Hypoglycemia, even in its milder form, affects mood, personality, and performance. As someone's blood sugar level drops, they can become anxious and agitated, confused and irrational. They feel out of sorts, out of control, and disconnected. When this occurs repeatedly, it drives them and the people around them crazy. At first others may not realize what's happening. A parent or the police may suspect instead that a teenager is high on drugs or alcohol. A spouse asks a question and gets no response. Then the spouse suggests that it's time for a glucose tablet, only to get an angry denial. Now the spouse is left wondering if the anger is a reaction to nagging or yet another sign of hypoglycemia. Understandably, relationships may deteriorate.

Friends and family members who have watched their loved one lose consciousness will tell you there's not much that's worse. Imagine waking up in your bed, watching in terror as your partner convulses next to you. Or think what it's like for parents to see their young child fall off a chair and stare at them, unable to speak. No wonder that from then on they can't shake the fear that some day hypoglycemia will strike and no one will be there to rescue the person they love.

On top of everything else, hypoglycemia is the prime rationale for the workplace discrimination I discussed in Chapter 5. Whole industries are unwilling to employ people with diabetes out of concern about hypoglycemia: perhaps low blood sugar will render a firefighter incapable or a truck driver dangerous on the road.

IN MY OWN HOME

I know what it's like to live under the cloud of severe hypoglycemia because Lance, one of my patients, became like an adopted son to me. I met Lance when I was a fourth-year medical student. He had developed type 1 diabetes at age nine, while he was attending Boy Scout camp in the Southern California mountains. He'd been feeling unwell at camp, with constant thirst and frequent urination. Later, when he knew me better, he told me that he'd even wet his bed. But he didn't mention any of this to the camp nurse. Maybe he blamed the problems on the fact that he was in a strange environment. Or perhaps he was reluctant to draw attention to himself because he was the only African American at the camp. But one morning he could not get out of bed. By noon, he was in a coma. The camp rushed him to the local hospital, which telephoned us for help. I was on call with the medical center transport team that flew by helicopter into the mountains to get him.

I was excited as I boarded the helicopter filled with emergency medical equipment: IVs, endotracheal tubes, medications, and solutions that I was sure could bring life back to anyone. The helicopter whirled off the roof of Childrens Hospital Los Angeles, sped through mountain passes, and landed on a rural high school football field on the forty-yard line. An ambulance met us and whisked us to the nearby hospital.

Lance lay on a gurney in the hospital's antiquated emergency room. He was emaciated and clearly dehydrated. Even though his body lacked adequate fluid, urine soaked through the sheet upon which he lay. We administered liquids and insulin immediately. Then we loaded him into the ambulance, drove back to the helicopter, piled Lance and ourselves inside, and took off. I remained at his side during the flight back to Los Angeles, watching as he improved from the solutions being dripped into his body.

I followed Lance in my medical student clinic; I continued to see him with the staff endocrinologists when I was an intern and resident. I was his doctor when I was an endocrine fellow, and he remained my patient once I was a fully trained endocrinologist. My staff and I helped get him into the best public schools possible, where the academics were excellent and the nursing coverage was more than just adequate. I secured the latest diabetes equipment for him and tried to help him keep his blood sugar in the acceptable range. When it went off track, I patched him back together. And he and I were rewarded. Lance sailed through high school; in fact, he was a star. He led the debating team and the chess club. After his senior year, he went off to college on a scholarship. By then he was old enough to see an adult endocrinologist rather than a pediatric specialist. But we'd gone through a lot together, and neither of us was ready to sever the ties.

One day in 1984 Lance arrived in the clinic for one of his every-three-month appointments. I was exhausted from lack of sleep. My sons were four and six, and we were in the middle of yet another babysitter crisis. But seeing Lance was always a pleasure. "So, Lance, how's school?" I asked him.

"Well..." He hesitated. "Things could be better. I'm having a lot of trouble with my diabetes, and classes are a lot harder than I ever thought they would be, especially math." His voice lowered and he looked away from me as he spoke. "I just don't know if I can hack it. I think I'll lose my scholarship, 'cause my grades suck." My heart sank. The deep level of concern in his voice made me nervous. All that work. And he had done so well in high school.

"Lance, how can I help make it better?" I implored. There were dark circles under his eyes, and his eyes were red. I couldn't tell whether this was from lack of sleep or because he'd been crying.

He shrugged. "I don't know. Two weeks ago my roommate came in the dorm in the middle of the day and said I was really out of it. Thought I was on drugs or drunk or something. But then he remembered my diabetes and called the dorm assistant. They had to stuff sugar down me. I woke up with this granulated crap all over my face and I don't remember it, not one damn thing. Scary, huh?"

Lance had hypoglycemia unawareness: he had lost his ability to sense that his blood sugar level was dropping. I tried to imagine how tough it was for him, dealing with diabetes, poverty, difficult classes, and a twenty-hour-a-week job. I wondered how he did it, how anybody could do it. No wonder he was having trouble.

"Well, let me see your blood sugar diary," I said. "Are you adjusting your insulin frequently?"

He handed me a ragged book filled with numbers representing his blood sugar tests over the preceding three months. Next to the numbers were comments like "worked late," "basketball," "pizza," and "date." At the beginning of each day's recordings, he had written down his insulin doses. A teenager with well-controlled diabetes might have blood sugar numbers ranging from 70 to 180 mg/dl on any given day. But Lance's numbers dipped as low as 40 mg/dl, then soared to 400 mg/dl twelve hours later. I stared in amazement at the extremes of his blood sugar excursions. A person could lose consciousness if his blood sugar fell below 40 mg/dl. "Lance," I said, deeply concerned, "this is really horrible. What's going on?"

"I do okay for a couple of days," he responded. "Then I have to work all night and that throws me off."

"Could you get a job during the day?" I asked.

"Yeah, but I would have to work even more for the same amount of money. Then I'd have no time to study." He hung his head, engulfed in despair.

At that moment, I had a thought. The idea crystallized in my mind, then leaped from being just a suggestion to becoming a full-fledged solution, a clear solution to everyone's problems—his need for stability and my family's need for a babysitter. I quietly explained, "Lance, listen to this and tell me what you think. If you don't like it, that's okay. You can just pass it off, no problem." He stared at me. I continued. "Transfer to school in LA and live in my house. Help me with my kids, mainly by just being there. Be there at night if I have to go into work, be there when they get home from preschool and kindergarten. You won't be a maid, but more like a big brother."

He looked at me with amazement as I went on: "We really need somebody to help us, Lance. We don't want to have someone we don't know live in our house. But we need somebody at home to be with our children. We'll pay you. Room and board will be free. It will give you a chance to finish school, and you'll have more time to study. I'll help with your diabetes—maybe we can get rid of those lows."

He interjected, "Hey, I don't know anything about little white kids."

"They don't know anything about big black guys," I replied. "So you're even."

He smiled. "Know what?" he said. "It might work."

Lance came to live with my family. He was a wonderful addition to all of our lives. My boys adored him and called him "Bro." He taught them karate moves; he introduced them to chess. He brought us laughter and love. And one morning he brought us severe hypoglycemia.

I had knocked on Lance's bedroom door, as I did every morning to awaken him. But that day there was no response. I knocked again. This time, I heard moaning and then a scream. The scream was primal. It came from Lance's room, but it sounded as if it had traveled from another universe. I knew immediately he was having a hypoglycemic convulsion. I needed to get to him right away, but the door was locked. I pounded on the door and screamed, "Lance! Lance!"

More moans. I had no idea where the key was, and there was no time to look. My husband had already gone to work. I yelled for help.

Adam, my six-year-old, and Jonah, who was four, came running. "Mommy! Mommy! What's wrong?" Adam asked.

"Bring me a knife from the kitchen," I told him. "The big sharp one that's near the sink." His eyes widened as he realized I was telling him to break the family rule about boys and sharp knives. I continued banging the door and shouting Lance's name, hoping to keep him from slipping into deeper unconsciousness. When Adam returned, I pried the knife between the door and the lock. Somehow, as I pushed and shoved, the door popped open.

Lance was on the floor, covered with frothy vomit, shaking violently. His head was tilted to the left, and his eyes were deviated upward and to the right—they looked like they were possessed by an incoherent spirit. Adam stared; Jonah burst into tears. I felt terror and panic.

"Get the sugar bowl, fast! Run!" I yelled to Adam. "Then get my doctor's bag out of the car." I turned Lance onto his side so that if he vomited again, he wouldn't inhale it into his lungs. Adam dashed back with the sugar bowl, half full now because of what he'd spilled on the floor en route from the kitchen. I shoveled sugar into Lance's mouth and rubbed it into his gums. Jonah tried to help, but in his convulsions Lance almost bit Jonah's finger. When Adam returned from the car with my medical bag, I ripped open the box that contained our salvation: glucagon. Injected into his muscle, glucagon would travel with lightning speed to Lance's liver to release all his stored glycogen and replenish his fuel supply.

I filled the syringe, my hands shaking, my pulse audible in my own ears, and my mind feeling as if I had been lifted out of my body. I've always gotten that out-of-body feeling during dire emergencies: when I've done cardiopulmonary resuscitation on babies; the first time I placed a tube into the chest of a newborn, knowing that if I missed the right spot, the infant could die; when I placed a large-gauge needle into the trachea of a three-year-old dying from a hot dog lodged in his airway. In all those instances I watched myself perform these tasks as if I were a distant observer.

With my mind and body disconnected, I managed to inject Lance with the glucagon-filled syringe. As I withdrew the needle, he stopped breathing for fifteen seconds, a near eternity. I poised myself to begin mouth-to-mouth resuscitation, to place my lips upon his vomit-filled face and mouth. Suddenly he sighed a cavernous sigh and began to breathe on his own. His violent movement ceased, but then he stopped breathing once again. Another eternity. A few seconds later, he began breathing normally. After a few minutes, he began to recover. Still somewhat confused and dazed, he asked me what had happened. Why was he on the floor? Were the kids okay? I touched his arm and told him to rest, and then I hugged my boys. Their bodies, like mine, were limp with relief.

After that terrifying episode, we became even more vigilant with Lance's blood glucose checks. He began testing himself in the middle of the night. And he never locked his door again.

Less than 20 percent of people with type 1 diabetes will experience the kind of severe hypoglycemia—with convulsions or coma—that Lance had. The problem is much rarer in type 2 diabetes, affecting less than 5 percent. But the fear of hypoglycemia limits how far all people with diabetes will push their treatments.

It's another tough balancing act: bringing blood sugar down to the normal range, while avoiding hypoglycemia. In the Diabetes Control and Complications Trial, which I described in Chapter 4, the group that controlled their diabetes strictly had a two- to three-fold increase in severe hypoglycemia. For this price, they received outstanding reductions in their risk of serious long-term complications. But not everyone is willing to make the trade-off. Many people pull back on treatment when they experience hypoglycemic symptoms. They sacrifice their future health—which is dependent on avoiding high glucose levels day in and day out over years—to feel safe in the moment.

THE BETTY CROCKER OF DIABETES

Early in 1993 I went to San Diego for a meeting to explore new ways to prevent hypoglycemia in patients with diabetes. I went to this meeting because I was sick of all of the hypoglycemia I had to deal with in my practice and at diabetes camp.

The meeting was packed with diabetes specialists. We'd all been hearing about the early results from the Diabetes Control and Complications Trial, and we'd intensified the management plans for our patients to keep their blood sugar levels closer to the optimal range. We knew this would benefit them in the long run. But now we were seeing more hypoglycemia. All of us were eager for practical solutions, but the speakers at the meeting described one arcane high-tech approach after another. Each of these approaches would cost a minimum of $100 million to create and would require many years to test and bring to market.

As I sat in that meeting, a decidedly low-tech idea popped into my head: uncooked cornstarch. I'd just read a study describing how eating large quantities of uncooked cornstarch right out of the box could help children with rare diseases that cause unremitting, severe hypoglycemia. Raw cornstarch serves as a reservoir of glucose in the intestinal tract because it's digested very slowly, over a period of six to eight hours. That's just the right amount of time to maintain a steady supply of glucose in the bloodstream through the night. Cornstarch was simple, available, and cheap—and if it worked in rare diseases that caused hypoglycemia in children, it might work in people with diabetes.

On the way home from San Diego I kept thinking about using cornstarch to prevent hypoglycemia during the night. I assumed it must have been tried long ago and had failed, because I couldn't believe I'd be the first to think of something like that. When I got back to Los Angeles I went to the medical school library and did a search. Nothing came up.

Over the next few weeks I couldn't get cornstarch out of my mind. What if a small amount of uncooked cornstarch could help prevent the night-time hypoglycemia that occurred in so many patients with diabetes? It was readily available and inexpensive. Also, because it was an ordinary food product, it wouldn't require approval by the U.S. Food and Drug Administration. So patients could benefit quickly, without the delay required by a drug trial.

Lance was living on his own by then. He had graduated from

college and gone to work in the financial world—he'd always been talented with numbers, perhaps because he'd had so much practice with blood sugar readings. He was married to a wonderful, supportive woman. Since that terrifying incident in 1984, he'd successfully avoided any further severe hypoglycemic episodes by conscientiously waking himself in the middle of every night to check his blood sugar. But the readings were sometimes low, which concerned all of us.

I called him and asked if he'd be willing to return to his old room for a few nights and try taking cornstarch before he went to bed. "No more middle-of-the-night lows," I informed him. "All it takes is a little cornstarch in some milk."

"Sounds disgusting," he said. Then he relented. "I'll give you one night," he said.

Now I panicked, because I had no idea how much to use. How much glucose would a person need overnight? I filled a notepad with calculations involving grams of cornstarch and milligrams of glucose. Five grams of uncooked cornstarch—approximately 2 teaspoons—seemed about right, I decided.

Lance and I decided to try our experiment on a Friday night, because neither of us would have to go to work the next day. That night I measured the cornstarch into a glass of milk. I stirred, but the powder and the milk wouldn't blend together. I added ice and emptied the glass into my electric mixer. Finally the powder disappeared into the milk. Lance checked his blood sugar, which was normal. I handed him the glass and said, "Gulp it down."

He did, and then he made a face. "This will never catch on," he said. "It's gross."

"Tough," I retorted. "If it works, you'll drink it no matter what."

I checked his blood sugar levels at hourly intervals through the night and into the morning. Hypoglycemia was my chief concern. But I also wondered if the cornstarch would push his blood sugar too high. To my delight, the numbers ranged from 110 mg/dl to 137 mg/dl, normal readings for someone with diabetes. The next morning Lance woke up feeling great. I was exhausted, but elated.

Lance gave me more than one night. He drank the cornstarch slurry again on Saturday and Sunday. I measured his blood sugar levels at midnight, 3:00 a.m., and when he awoke in the morning. The results were the same: normal blood sugar. In the process of avoiding lows, this small amount of cornstarch had not caused highs.

I called three more patients with a history of hypoglycemia who I thought would be willing to try cornstarch at night. All of them were delighted by the results. Even Lance was convinced. He ate cornstarch every night, though he continued to complain about the taste.

Now I was eager to do a more formal study. I wrote a protocol to submit to my institutional review board at the hospital, the group that approves and monitors research in human subjects. I figured that the approval process would be simple, but I was wrong. The informed consent—the statement made to participants, which they must sign—needed to be rewritten three times before the board was satisfied. I had to tell patients that cornstarch might make their blood sugar too high, or make them sick. I had to tell them that if it did, the hospital would not assume any liability, even though one of their agents—me—had caused the problem. Finally, the board granted its approval.

I enrolled thirteen patients who had frequent episodes of nighttime hypoglycemia. For two weeks they ate their usual bedtime snack, a bowl of cereal with milk. They measured their blood sugar levels each night at 2:00 a.m. and each morning at 7:00 a.m. Then for the following two weeks they did the same measurements, but 5 grams of uncooked cornstarch replaced some of the carbohydrate in the cereal-and-milk snack.

During the two weeks when they ate plain cereal and milk, the patients had an average of four low blood sugars. But in the two weeks when cornstarch was added, the average dropped to just one low blood sugar. Meanwhile, there was no increase in the number of high blood sugar levels. I couldn't believe that such a simple measure produced such excellent results! I started to advise all my patients to add uncooked cornstarch to their bedtime snack—and I got fewer phone calls in the middle of the night. When I published my findings, I received letters from around the world thanking me.

That summer I conducted a more sophisticated study at diabetes camp. Once again I had to rewrite the informed consent three times before I could obtain institutional review board approval. Half of the campers agreed to enter the study. One problem remained. How would I weigh so many doses of cornstarch? I didn't want to bring our expensive laboratory scale to camp, so I went to Hollywood Boulevard and found a "boutique" that sold equipment to weigh and package other white powders, mainly of an illegal nature.

The salesman wore a sleeveless black T-shirt. Large tattoos covered both of his muscular arms, and his lower lip was pierced with a diamond stud. "I'm doing a study at a camp I run for teens," I explained nervously. "I need scales to weigh out five grams of cornstarch every night to give my campers."

He looked at me incredulously, as if he were thinking, "Sure, lady. Cornstarch. That's what they all say." He showed me scales that could measure in grams; the prices ranged from $12 all the way up to $240.

"I'll take five of the twelve-dollar scales," I said. "I also need little bags to keep the cornstarch in." He gave me a package of twenty-five. "But I need three hundred and fifty of them," I informed him.

He counted out fourteen packages, each containing twenty-five little bags, and put them in a shopping bag with the five scales. As he handed me the bag, he asked, "So, how do I sign up for this camp?"

Sixty-five teens enrolled in our study. Each night they ate a bedtime snack of pudding. Half of the time the pudding contained uncooked cornstarch. But when we added the cornstarch, the pudding became thick and gummy. Since we didn't want the kids or the doctors to know which version they were consuming, we altered the regular pudding to make it thick and gummy, too. All the campers grumped and groaned about the terrible pudding. We had to watch them to be sure they consumed the entire snack and didn't spit it out or throw it away. We reminded them they had agreed to participate in a clinical research study. But they knew from the informed consent that we couldn't force them to continue if they didn't want to.

As camp progressed, we lost some participants. Eleven children went home from camp early; three girls dropped out of the study because they were dieting and wanted to skip the evening snack all together. One of the dieters experienced a middle-of-the-night convulsion a few nights later.

Despite the setbacks and difficulties, the study was a success. Our findings confirmed the results of the pilot study: ingesting a small amount of uncooked cornstarch as part of the evening snack reduced by a factor of three the amount of hypoglycemia at midnight and in the morning, without increasing hyperglycemia. And if it worked in teens, it was likely to work in anyone with diabetes.

The staff and I were thrilled by the results. But to our dismay and astonishment, not one of the teens in the study said they would eat cornstarch when they returned home. "It tastes really bad," they said. "It's not convenient. And it's just too weird." As Lance had warned me, this simple and inexpensive intervention would not catch on until we found a better way to present the cornstarch.

I donned an apron and began experimenting in my kitchen. How could I disguise the taste of the cornstarch without cooking it, which would destroy its ability to act as a glucose reservoir? I tried mixing it into drinks; I mashed it with peanut butter. But those concoctions were even worse than the pudding. Eventually, I devised a snack bar containing chopped peanuts, crisped rice, and other ingredients along with the uncooked cornstarch. The following summer we repeated the study at diabetes camp, using the new snack bars instead of the terrible-tasting pudding. The bars had the same benefits and the kids loved them.

A few years later, the cornstarch bars were in commercial production. My sons came up with a great name for them: ExtendBars, because they extended the absorption of glucose overnight. ExtendBars are still sold today, in pharmacies and online. And I still receive mail and e-mails from people all over the United States and Canada thanking me. In 1996 *USA Today* wrote an article about how I found a simple answer to a complex problem. They referred to me as the "Betty Crocker of diabetes."

Hypoglycemia continues to limit us—patients and doctors—in the battle against diabetes and its long-term complications. Researchers all over the world struggle to understand why it occurs, what parts of the brain are affected by severe hypoglycemia, and why people with diabetes cannot defend themselves against it as effectively as those without the disease. This effort is well worth the time and money. One day we will beat hypoglycemia. When we do, people with diabetes will be more willing to control sugar aggressively, so they'll stay healthier. And they and their loved ones will sleep a whole lot better at night.

SEVEN

The Long Haul

I first met Jack during my internship at Childrens Hospital Los Angeles in 1976, a year after I moved to California. He was the pharmacist at the drugstore down the street from our house. If my husband or I needed medication, Jack dispensed it. He was about fifty-five years old, a jovial, fun-loving, and all-around great guy. He joked about having diabetes and about being overweight. "I'm the sweetest man in town," he'd say to everyone who entered the store. He'd offer them a chocolate kiss from a jar on the counter, then he'd unwrap one for himself and pop it into his mouth.

After I started my fellowship in endocrinology, I tried to cajole Jack into taking better care of himself. The problem was that Jack loved to eat. He loved pie; he loved steak and potatoes; he loved pasta; he loved ice cream—and he loved all of them in large quantities. Most of all, he loved candy. I tried to convince him that snacking on candy all day was a bad idea. To get back at me for pestering him, Jack would slip a candy bar into my shopping bag. "That's one less for me," he'd say with a laugh. Over the years Jack gained more and more weight—and I grew increasingly concerned about him. His sparkle wasn't quite as bright; the smiles and the jokes came less frequently.

By the time Jack neared sixty-five, he'd had type 2 diabetes for almost twenty-five years. He looked paler than before and had become puffy around the eyes, a sign that he was retaining fluid. He moved more slowly and seemed short of breath. Instead of standing, he sat on a stool behind the counter. "My legs are killing me," he'd explain. I could see that his ankles were swollen. Jack was dispensing drugs to other people to make them well, but he was getting sicker and sicker. Meanwhile, the candy jar hadn't budged.

As a pharmacist, Jack knew that the cornerstones of successful diabetes management were controlling blood sugar, eating right, and getting plenty of exercise. But self-control and Jack were just not on the same page. I harangued him: "Get your blood sugar down!"

"It's too late," he'd say.

"No!" I insisted. "There's still time."

Within the year, Jack's kidneys failed and he went on dialysis, using equipment to do the job his kidneys could no longer do. Now Jack came to the pharmacy only on Saturday mornings. My heart broke when I saw him attempting to cover up how tough his life had become. Only when I pressed him did he admit the truth. And when he did, tears welled up in his eyes and mine.

"Dialysis is terrible," Jack told me. He described the complicated, time-consuming peritoneal dialysis routine that he performed at home. It was a poor substitute for his failed kidneys. A permanent catheter had been placed in his lower abdomen; it was uncomfortable most of the time. Every evening, Jack hooked up a bag of dialysis fluid to the catheter. He sat as the liquid drained into his abdominal cavity, where it would cleanse his blood overnight. Then he went to bed, feeling bloated. In the morning, he opened the catheter and drained out the liquid, which now contained the toxins and waste products that made him feel weak and nauseated much of the time. "I've stopped eating candy," he said. "My blood sugar numbers are perfect." But he sounded sad, not triumphant. Now it really was too late. Within the year, Jack was dead of kidney failure associated with years of poorly controlled diabetes.

The complications of diabetes can be devastating and life-threatening, but they don't appear overnight. This disease slowly permeates the body, changing life and robbing health. People like Jack, who don't keep their blood sugar under good control, typically start to see symptoms of damage about a decade or two after diagnosis. The impact of diabetes is pervasive because it affects both the circulatory system and the nervous system. These intricate networks reach every part of us, from our toes to our scalps.

When I first tell people they have diabetes, I always wonder just what to say about possible complications. I know that if they follow a complex and demanding daily routine—testing their blood, adjusting their medicine, planning their exact food intake and exercise, and keeping detailed records of all of this—they can likely avoid complications and live a long, healthy life. I also know that if they cannot manage this arduous task day in and day out, year after year—if they chronically overeat and fail to match their food intake with their medication, if their lives are too disorganized, or if they somehow deny that this is about them and their bodies—then they most likely will face serious, even lethal, health problems. How much of the negative should I reveal?

Talking to teens right after they're diagnosed with type 2 diabetes is particularly difficult. It's tough enough to convey to them and their families what diabetes means here and now. Trying to focus them on what might happen twenty years from now is futile at this point. I have to wait, gain their confidence, and show them the immediate benefits of good diabetes control. Then I can gradually explain the perils that await two decades hence.

Since type 2 is a new condition in youth, we have only limited data on what they can expect. But the information we do have is devastating. Dr. Heather Dean of Children's Hospital of Winnipeg—who has studied diabetes among youth of the First Nation, descendants of Canada's native people—reassessed the health records of youngsters who had been diagnosed with type 2 diabetes at least ten years earlier, before they were eighteen years old. The patients in the study ranged in age from eighteen to thirty-three. Despite their youth, a shocking 9 percent of them had died; 6 percent of them were on kidney dialysis. First Nation people, like Native Americans in the United States, have a much higher rate of diabetes than that of Caucasians; they also suffer higher rates of complications. Nevertheless, these numbers suggest the toll that diabesity can take when it strikes early.

Usually, I go slowly during my initial meetings with newly diagnosed patients. I want them to understand the risks, but I don't want to overwhelm them and plunge them into despair. The messages I try to convey are that the complications of diabetes can be prevented, or at least delayed and lessened, if they can control their blood sugar—and their diabetes treatment team is behind them to help them succeed.

TO THE HEART OF THE MATTER

The most serious complication of diabetes is cardiovascular disease. Heart attacks and strokes kill about three-quarters of people with diabetes. When you have diabetes, your risk of a heart attack is just as high as the risk faced by someone without diabetes who has already had a heart attack. Diabetes elevates heart risk even more for women than for men, according to a 2004 report in *Archives of Internal Medicine*. Having diabetes increases the risk of a heart attack by 150 percent in women but only 50 percent in men. So it's particularly important for women with diabetes to control blood sugar and reduce other risk factors for cardiovascular disease, especially high blood pressure and high cholesterol.

Diabetes raises cardiac risk because of a process called glycation. As I mentioned in Chapter 2, insulin is not required for glucose to enter the cells of the nervous system, including the brain; nor is insulin needed to allow glucose into red blood cells or into the endothelial cells that line the blood vessels. When too much sugar is circulating in the blood, some of the excess attaches to proteins and molecules in the red blood cells and endothelial cells—this is glycation. The destructive effects of glycation are similar to what happens to fruit as it ripens: first it becomes sweeter and sweeter, then at some point it begins to deteriorate and rot.

Chronically high blood sugar causes inflammation in the large blood vessels of the heart and brain. Glycation swells the endothelial cells that line the blood vessels. Over time, blood flow to vital organs becomes impaired. The problem is exacerbated if a person with diabetes is overweight, because chemicals secreted by fat cells promote inflammation. If the person also has metabolic syndrome, with elevated cholesterol and elevated blood pressure, cardiovascular problems become even more likely.

Despite the grim statistics, many people with diabetes, and even their healthcare providers, don't fully understand the risk. That's why the American Diabetes Association and the American College of Cardiology have begun the campaign called Make the Link, designed to reveal the association between diabetes and heart disease. The National Diabetes Education Program (NDEP) has developed Know Your ABCs. This program emphasizes the importance of knowing your A1c (the test known as the diabetes report card, which indicates blood sugar control over the previous three months), your blood pressure, and your cholesterol level—and attempting to normalize all three of them.

Women are especially likely to underestimate the danger of heart disease; many assume it's a problem only for men. In a 2003 survey of more than a thousand women, sponsored by the American Heart Association, fewer than half of the women correctly identified heart disease as the leading cause of death in women. As a result, women may not take the threat as seriously as they should—especially if they have diabetes.

Sylvia, one of my mother's bridge partners, is an unfortunate example of what can go wrong. Sylvia was a widow who doted on her only child, a lawyer whose attentiveness to her won him the approval of the bridge club. She was diagnosed with diabetes at age sixty-six, and my mother gave me regular updates about her condition over the next two years.

Sylvia thought her doctor had made a mistake when he called after her annual physical to tell her she had "mild" diabetes. Her fasting blood sugar was 150 milligrams per deciliter (mg/dl), over the diagnostic threshold of 126 mg/dl. "That's impossible," she told him. "I don't have any symptoms." True, she was urinating more often and needed to use the bathroom in the middle of the night. But my mother and the other bridge club members didn't have diabetes and all of them reported problems with their genitourinary tracts: urinary incontinence, urinary tract infections, and sagging vaginas. These difficulties, they agreed, were caused by childbirth, menopause, and aging.

Sylvia was about thirty pounds overweight. Her cholesterol and blood pressure were slightly elevated. Her doctor advised her to go on a diet and to get more exercise; he arranged for her to see a nutritionist. "If your blood sugar levels don't come down, you'll have to take medicine," he warned. "I'd start you on pills first. But Sylvia, if you don't take care of yourself, you might eventually have to go on the needle."

Sylvia didn't want to take medication; she wanted to be "natural." So she followed the nutritionist's advice. She started walking to her bridge club, and she put the entire club, including my mother, on a new regimen. Instead of eating cake, they snacked on fruit and cut-up vegetables as they played bridge. She also tried different herbs and teas and homeopathic remedies.

Several months later, Sylvia went back to her doctor for a checkup and a battery of tests. He told her, "Sylvia, you're doing a great job. You've lost a few pounds. Your blood sugar is better, and so is your blood pressure; your cholesterol has come down, and your electrocardiogram looks pretty good. But the numbers are still a bit high, and I keep debating with myself whether to put you on medications. But I know how you hate pills, so just keep up the good work."

Over the next year, Sylvia gradually returned to her old ways. She regained some of the weight she'd lost; her blood sugar, blood pressure, and cholesterol levels rose slightly. Now her doctor suggested medications a little more strongly, but he didn't push her. Sylvia still thought he was overreacting. I was concerned when my mother told me about this, but my mother reminded me that Sylvia's doctor hadn't insisted.

One morning, a little more than two years after Sylvia had been told she had "mild" diabetes, she woke up at 4:00 a.m. with nausea and pain in her left shoulder. Heartburn, she thought. She got out of bed, took a Tylenol and a Tums, and made herself a cup of herbal tea. At 6:00 she drew a hot bath, but the hot water made her feel worse.

By 7:00 that morning she was ready to call her doctor. A recording asked her to press 1 if she was having a life-threatening medical emergency, but she didn't do that. Instead, she left a message: "This is Sylvia. Ask the doctor to call me when he gets a chance. Not to worry—I just want to tell him I don't feel so well today." Then she called her son and told him about her symptoms. Sylvia often called her son in the morning, frequently with minor health complaints. He didn't realize that shoulder pain and nausea might be symptoms of a heart attack, but he encouraged her to see her doctor.

At 8:45 a.m. the doctor returned Sylvia's call. She told him she was nauseated and having the worst case of heartburn ever. "Sounds like a pretty bad episode," the doctor responded. "Any chest pain?" he asked. Sylvia wasn't having chest pain. She didn't tell him about the shoulder pain she'd had earlier, and he didn't ask. "I want to see you this afternoon," the doctor said. "There are good medications for heartburn and you won't need them for long."

Sylvia never made it to the doctor. Her son called her at 10:00, but there was no answer. Assuming she'd gone to the doctor, he waited until noon to try again. When there was still no answer, he left work and went to her apartment. Sylvia was on the floor, lifeless, halfway between her bathroom and bedroom. The scene that greeted her son hinted at her terrifying final moments. The nausea must have grown more intense. She vomited on the way to the bathroom. Afterward, she probably felt faint. The pain in her left shoulder must have returned, this time more severe. She started back to her bedroom, trying to reach the nearest telephone. By then she was probably staggering, barely able to stand, struggling to breathe. As her oxygen-deprived heart began to die, the crushing chest pain must have overwhelmed her and she collapsed.

When my mother told me how Sylvia died, I felt sad and frustrated, but not surprised. Had Sylvia been willing to take medication to control her blood sugar, cholesterol, and blood pressure, she might have avoided the heart attack that took her life. An insulin sensitizer might have brought her blood sugar down to a normal

range; a statin could have reduced her cholesterol; and an ACE inhibitor might have normalized her blood pressure. A baby aspirin
would have helped, too. These commonly used drugs, which have
minimal side effects, are proven lifesavers. I wished Sylvia's doctor
had been more vehement in trying to persuade her. But I know it's
not always easy to convince people to take medication.

The problem was compounded by the fact that Sylvia's cardiac
symptoms were atypical. Usually, the first sign of a heart attack is
chest pain on the left side radiating down the arm. But sometimes a
heart attack is heralded by nausea, severe fatigue or malaise, or
heaviness in the chest rather than pain. This kind of atypical presentation is more common in women than in men. Even healthcare
providers can't always differentiate a heart attack from something
less serious—especially from a description over the telephone.

WHEN DARKNESS DESCENDS

Blindness is one of the most feared complications of diabetes. Fortunately, most people with diabetes are able to preserve their vision
by controlling blood sugar and having regular checkups, so they can
be treated promptly for any difficulties that threaten their eyes.

I still remember the first time I saw the inside of someone's eye
when I was in medical school. My patient—a healthy woman in her
fifties who was having a routine checkup—sat in an examining chair.
I sat opposite, awkwardly holding the ophthalmoscope, a viewing
instrument that looks like a flashlight. At the top, along with the
light, was a dial that let me select a lens through which I could look
into her eye. I spun the dial with my thumb while I tried to steady
my hand against her cheek so that I could see past the clear cornea at
the front of her eye, through the fluid-filled center, and to her
retina, the light-sensitive membrane at the back of the eye.

Finally I found the correct position. The glistening pale pink
retina filled the peephole through which I looked. I was amazed. I
felt as if I was viewing the mirror to her soul. Coursing against the
pink of the retina, bright red blood vessels curved and fanned out
from a central point, the optic disc. I knew that the twists and turns

of the retinal blood vessels could tell me about the health of my patient. And the flattened, ringed optic disc—the area of the retina where nerves converge and lead into the brain—could provide clues about how the brain behind that disc was functioning. To become the doctor I hoped to be, I had to learn to read their signals, the cryptic messages the retina was conveying.

Diabetes can damage cells in all parts of the eye. People with diabetes are 60 percent more likely to develop cataracts, a condition in which the clear lens of the eye becomes cloudy, dimming vision like frosted glass. Though cataracts are common in the elderly, people with diabetes may develop them in middle age. Treatment involves surgery to remove the lens; sometimes it's replaced with an artificial lens.

Glaucoma—dangerously elevated pressure inside the eye—is 40 percent more common in people with diabetes. Sometimes drugs can reduce the pressure; the problem may require surgery to drain fluid from the eye. Untreated glaucoma can damage the retina and cause blindness.

If diabetes is poorly controlled, sugar attacks the tiny blood vessels at the back of the eyes, which weaken and become clogged. Through the ophthalmoscope, the clogs appear as dots sprinkled throughout the retina. This is the first sign of retinopathy, abnormality of the retina. As retinopathy advances, some of the tiny blood vessels begin to break and bleed. The eye tries to grow new blood vessels to take their place. But the new vessels do not grow normally. Instead, they damage the eye further.

At first, if just a few blood vessels break, the person might not notice any changes. With more broken vessels, vision can be affected. Bleeding in the eye can be stopped by laser treatments. These treatments don't cure the problem; they merely cauterize the affected blood vessels to stop the bleeding and contain the damage that has already occurred. If vision has deteriorated, laser treatment may help restore it somewhat and delay further loss. With more advanced retinopathy, blood vessels may bleed into the liquid center of the eye. Or the growth of new blood vessels may detach the retina from the back of the eye, which means that visual images can no longer reach the brain. At that point, vision may be lost altogether.

I look at the retinas of my young diabetes patients during every checkup, and once a year they have a full eye examination, with their pupils dilated. Fortunately, none has ever lost vision, and only a few have required laser treatments for eye disease. One of them was Jennifer, who was brought to me by Los Angeles County's Protective Service Agency. As a pediatrician and as a mother, I feel sick when I see a child denied the most basic of needs, the need to be loved and protected. That was how I felt when I first met Jennifer. At ten, she was so small that she looked like a six- or seven-year-old. She was withdrawn and didn't make eye contact. Her blue eyes were fixed on her lap, so I could barely see the dark circles beneath them, dark circles from sleepless nights and tears. A wisp of unkempt blond hair matted against her forehead. I wanted to run to her, push the hair from her eyes, and hold her.

Jennifer was diagnosed with type 1 diabetes as a baby. She'd spent her entire life in chaos. Her mother was a drug addict and a prostitute. Jennifer had lived in four states and had been in and out of protective services in every one of them. The day before she was brought to my clinic, she had come to school sick and vomiting. She hadn't been able to take insulin for two days because her mother forgot to buy it.

Jennifer's teacher and the school nurse had been concerned about her for several months. Her size, her appearance, and her withdrawn behavior all suggested neglect or even abuse. But when they questioned Jennifer about her life at home, she always insisted everything was okay. And she had no bruises or other external signs of abuse. Now the teacher and nurse had reason to believe that Jennifer was in danger. They called Child Protective Services, and the County of Los Angeles removed the girl from her home.

While she waited for foster placement, Jennifer spent four days at Childrens Hospital Los Angeles to get her diabetes under control. I reconstructed her past based on what Jennifer could tell me, plus detective work and educated guesses. I was outraged to see what inadequate care had allowed diabetes to do to a child.

On the first day she lay in bed, attached to IVs. By the second day, her condition had stabilized and she was able to walk. Our nurses and nutritionists taught her about diabetes. As they did, they showered her with affection. They brushed and braided her hair. When they brought her a new glucose meter and other supplies, they also brought toys from the hospital toy room. Despite all the attention, Jennifer remained guarded and melancholy. On the third day, when her new foster mother arrived to meet her, she became even more sullen.

In foster care, Jennifer's life was less chaotic and her blood sugar was well controlled. She looked happier and began to treat the clinic staff like old friends. After six months, Jennifer's A1c had dropped from an alarmingly high 13 percent down to 7.8 percent, well within the goal we had set for her. But three years later, when Jennifer was a rebellious thirteen-year-old, her A1c soared again. At her checkups, she wouldn't look at me; she responded to my questions with monosyllables. Was she keeping a blood sugar diary? Yeah. Where was it? Forgot to bring it. Did she take her insulin shots regularly? Yeah. Was she following her food plan? Yeah. Her foster mother shook her head and silently mouthed, "She's lying." I tried to connect with Jennifer, but nothing I said could penetrate the wall between us.

The last time I saw Jennifer, she was sixteen and had just completed her second set of laser treatments for retinopathy. When I looked into her eyes with my ophthalmoscope, I didn't see twisting and turning blood vessels standing out against the glistening pale pink background of the retina. Instead, I saw white scars and swirls, black and red dots. There were no landmarks; it was difficult to see the vessels emanating from the flattened optic disc. The discs in both eyes had thousands of dots around them, scars from the laser. I felt as if I were looking into outer space. The sight made me fumble with the ophthalmoscope as I had during my first days in medical school.

Jennifer's body can never recover from ten years of poorly controlled diabetes plus three years of teenage rebellion. Though we've saved her vision for now, her future is uncertain. And I know that the scars in her eyes are small compared to the scars her mother left in her heart.

THE KIDNEYS ARE CRITICAL

I met Yolanda and Berta in the summer of 1998 during a question-and-answer period at a health fair sponsored by the University of Southern California (USC) and the *Los Angeles Times*. This is a huge outdoor fair held annually on the USC campus in the heart of Los Angeles to provide information to those with limited access to health care. The campus is magnificent, filled with impressive buildings and grassy courtyards. Thousands of people of all ages, shapes, and colors—students, young adults, families with small children, elderly couples—attend this two-day event, and perhaps a hundred health organizations and companies have booths.

On the day I met Yolanda and Berta, my job at the fair was to answer questions about diabetes in one of the indoor lecture halls. I stood at the podium in an amphitheater. In front of me sat hundreds of people in a semicircle of ascending rows of seats. There was a second microphone in the audience. Behind it, those with questions formed a long line.

I began by presenting a few statistics about the growing epidemic of diabesity. Next, I talked briefly about diabetes, describing its complications and explaining how they can be prevented with medications and lifestyle changes. Then I took questions. One by one, people in the line took their turn at the microphone. Their questions were never about general points of information, such as why one medication is better than another for people with diabetes. No, their questions were about specifics: "Why has my doctor told me to take two pills, rather than one, every night?" or "My friend Gladys has to take the needle. Why?" I wanted so much to help. But without knowing the details of their medical condition, how could I possibly answer these questions?

I noticed a woman in a long, traditional Mexican skirt and blouse waiting patiently in line. She appeared to be about fifty years old. Her name, I learned later, was Yolanda. Finally, she reached the microphone. "Doctora," she began.

"Sí," I replied into my microphone, wishing I were fluent in Spanish.

"Doctora," Yolanda continued, "mi sister, Berta, she not good. Her doctor, he say Berta has azúcar, the sugar. She need una máquina for her riñones." A machine for her kidneys. I was relieved that I could understand her easily. She pointed to a woman who was sitting in the audience. Berta appeared to be much older than her sister, possibly in her sixties or seventies; she was pale, puffy, and wrinkled.

"How long has Berta had diabetes?" I asked, not sure what I could do with the answer.

"Just now she told about the azúcar and about la máquina," Yolanda replied. If Berta was in kidney failure at the time of diagnosis, that was a bad sign. It meant she'd had diabetes for many years, but no one knew it—all those years without treatment. The long course of the disease meant she must have type 2 diabetes. Yolanda continued: "Doctora, Berta need una especialista. Is possible Berta come to you?"

I started to tell her that I'm a pediatric diabetes specialist, that I don't treat adults. But she looked so desperate that I blurted out an offer: "Your sister needs a specialist for her diabetes and kidneys, and I think I can help you find one." That was a big promise. As soon as I said it, I had misgivings. I didn't know anything about Berta—if she had insurance, if she was in the United States legally, if she would even show up if I found someone for her to see.

"Dios, mi Dios," Yolanda said quietly into the microphone. As uncertain as I was, I was the answer to her prayers.

At the end of the question-and-answer period, I beckoned the sisters to the podium to ask a few questions. I was astonished to learn that Berta, who looked elderly, was only forty-five years old. Yolanda told me that her sister had been heavy when she was diagnosed with diabetes, but she'd lost weight as she got sicker. I asked what medications she had been put on. Berta pulled a brown paper bag from her large purse. In it were bottles of pills. I looked at the labels. She was taking diabetes pills that were inappropriate for people with kidney failure, because one of their side effects made kidney function worse; if the kidneys were already compromised, the medication was a further insult. She had blood pressure pills that weren't used for people with diabetes, because the drug usually wasn't powerful enough to be effective in someone with the disease. Berta's brown bag also contained a diuretic—a pill to increase urine output. This pill required close monitoring of blood salts, something that I doubted was being done. Not exactly state-of-the-art treatment.

The medications came from a local family clinic. I knew that some of its doctors were wonderful and caring, but others were uninformed and dangerous. Berta must have seen one of the latter, because the medications in the brown paper bag would not make her well but actually make her sicker. I told Yolanda that Berta needed to see doctors at "the General," the county hospital associated with the University of Southern California where I teach. I would arrange the appointments for a day when I could be there and help her navigate the system.

Two weeks later Berta and Yolanda met me in the lobby of the General. The place is huge and daunting, filled with hurrying staff, people with medical appointments, and confused visitors there for the first time. Colored lines on the floors point the way to the emergency department, to the pharmacy, to radiology, or to one clinic or another. If you were color-blind, you could spend years wandering the halls. But I know my way around, and the three of us set off to see my version of the wizard.

The waiting room of the Endocrinology and Diabetes Clinic was overcrowded with people who looked really sick. We were taken to an examination room. I watched the nurse take Berta's vital signs. Her blood pressure was 210 over 165 (210/165). The first number represents the systolic pressure, blood pressure while the heart contracts; the second number is the diastolic pressure, when the heart rests between beats. A normal reading is 120/80 at the most; anything over 140/90 is considered significantly elevated. At 210/165, Berta's blood pressure was high enough to kill her. They measured her blood sugar: 318 mg/dl. That was also much too high. I worried that it might be too late to save Berta.

We had an appointment with the head of the clinical diabetes department, a man famous for his devotion to his patients and to his specialty. I was proud to be his colleague. He greeted Berta and Yolanda, then asked them a multitude of questions, like we all did, in

English and in pidgin Spanish. But we understood each other. Slowly he put the whole story together.

Berta had not been well for two or three years. She had gone to folk healers, but the medicines they gave her didn't make her feel better. She'd been urinating many times through the night. Sores on her legs oozed clear fluid and occasionally bled but would not heal. Her feet burned, her vision was blurry, and her heartbeat was irregular. She suffered from heartburn and frequent stomachaches. Her appetite had disappeared, and she'd lost thirty to forty pounds. Her skin hung, as if she were wearing a suit that was much too big.

Respecting her modesty, my colleague examined her. He prodded and probed and asked if this or that hurt. He was a master. I felt grateful for his humanity and his brilliance. He examined the brown bag filled with medicine and looked at me; I could guess his thoughts.

In a firm voice he told Berta: "I'm going to put you in the hospital. We need to do a lot of tests. I'm going to start giving you insulin injections." He pointed his right index finger to his left forearm as if he was giving himself a shot with a syringe. "Berta," he said, "I think we can save you; I think we can save your kidneys. But you will have to work hard. We will have to work hard together." Berta and Yolanda began to cry. And I did, too.

Berta was admitted to the hospital's diabetes unit and hooked up to IV lines. During the next two days, she underwent multiple tests to evaluate her kidneys, her blood fats, her blood count, her blood chemistry, and her liver. X-rays were taken of her heart, lungs, and abdomen. She took a heart stress test. She had two 24-hour urine collections. In between tests, a nurse educator, a nutritionist, and a social worker—all Spanish-speaking—visited her.

Her new medical regimen began. To control her blood sugar, Berta would need insulin injections. She told me she was trembling when they gave her the first shot, but it didn't hurt. Within a day, she was administering the injections herself. She was given a new glucose meter, one with a memory, so she could show the doctor her sugar numbers on her return visits. Berta's medical team met to discuss the best combination of drugs to address her multiple problems. In addition to insulin, she would require medications to improve her kidney function, control her blood pressure, and lower her cholesterol and other blood fats. When she returned home, she needed two brown bags for all her bottles of pills.

Over the following weeks, Yolanda called me every few days with progress reports. Berta was so much better now; her energy had returned. After a few weeks she could walk to the market and then make dinner, which she hadn't been able to do for several months. A month after Berta left the hospital, Yolanda took the bus to visit me. She brought me homemade tortillas with chicken and rice. On the top of the chicken was guacamole. She told me I had saved her sister's life and that she would thank God every night as long as she lived for the day she met me. I told her I was glad to help, and I was.

Berta is not alone. Between 10 and 21 percent of people with diabetes suffer from kidney disease. Diabetes is the leading cause of end-stage renal disease (ESRD). Approximately 43 percent of new ESRD cases are attributed to diabetes. Our two kidneys are busy organs. They make hormones that control blood pressure; they regulate our body chemistry; and they stimulate the bone marrow to make red blood cells. But their main jobs are to get rid of excess water and cleanse the blood of toxins. All of our blood passes through our kidneys many times during the day. The kidneys use their huge network of small blood vessels as filters. Tubes, called ureters, carry unwanted substances and excess water from the kidneys to the bladder, so we can dispose of them by urinating.

Excess sugar in the blood damages the kidney's blood vessels. Regular screening for kidney involvement is essential because there are no symptoms at the very early stages—the time when intervention can reverse the process. The first sign of damage is the presence of protein in the urine. Normally, the urine contains little or no protein. The kidneys don't filter protein molecules from the bloodstream, because most of these molecules are too big to pass through the blood vessel walls. But if the kidney's blood vessels are damaged, protein begins to spill into the urine. Routine urine tests can detect the high concentrations of protein found if kidney damage is significant. But abnormal amounts of protein can be detected much earlier—before symptoms appear—by a special urine test called the microalbumin test. This test is performed yearly to check for early signs of kidney damage.

The first symptom of kidney trouble that patients notice is usually edema. Ankles and legs swell; the face becomes puffy, especially around the eyes. As kidney damage progresses, excess fluid accumulates elsewhere in the body. Edema distends the abdomen, causing discomfort and making clothing tight. The lungs fill with fluid, producing breathlessness. Blood pressure rises, causing headaches and fatigue, and heart problems may develop.

When the kidneys don't function properly, the entire body is affected and the quality of life deteriorates. Toxins accumulate in the blood, causing a wide range of symptoms, from itching and nausea to mental confusion and seizures. Anemia develops because the kidneys can no longer stimulate the bone marrow to make red blood cells. The result is chronic exhaustion and weakness.

Controlling blood sugar is the best way to prevent kidney damage in diabetes. In the early stages of kidney failure, medication can improve blood flow in the kidneys. This helps preserve them, or at least delays their deterioration. But as kidney disease advances and symptoms become more severe, medication can no longer help. At that point, patients must start dialysis, as my pharmacist friend Jack did. The only other option is a kidney transplant. But there aren't enough available kidneys to go around, and not everyone can withstand the surgery and the immunosuppressant drugs they will need to take for the rest of their life if the transplanted kidney is to survive.

THE BODY'S INFORMATION HIGHWAY

Diabetes attacks the nerves through the glycation process—similar to fruit ripening and rotting—that I described earlier. Sugar attaches to proteins in nerve fibers and in the insulation that surrounds the nerves. Damaged nerves can't transmit information properly. About half of people with diabetes have some damage to their nerves. Though the symptoms are not always severe, nerve damage can cause terrible pain and disability.

Our peripheral nervous system—the nerves outside of the spinal canal and brain—enables us to move; it enables us to touch and feel, taste and smell. Thanks to our peripheral nervous system, we can wiggle our fingers and toes, and we know if we've injured them. Nervous impulses are transmitted to our brain from every inch of our skin, muscles, and bones—and then back again from the brain. Damage to the peripheral nervous system, called peripheral neuropathy, causes numbness or burning pain in the extremities: the arms, hands, legs, and feet. Sometimes peripheral neuropathy is merely a mild annoyance. But loss of sensation can have disastrous consequences.

When I was in medical school, I took care of Stan, a decorated World War II veteran whose diabetes had been diagnosed at age thirty-two, right after he returned from the European battlefields. Now, almost thirty years later, he had come to the clinic at a Veterans Administration hospital for one of his routine checkups. When he saw me, his expectant expression changed to a look of dismay. I could tell that he was unhappy about the prospect of being examined by a young woman. I understood his concern, because I felt uncomfortable, too. This was the first time I'd performed a complete physical on a man, and he was old enough to be my father.

Stan sat on the examining table in his hospital gown and socks; I stood in front of him in my white coat. To break the awkward silence, I introduced myself and asked him how he was feeling. "Not bad, ma'am," he replied. I couldn't remember ever being called ma'am before.

After I took his medical history, I began the examination. I looked in his eyes and ears, felt his neck, and peered into his mouth, my flashlight illuminating the dark recesses as he said "Ahhhh." I listened to his heart and lungs with my stethoscope. Then I asked him to lie down. This made both of us uneasy because we knew I would have to examine his stomach and his genitalia. Somehow, both of us got through that part of the exam. All that was left were his legs and feet. I tapped his knees to test his reflexes. "May I remove your socks?" I asked.

"I left them on because my feet smell bad," Stan said apologetically.

"I need to have a look," I said, and pulled off his socks. The sight and smell that greeted me almost made me vomit. There was a huge, gaping hole at the bottom of Stan's left foot. The tissue of his sole was eaten away, leaving a gray, putrid sore. Blackened dead skin surrounded the edges. Stan had gangrene, tissue death and decay. I had seen pictures of gangrene in medical textbooks; I'd read about it; I'd heard lectures about it. Now I was seeing it for the first time, but there was no doubt in my mind what it was. I tried to conceal my reaction. "How long have you had this sore?" I managed to say.

"What sore?" Stan asked. He knew his feet had begun to smell particularly bad, but he had no idea that the reason was an infected, gangrenous sore. This extensive wound didn't hurt—even when he walked on it—because Stan's nerves could not transmit the necessary signals between his foot and his brain. Long-standing diabetes in poor control had compromised his circulatory system, too. His poor circulation meant that the nutrients needed for healing hadn't been brought to the injured tissues. So the infection had proliferated. Intravenous antibiotic treatment was started immediately. But without adequate blood flow, antibiotics can't reach an infection. The gangrene continued to advance, despite medication. Two months later, Stan's left foot was removed so that the infection would not destroy his entire leg.

Amputation is the most terrible consequence of peripheral neuropathy. People whose feet are numb don't notice a blister or a stone in their shoe; if a sore develops, they may not realize it unless they're vigilant about checking their feet. If the problem isn't addressed, the sore may enlarge and become infected, as happened to Stan. These days, we still use antibiotics to combat gangrene. In addition, we have novel and experimental wound treatments, such as tissue growth factors—medicines to stimulate wound healing—and hyperbaric oxygen, in which the tissues are exposed to 100 percent oxygen. But once gangrene sets in and the damage is advanced, it's too late to reverse. At that point, the only way to stop the destruction is to amputate the areas of infection and gangrene. Each year, approximately 82,000 people with diabetes lose one or more toes, a foot, or even a leg.

Every summer at diabetes camp I make a special point of talking to the campers about their feet. This is an ideal opportunity, because they all take off their shoes at the pool and in their cabins. I explain that they need to examine their feet every day, checking their soles and looking between their toes. At this, the teenagers roll their eyes and mutter, "Whatever." I ignore their reactions and continue: If they find a sore that doesn't heal quickly, they should see their healthcare provider so any infection can be eradicated before it has a chance to spread. I tell them: "An ounce of prevention is what saves people's feet."

In addition to causing peripheral neuropathy, poorly controlled diabetes damages the autonomic nervous system, the part of the nervous system that controls some of our body's functions without our awareness, such as our heart rate and the flow of food through our digestive tract. Without the ability to auto-regulate, internal havoc ensues. For example, as I mentioned in Chapter 6, some people with diabetes become unable to correct hypoglycemia if it occurs. That's because their autonomic nervous system—which normally coordinates the release of adrenaline and glucagon as blood sugar falls, leading to the release of stored glucose—no longer performs this essential task. Deterioration of the autonomic nervous system also leads to hypoglycemia unawareness, an inability to detect that blood sugar is becoming dangerously low.

The gastrointestinal problems that afflict some people with diabetes are yet another consequence of nerve damage. A myriad of nerves control the involuntary processes involved in digestion, from our swallowing reflexes to the contractions that move food out of the stomach and through the intestines. When these nerves are damaged by diabetes, the stomach may empty too slowly, causing stomachaches, abdominal bloating, or even vomiting. Damaged nerves may prevent the intestines from functioning properly, resulting in pain, excessive gas, constipation, or diarrhea. The diarrhea can be so explosive that it results in soiling. This is a devastating symptom. If it happens frequently, a person may become fearful about leaving home and might even quit work and become socially isolated. Medication can help somewhat, but most people who develop autonomic neuropathy affecting the gastrointestinal tract do not find complete relief. These symptoms would be bad enough for anyone, but digestive problems are disastrous for people with diabetes because sugar control becomes even more difficult. With inconsistent absorption of food, they may experience wide and dangerous swings from extremely high to extremely low glucose levels.

LOVE, MARRIAGE, AND SEX

Diabetes has life-altering complications at any age. But there are special issues for young adults as they fall in love and think about marrying and starting a family. When I talk with a youngster who has just been diagnosed—whether with type 1 or type 2 diabetes—I think of Steve, one of my patients, and his wife, Mia.

Steve was diagnosed with type 1 diabetes in 1976, when he was eight years old. At the time, it wasn't possible to monitor blood glucose at home. Even with daily urine tests, Steve couldn't control his blood sugar well for the first five years he had diabetes—and for the next five, he and his family lived out of the country because his father was working in Chile. Steve had better medical supplies for his diabetes than anyone else in the entire country; he returned to the United States twice a year for medical checkups. Still, it was difficult to manage his disease as aggressively in Chile as he would have in the United States.

By the time Steve was twenty-three, his kidneys had failed. His father donated one of his kidneys so that Steve could have a transplant. A year later, the transplanted kidney began to fail. But one night during that unhappy period, Steve encountered Mia at a party. Spotting each other across the room, there was instant mutual attraction. At that magical moment, Mia didn't notice that Steve was pale and his eyes were puffy. Her quiet strength and joyous laugh captivated him. They talked. He told her of his illness, but his disease was of no concern to Mia. Steve's warmth and humor won her over. In the following weeks and months, they did not leave each other's side.

At our regular medical appointments, I rejoiced at Steve's radiance when he spoke about Mia. But I was filled with dread as I read his medical reports. The donated kidney failed. He received another kidney transplant from a car accident victim. Steve had tremendous difficulty tolerating the immunosuppressant drugs required so his body would not reject the new kidney. When we gave him the standard doses of these drugs, he had catastrophic side effects and infections. But when we decreased the doses, his kidney function deteriorated. It was a balancing act, and Steve was teetering on the edge.

Meanwhile, Mia and Steve decided to get married. Everyone tried to talk Mia out of it. They told her Steve might die and she could become a widow. Even Steve said it was more than he could ask. But no one could change her mind. And after a while, no one continued to try.

Shortly after his marriage to Mia, Steve fell into the abyss. The immunosuppressant drugs had left him vulnerable to infection. Bacteria invaded his lungs, causing copious secretions that made him feel as if he were drowning. He developed recurrent fevers with shakes and chills. We admitted him to the hospital and gave him very strong antibiotics. Once again, we manipulated his immunosuppressant drugs. But when we did, Steve's second transplant failed. At this point, he was so weak and debilitated that he could no longer tolerate dialysis. Another transplant was out of the question.

Mia sat by his side the entire time. She fed him medications. She spooned what little food he could tolerate into his mouth, and helped him sip the liquid meals we prescribed for his sustenance. When he turned blue with ravaging infection, she cleaned him and caressed him. She saw him cough up pus. She watched him slowly suffocate and drown in his own secretions. She heard him rattle with death. I asked Mia how she could bear it, how she could do all she did. "I do it because I have no choice," she said quietly. "I knew when I met Steve, when I fell in love with him, and when I married him that I could not change what was to happen. I knew Steve would never be well and I would be a widow. It didn't matter. I wanted to be his wife, to be with him, even if it was only for a day."

Steve and Mia never slept blissfully or peacefully through the night. They didn't take any trips, not even a honeymoon. They lived with buckets of medications, insulin shots, blood sugar checks, breathing treatments, special diets, and hospital rooms. There was no escape, not even for a minute, from his illness.

Steve died in Mia's arms. They had been husband and wife for less than a year, and he was gravely ill for the entire time. When it was over, Mia thanked us for letting her be there. "May I lie with him? Can we be alone?" she asked me. Tears streamed down her face.

"Of course," I said, barely able to talk. We moved the equipment and helped Mia lie down next to Steve in his hospital bed, her body lightly touching his. Then we left them alone for the last time.

Steve and Mia hadn't planned to have children. I never questioned them about their intimate relationship, nor did they volunteer details. But sexual dysfunction and infertility are among the cruel complications of diabetes. Within ten years of getting diabetes, most men notice changes in sexual performance. By age sixty, more than half of all men with diabetes experience erectile dysfunction (impotence); it occurs in 9 percent of those in their twenties. The cause, once again, is excess blood sugar, which damages the nerves and blood vessels of the penis. Normally, an erection is triggered when sensory information from the nerves causes blood vessels in the penis to become engorged with blood. But when the nerves are damaged, they cannot communicate the necessary information to the penis. And poor circulation means that blood flow is inadequate to cause and sustain an erection.

Good blood sugar control can prevent erectile dysfunction and, at an early stage, can help reverse symptoms. Once the problem develops, medication—such as sildenafil (Viagra) or related compounds—can help men to resume pleasurable sexual function. If damage progresses and medication no longer works, penile implants and vacuum devices can get the penis erect. Psychological counseling also may be helpful.

Healthcare providers struggle with how and when to tell male patients about this particular danger of poorly controlled diabetes. In my experience, threatening young men with a nonfunctioning penis has never seemed to work. At diabetes camp, where we talk about sexual issues a lot with teenagers, the boys already know this is a risk. What proves most motivating is educating them about how an erection occurs and explaining—in a nonthreatening manner—how that process is damaged by poorly controlled diabetes.

Adolescent girls and young women with diabetes also worry about sexual function. I explain how diabetes can interfere with this part of their lives. High sugar levels can cause yeast infections and vaginal inflammation that rob women of sexual enjoyment. If diabetes complications involve the nerves and circulation to the woman's genital tract, she may be unable to experience the normal pleasure associated with sexual stimulation. But I can also reassure women that all these problems are much less likely to occur if blood sugar is well controlled.

DIABETES AND FERTILITY

Diabetes may lead to infertility in women. When the disease is poorly controlled, adolescent girls and women may have irregular periods and fail to ovulate regularly. This makes conception more difficult or even impossible. And if a woman does become pregnant, her diabetes markedly increases the risk for both her and her baby.

Sugar travels across the placenta to the developing baby. High maternal sugar levels increase the probability of damage to the fetus. One of the long-term dangers—particularly if the mother's diabetes is not well controlled during pregnancy—is that her child will have an increased risk of developing the disease. Fortunately, if a pregnant women is meticulous about her blood sugar control, she can usually have a healthy pregnancy and a healthy baby.

At camp and in my clinic, I remind teens of both sexes about the importance of preventing unplanned pregnancies. I'm always concerned when one of my teenage patients with diabetes gets pregnant. If the pregnancy is unplanned—as it usually is—her blood sugar level was probably dangerously high at the very earliest stages of fetal development. The fetus may be malformed before she even knows that it exists. Three of my teenage patients with diabetes have had unplanned pregnancies with extremely poor results. One baby was born with one leg missing; another had a serious heart defect;

and a third suffered from a malformed gastrointestinal tract and was unable to eat.

With these three tragic cases in mind, I panicked when Etta, one of my fourteen-year-old patients with poorly controlled diabetes, became pregnant unexpectedly. I first met Etta when she was twelve and already a rebellious adolescent. When I told her what she needed to do to take care of her diabetes, she wouldn't look at me. She picked at her nails, fidgeted in her chair, and shut me out. I put my hand lightly on her shoulder, trying to reach out to her. She jerked back. I tried to lighten the situation with a little joke. She didn't smile.

Over the following two years she did turn up for her regular appointments, but there wasn't much improvement in our relationship. When Etta became pregnant, she told me that she wanted to have the baby. "I'm concerned," I told her. "Your A1c test is so high that it's off the scale. There's been a lot of sugar in your bloodstream—so much that it's not only hurting you but also hurting the fetus that you're carrying."

"I don't care what you say," Etta told me. "I'm gonna have this baby." We talked some more. Etta told me she wanted a child, someone she could love and who would love her back. It didn't matter to her that her body would be strained by carrying a pregnancy while she had poorly controlled diabetes and while she was still developing herself. After all, she was only fourteen years old.

I asked Etta if I could talk to her mother; reluctantly, she gave me permission. I didn't feel optimistic. Etta's mother, Grace, hadn't been able to help over the past two years when her daughter failed to take care of her diabetes. I knew Grace had tried, but Etta kept her at a distance. It was not easy for any adult to be part of Etta's life.

When I finally reached Grace by phone, she told me she had no control over what her daughter did. She seemed resigned, as if there was nothing she could do to influence anyone or anything, including her own daughter. As we talked about Etta's pregnancy, Grace's voice became shaky, and it sounded as if she was sniffing back tears.

During her pregnancy I saw Etta every few weeks. She became more receptive as her body changed. Each time I talked with her,

she seemed to trust what I had to say a little bit more. She took better care of herself and her diabetes improved. She paid more attention to her diet, and she began walking to and from school, which
was two miles from her home. Eight times a day she checked her
blood and adjusted her insulin. She agreed to use an insulin pump—
something she'd never been willing to do before—because that was
the best way she could care for her diabetes during pregnancy. Her
insurance company was willing to pay for the pump, because they
realized that meticulous diabetes management would save them
money in the long run.

Etta's relationship with her mother improved, too. At her
twenty-four-week checkup, Grace and I accompanied Etta for her
ultrasound. I watched in fascination as I saw this baby growing inside a mere child. All three of us marveled at its heart beating—beating, I was relieved to see, without apparent defects.

When Etta went into labor prematurely, Grace was by her side,
wiping her forehead and squeezing her hand. The baby—a girl, who
Etta named Tawnee—was large but normally formed. Tawnee experienced respiratory distress and required some extra oxygen. But her
lungs recovered, and after a few days she went home with her mother
and grandmother. I was thankful that I did not have to add Etta's baby
to the statistics on teenage pregnancy complications.

When I speak with patients who have just been diagnosed with diabetes, I tell them, "You must take one day at a time." I tell them,
"We will teach you what each blood test means, how your medicines
work, and how to find a balance." I tell them, "You will have some
high blood sugar numbers and some low numbers. You need to try
to figure out why they are high or low and then you need to try to fix
them. Sometimes, no matter what you do, your tests will be abnormal." Then I add, "But don't look at any one number and feel
doomed. Don't think, 'There go my eyes' or 'Now my kidneys are
damaged.' It doesn't work like that. Managing diabetes is about doing the best you can. But it's also about living your life and following
your dreams. The most important thing to realize is diabetes is
about the big picture. It's about the long haul."

When I tell them this, I sit close to them. I look directly into their eyes. I want them to take care of themselves—but I also want them to enjoy life and to make plans for the future. I know I've done my job when they realize all those "one days" put together will determine their risk of developing the devastating long-term complications that diabetes can bring. Once I see them performing their blood tests, taking their medications, balancing their food and activity, going to school, working, climbing mountains, playing the guitar, and taking tennis lessons—going on with their lives with diabetes—then I know they will succeed.

PART 2

The Evolution of Our Destruction

EIGHT

Designed for Feast or Famine

When I became president of the American Diabetes Association in June 2002, I knew that at our next annual meeting I would be expected to stand on a podium in front of thousands of people and give a presidential address. I'd attended twenty-five previous presidential addresses, and had truly enjoyed and learned from them. My many predecessors, all but one of whom had been men, gave inspiring and informative talks about funding for diabetes research, the future of diabetes care, diabetes across the globe, and the people and the concepts that have moved diabetes treatment forward. But now the diabesity epidemic loomed. I wanted my speech to be a call to action against diabesity. To do that, I would have to explain the origins of this epidemic.

I started having trouble falling asleep. I would lie awake contemplating a question that seemed to me to be of cosmic proportions: why are some people overweight while others are not? Is it because obese people have high-risk genes? Can we blame the toxic environments they live in? Or are they obese because they lack the will to adapt healthy lifestyles? I would think about the children I'd seen recently. I'd picture girls who weighed less than 100 pounds and others who weighed over 200; I'd ask myself why one boy was scrawny while another packed so many pounds around his midsection. And I'd think about their parents, whose shapes usually were similar to those of their children.

For hours, I would argue with myself, taking all sides. There was no doubt in my mind that genes played an important role. Since genes are critical, how could anyone be held responsible for their obesity? But even with high-risk genes, people still had to eat too much and exercise too little to gain weight, implying they had personal control. After all, I routinely told my overweight patients to lose weight—and many of them did. Then I would remember why others, seemingly just as intelligent and motivated, could not follow their diets or meet their exercise goals. Many of them lived in neighborhoods where outdoor exercise was unsafe and appropriate food choices were hard to find; their families were poor, and sugar and fat were cheaper than fresh fruits and vegetables. As I argued with myself into the early morning hours, I came to believe that obesity is rooted in all three: genes, the environment, and individual choice.

I also struggled to understand how diabetes became a human disease. Why have genes for obesity and type 2 diabetes persisted through human evolution? What possible survival advantage could they offer? And how do they explain why diabesity, which was not a problem of epidemic proportions in the past, is exploding now?

As I thought about these issues, I read many books and articles; I talked with experts in a variety of fields, from paleontology to anthropology, from geology to genetics. I felt as if I were back in medical school. It was an arduous experience, but it crystallized my thinking about why we are in the midst of a diabetes epidemic and what we must do to reverse it.

To understand diabesity, we must start with our genes. Scientists haven't yet agreed on the total number of genes that constitutes the human blueprint, but the latest estimate is around 24,000. Scientists have pinpointed over 250 genes in humans that may help determine what we weigh. These genes influence our appetite, explaining why some babies are indifferent to food while others eat eagerly. They affect our metabolism, making some people seemingly able to eat a great deal without gaining weight, while others cannot. Certain genes influence our storage of fat, whether we'll be shaped like apples or pears. Other genes affect the odds of developing insulin resistance and type 2 diabetes. As the number of adverse genes piles up, the balance tips, making excess weight and type 2 diabetes far more likely.

IN THE BEGINNING

About 40,000 years ago, on some savanna, a Paleolithic man and woman emerged to become the great, great, great...grandparents of us all. Their Paleolithic genes still inhabit our cells; we continue to pass them from one generation to the next. And these genes shape our metabolic pathways. We must look to our Paleolithic ancestors to understand the modern-day problem of diabesity. We must look to them to know why the environment we have created is so toxic to our essential well-being. We must put ourselves in their place and in their lives to understand how the genes that must have been advantageous in the past are killing us now.

Our Paleolithic ancestors were hunters and gatherers. The men traveled long distances in search of food. They tracked wild creatures—predecessors of the bison, bear, and other large mammals that inhabit our earth now. They killed their prey with rocks and primitive spears. After the men feasted on the carcass, they hauled the remains home to feed their families. But sometimes the hunt was unsuccessful and they went hungry. In the presence of an unreliable food source, no one ever knew exactly when or where they would get the next meal. When food was present, especially the rarer and more precious fat and protein of animal products, gorging and trying to store calories within the body was a wise strategy.

Paleolithic men were lean, muscular, and strong. Their bodies evolved to withstand the perils that hid behind every tree and boulder in their ancient landscape. Between hunting, nomadic migration, and chasing off perilous intruders, they rarely had time to sit and relax. Their day was spent in vigorous physical activity. Insufficient food was a constant risk.

Women—the childbearers and nurturers—stayed closer to home. Like the men, they were physically active, but their work required more cunning than strength. They kept the fires burning and taught their young about danger and survival. To supplement whatever prizes the men brought back, the women foraged. They gathered nuts, berries, fruits, vegetables, and roots. Obesity was probably unheard of, because the food supply was so unreliable. But the women undoubtedly had a higher proportion of body fat than the men did, as is true for women today.

Our Paleolithic ancestors enjoyed a varied diet. When the supply of game or vegetation ran low, the community moved to more promising land. Over the year, as seasons changed and they migrated in search of food and easier survival, they could consume up to a hundred different varieties of fruits, nuts, and vegetables. Children were nursed until age two or three. After weaning, their main beverage was water.

Our own dietary preferences reflect the needs of our Paleolithic ancestors. They could not have survived without receptivity to new foods; flexibility enhanced their ability to endure in changing environments. We share a built-in preference for variety. That's why we're more tempted to overeat at a buffet than when we're offered just a single option. Indeed, the success of some modern weight loss diets rests mainly upon the appetite-reducing effects of restricting food choices.

There is no doubt that our attraction to sweets is rooted in our genes. In Paleolithic times, plants with sweet fruit provided quick energy and were safe to eat. Since bitter plants were often poisonous, they were best avoided. Human taste evolved to prefer sweet foods because those were without peril in our ancient landscape.

We can't be certain, but our best guess is that the Paleolithic diet was approximately 30 percent protein. The chief protein sources were fish and meat. We can assume that the mammals our ancestors ate were lean. These beasts didn't live in feedlots or graze on carefully managed pastures. They had to exert themselves to obtain nourishment and to avoid becoming the meal of some other creature. So like the hunters who hunted them, they were largely muscle.

Probably about 50 percent of our ancestors' diet consisted of nuts, seeds, fruits, roots, and vegetables. Vitamins and minerals were abundant in these foods. Men and women consumed up to 100 grams of fiber per day—five to ten times as much as is typical today. About 20 percent of their diet was fat, mostly from nuts and seeds. The fat in nuts and seeds is the unsaturated kind, which actually helps keep blood vessels free of the damage that saturated fat can cause. Since the meat was lean, the Paleolithic diet included minimal saturated fat compared to today's diet.

Paleolithic men and women did not live long. If they survived birth and infancy, most died in what we would consider young adulthood. They were vulnerable to famine, predators, accidents, and infections; the women faced all this plus the risks of childbirth. But we can assume that our ancestors' health problems didn't include the obesity-related woes that plague us today. Their blood vessels presumably were free of fat deposits, so strokes, heart attacks, and high blood pressure were probably rare. Thanks to their high-fiber diet, their colons must have functioned well, without the modern woes of colon cancer and intestinal polyps, constipation, hemorrhoids, and fissures. Diabesity was unknown.

THRIFTY GENES

The genes that designed the bodies of our Paleolithic ancestors evolved for people who spent their days in physical activity and whose diet was low in calories and saturated fat. Evolution selected genes that could withstand a harsh reality: a tenuous food supply, barren winters, and recurrent droughts. In an influential article published in 1962, the late geneticist James Neel called them "thrifty" genes because they helped maximize the amount of energy that could be obtained and stored from every calorie consumed. One mechanism for accomplishing this was insulin resistance.

It's not hard to imagine how Paleolithic life selected who would live and who would die. Infant mortality was very high. In this harsh world, insulin resistance was an adaptive mechanism for babies, both before and after birth, enabling them to use meager calories more efficiently. In times when food was more plentiful, thrifty genes would enable them to eat heartily and stockpile body fat for the inevitable harder times. When famine came, thrifty genes would conserve those fat stores, slowing down metabolism and preserving the body's energy reserves as much as possible. Evolution favored those women able to accumulate body fat despite periods of famine, since they were more fertile and better able to endure the physical demands of pregnancy and nursing babies.

Thrifty genes were advantageous for Paleolithic life. But 5,000 to 10,000 years ago, much of the world began to change. Some bands of humans developed agriculture; others learned to domesticate animals. They abandoned their nomadic ways, settled down, and developed vast civilizations. These civilizations were able to grow crops rather than forage for them. They were able to raise animals in an enclosed space rather than hunt them. They were able to survive in larger groups because their food supply had become more reliable and they could store extra provisions. Famines and shortages, although not unheard of, became much less frequent. But there was a price to be paid for this progress. The balance that had evolved between humans and their nutritional environment was altered.

With agriculture came a huge dietary shift: the preeminence of grain and increased consumption of meat. With abundant grain and food products developed from grain, humans consumed less fish, fruits, and vegetables. Animals raised for human consumption were fatter than the lean prey eaten by Paleolithic people, and the saturated fat they contained was less favorable to the human metabolic and cardiovascular systems.

Achim Gutersohn, a German geneticist, has hypothesized that the thrifty genes became less important in stable societies with better climates and more abundant food supplies. His theory helps explain why diabesity is more common in some parts of the world than in others.

Thrifty genes are very common in Africans (and African Americans). Gutersohn estimates that 90 percent of those of African descent have thrifty genes. Since the food supply was not optimal in Africa, some of our ancient ancestors migrated to Eurasia. The food supply and climate were better in Eurasia, and the thrifty genes became less common in their descendants. Some settled in Asia, others in Europe. Perhaps 50 percent of Asians have thrifty genes, according to Gutersohn. But those who wound up in Europe made further improvements in food procurement. As the risk of starvation was reduced, more people who lacked genes to withstand famine could survive to adulthood and reproduce. That's why the thrifty genes are found in only 20 to 35 percent of Europeans and Americans descended from Europeans.

Meanwhile, in other corners of the globe, ancestors of the indigenous peoples of the Americas, Asia, the Pacific, and Africa continued to face a less-than-abundant food supply. Many still relied on hunting and gathering. Some farmed, but with less effective technology than that enjoyed by European farmers. Their thrifty genes remained important—and became all the more so when these peoples were conquered by a succession of European colonizers who decimated their lands, slaughtered their herds, and forced them to migrate across the planet under the most inhumane conditions imaginable.

CHANGING NATIVE WAYS: THE STORY OF THE PIMAS

Few peoples of the world more clearly show the effect of thrifty genes than the Pima Indians who live in southern Arizona. Their ancestors arrived in Mexico roughly 30,000 years ago. Some of the Pimas remained in Mexico, but about 2,000 or 3,000 years ago, others migrated north. The Pimas were skilled farmers. Those who came to southern Arizona established a sophisticated irrigation system that made the desert flourish with fruits, vegetables, and legumes. But their lives changed dramatically in the late nineteenth century, when white farmers came to the area and diverted their water supply. The Pimas' previously reliable agriculture faltered, leading to widespread poverty and malnutrition.

During the twentieth century, the Pimas adopted a more typical American lifestyle. Their traditional diet had been low in fat and high in starch and fiber; now their fat consumption increased significantly. They also became less active physically. Similar lifestyle changes affected the U.S. population as a whole. But the impact on the Pimas was far greater because they had more thrifty genes.

In the early 1960s scientists and doctors from the National Institutes of Health (NIH) came to the Pimas' Gila River Valley reservation in Arizona to study rheumatoid arthritis in the community. As they examined members of the tribe, they discovered that an astonishing number of them were obese and suffered from type 2 diabetes. Eighty percent of the people living in the Gila River Valley community were overweight. Over 50 percent of Pimas over the age of thirty—and a staggering 80 percent of those over age fifty-five—had type 2 diabetes.

This discovery inspired an extraordinary collaboration between NIH scientists and the Pima nation to study obesity and diabetes, a collaboration that has continued for nearly four decades. Ninety percent of people on the reservation have participated. They've been interviewed and examined; they've been weighed and measured for height. They've kept activity diaries, worn heart rate monitors, swallowed glucose solutions, and provided blood samples. Some have spent days isolated in special chambers so their metabolism could be measured precisely.

Thanks to their efforts, scientists have been able to map the genes shared by families whose members are especially likely to suffer from diabetes. These studies have helped us understand how insulin works in our bodies and how we process food and utilize energy. NIH researchers have also traveled to Mexico to visit a Pima community there. The Mexican Pimas share a genetic heritage with the Pimas from Arizona. But their lifestyle is very different. They live in remote rural mountains and still lead the physically active life of farmers. Their diet is low in fat and high in vegetables. Despite their thrifty genes, the Mexican Pimas have low rates of obesity and diabetes.

Out of decades of research about the complex interplay of genes and the environment comes the knowledge that being overweight is the single strongest predictor of type 2 diabetes. And we've also learned that increased physical activity and beneficial dietary change can delay or prevent diabetes, even in a population whose genes make them vulnerable to it. We all owe much to the Pimas' generosity.

One of my former patients, Dora, was part Pima. I had met her mother, Jo, at an American Diabetes Association public seminar in Los Angeles. I'd given a lecture about type 2 diabetes and obesity in children, and Jo had approached me afterward as I was standing in line to get a cup of coffee. I guessed from her high cheekbones, bronze skin, dark eyes, and black hair that she was Native American. She was wearing a simple blue dress with a striking silver necklace that included a single stone of the same blue. She looked about thirty-five or forty.

Jo told me she was fascinated by what I had to say about Native youth in Canada and in the United States. I had described their heightened risk for type 2 diabetes and mentioned that they had a poor overall outcome once diagnosed. "I'm Pima," she added. I was immediately eager to speak with her, to hear about her experiences with diabetes. We found a place to sit and drink our coffee. I asked Jo about her family, and the question opened a floodgate. This is not an unusual experience for a physician. Mostly I consider it part of the privilege of being a doctor.

Diabetes had robbed Jo of nearly everyone she loved. Her mother had become disabled from a stroke. Her father, before he died, had been on dialysis for several years. And her older brother, her only sibling, was taking two diabetes medications. Jo told me that she had developed gestational diabetes fourteen years earlier, during her pregnancy with her daughter Dora. This is a common problem for Pima women. She was already heavy, and once she became pregnant, additional weight came on quickly. By the time she was diagnosed with diabetes, in the middle of her second trimester, she had already gained twenty-five pounds. "I expected to gain weight, so I didn't realize that anything was wrong," she said. With dieting, exercise, and help from her healthcare team, she was able to stop gaining. Nevertheless, she needed to take insulin injections during her third trimester.

After Dora was born, Jo's obstetrician gave her a strong warning: unless she exercised and lost weight, she would develop permanent diabetes. The doctor had delivered many Pima babies and had seen how much devastation diabetes caused in the tribe. He told Jo, "You can choose to deny your genes their apparent destiny. It's up to you." He explained that if women got diabetes during pregnancy, their children would be at higher risk for the disease later.

After her delivery and while she was nursing Dora, weight loss was easier for Jo. And she'd made up her mind. "I decided I would not let diabetes steal my health," she said. At least three times a week, Jo took long walks around the reservation, pushing Dora in her stroller. She stopped eating between meals and cut back significantly on junk foods, like sodas and chips. Six months after Dora's birth, she returned to the doctor for a checkup. She had lost 28 pounds, and her fasting blood sugar level, which had reached 182 mg/dl during her pregnancy, was now down to 116 mg/dl—higher than normal, but under the 126 mg/dl cutoff for diabetes.

One year after she delivered Dora, Jo weighed 36 pounds less than she had when she became pregnant, and her blood sugar was normal. For the first time since she was a teenager, she was no longer overweight. Now, fourteen years later, Jo told me that she was still exercising regularly and eating well—and it was obvious by looking at her. She told me she was 5 feet 4½ inches tall and weighed 126 pounds. She stood up straight, and I could tell she was proud of her body and her commitment to it.

"Everyone on the reservation has relatives with diabetes. It's everywhere," Jo said. "But too many people ignore it. They eat the wrong foods; they don't exercise. They smoke and drink too much." Jo and her husband had moved to L.A. recently, in part because they wanted to live healthier lives. Now they were concerned about Dora. "She's gaining weight, and we're worried about diabetes," Jo said. "My husband is part Pima, too."

I told Jo to make an appointment for Dora to see me at Childrens Hospital Los Angeles. A few weeks later, I met with the three of them: Jo, her husband, Dave, and Dora, their fourteen-year-old daughter. Looking at Dave, there was no doubt he had Native blood. He was tall and dark, with deep-set eyes and high flat cheekbones. He was heavy; I guessed that he carried an extra 25 pounds. Though Dora was overweight, she was a striking girl. She had the glowing dark skin of a Native American. Her eyes were big and brown, and when she smiled, straight white teeth appeared. Her cheekbones were high, like her parents', making her face look some-what triangular.

Dora's blood glucose had been measured, and it was normal. Jo and Dave looked relieved when I told them that Dora didn't have di-abetes; Dora herself didn't react to the news. I took a full history. Dora had weighted 9½ pounds at birth. Full-term babies above 8 pounds 13 ounces (4,000 grams) are considered "large for gesta-tional age" (LGA). That means they're heavier than 90 percent of full-term newborns. Doctors take special note of LGA babies be-cause high birth weight might indicate a medical problem. An LGA baby may simply have unusually large parents. But maternal dia-betes is the most common cause. When a pregnant woman has dia-betes, her baby receives excess glucose. This stimulates the baby's pancreas to produce excess insulin. As a result, the baby grows larger than normal. The higher the mother's sugar levels during gestation, the greater the risk to the developing child.

Though Dora had been exposed to excess glucose in utero, she didn't have the panoply of other problems that could have occurred because of Jo's gestational diabetes. But as a diabetes-exposed baby, her risk of developing obesity and diabetes later in life was approxi-mately three times greater than that of a baby whose mother did not have gestational diabetes. We don't yet know why the risk is greater for these infants. But one possibility is that the developing pancreas is damaged by the abnormally high demand to produce insulin.

Dora had been healthy at birth, and she'd remained healthy as a child. Her growth and development, including her weight, had been normal. But once her periods started at age twelve, she began to grow and to gain weight rapidly. In one year she grew 2 inches. Such growth with a gain of 10 pounds would have been normal. But Dora gained 26 pounds that year. And the following year she grew 1 inch but gained 19 more pounds. At age fourteen, she was 5 feet 3 inches tall and weighed 150 pounds. A normal weight for a fourteen-year-old girl of that height is about 120 pounds. Dora's excess weight was mainly in her midsection. That meant she had excess visceral fat, fat inside her abdominal cavity—the kind of fat that's associated with insulin resistance and metabolic syndrome, a cluster of symptoms that includes excess weight, high insulin levels, high blood pressure, and high blood fat. Given her genetic heritage, her prenatal exposure to diabetes, and her excessive weight, she was at very high risk for diabetes.

"She used to play sports, but now she's just interested in talking on the phone and going to the mall with her friends," Jo said. Dora glared at her. "I try to get her to eat salad and fresh fruit," Jo continued, "but she fills up on doughnuts and fries." Dora looked away, her face angry. I suggested to the family that I speak with Dora alone; Jo and Dave went to the waiting room.

When we were by ourselves, I asked her, "Why do you think your parents wanted you to come see me?"

" 'Cause they think I'm fat," she answered, looking at the floor.

"Only because of your weight?" I asked. I wondered how much she understood about her risk of diabetes.

"My mom keeps telling me that I might get diabetes or something," she said.

"Do you know what diabetes is?" I asked, concerned Dora might not comprehend the gravity of the problem. I could tell by the grimace on her face that she understood the implications, but like most fourteen-year-olds, she responded with a shrug. So I began to tell her about diabetes.

After I had gone on for a minute, she interrupted. "Look, I know diabetes is bad. My grandpa died because of it, and my grandma had a stroke. Her face went funny and her arm stopped working. But you just said I don't have it."

"That's true," I said. "However, you're part Pima and you're at high risk for developing it." I told her about thrifty genes and how they'd helped her ancestors survive. Now she was looking at me. I talked about the Mexican Pimas, whose lifestyle helps them avoid diabetes. This seemed to interest her. "If you make some changes and lose weight, you can avoid it, too. How about if we make a plan to do that?" I suggested. She agreed.

I arranged for Dora and her parents to meet with a nutritionist and a psychologist. We would give her the information and skills she'd need to make significant changes in her behavior and eating habits. But that wasn't enough. We'd also need to motivate her—to draw upon her strengths and her desires, so that she would persevere. Jo and Dave would have to learn how to support their daughter in a positive way, without the criticism that had caused family tension before. It would be hard work for everyone.

Over the next two months, Dora and her family attended weekly meetings at the hospital. Plans were geared to Dora's preferences. She selected the foods she would eat and the physical activities she would pursue. Her eating habits quickly improved. At one meeting, she proudly told the nutritionist that she hadn't touched sweetened soda or candy for ten days. When a local health club started a program for teenagers and two of Dora's friends joined, Jo and Dave agreed to pay for a membership. At the end of two months, Dora had lost nine pounds. Her body was not only slimmer, but also more toned.

As her program continued, Dora decided to learn more about what the Pima people ate in the times of her ancestors. Cactus and jicama—foods she hadn't eaten since she left the reservation—returned to her diet. Jo told me privately that Dora was now willing to eat salad. Over the next year, Dora grew another inch and she lost a total of 19 pounds. At 5 feet 4 inches, her weight was 131, within the normal range. She no longer carried excess fat around her midsection, and her blood pressure was at a healthy level. Like her mother, she had greatly reduced her risk of diabetes, despite her genetic heritage.

THE LONG SHADOW OF EARLY LIFE

Our body's tendencies to become obese and to develop type 2 diabetes are affected not only by our genes and our lifestyle, but also by our early development. The concept that nutrition in the womb and the cradle helps determine risk for some adult diseases is known as the Barker hypothesis, after the pioneering work of Dr. David Barker, a distinguished British epidemiologist. Barker's theory, first proposed in the 1970s, is that before birth and during infancy, when a developing baby is most vulnerable—and also most easily changed—nutrition can have lifelong effects.

To test this idea, Barker undertook a search for medical records of babies born in the early 1900s. He's described how the search took him and his staff to hospital archives, sheds, boiler rooms, and flooded basements throughout England. But most of what they found was not sufficiently comprehensive. Then they discovered the ledgers left by Ethel Margaret Burnside, the first chief health visitor and lady inspector of midwives in Hertfordshire, a county just north of London.

Appointed in 1911, Burnside led an army of trained nurses and midwives who attended births and followed the babies' progress afterward. Contemporaries described her as a formidable woman, tall and thin, with a penetrating voice and dominant personality. To supervise the nurses, she traveled across the county by bicycle, logging nearly 3,000 miles in a single year. At a time when babies' weights were often merely guessed, Burnside insisted that nurses weigh each infant on a scale. The weights were recorded—at birth and at one year of age—along with other information about the baby's health and development.

Barker used records from England's National Health Service to trace 15,000 men and women who had been born in Hertfordshire before 1930. Then he matched information about their current health to the infant data that Burnside's nurses had collected more than half a century earlier. Looking first at male deaths from coronary artery disease, Barker discovered that men who had been small at birth, and who were still small at age one, were at highest risk.

A full-term baby who is under 5½ pounds—which is smaller than 90 percent of full-term newborns—is considered "small for gestational age" (SGA). Premature babies who weigh less than 5½ pounds at birth are not necessarily SGA; it depends upon how their weight compares to their gestational age. As with some babies who are unusually large, SGA babies may be small because of their parents' size. But their growth may have been limited by their mother's malnutrition or by other conditions that deprived them of nutrients in the womb.

Barker concluded that undernourishment in utero and in the first year of life has permanent effects on physiology, with lifelong consequences. All babies begin life with a *genotype*—the collection of some 24,000 genes that form the code for their development. But these genes may manifest themselves differently, depending upon the environment in which they live. That manifestation—how the developed person turns out—is the *phenotype*. For example, the typically obese Pimas of Arizona share a genotype with the typically lean Pimas of Mexico. But their different phenotypes reflect their divergent lifestyles. Though early nutrition doesn't affect the genes themselves, it can alter the phenotype.

Heart disease is not the only later risk from low birth weight and low weight at age one. Subsequent research by Barker and others, in England and throughout the world, has found similarly strong associations between early malnutrition and both obesity and type 2 diabetes. Being born too small is even riskier than being born too large. There is an extraordinary sevenfold increase in risk for diabetes for SGA babies compared to those with normal birth weights.

How can it matter fifty or more years later that a person was born small? One explanation is that the baby's developing body, faced with insufficient nourishment, devotes its limited calories to the most essential organs, such as the brain and the heart. Thus the beta cells of the pancreas, which produce insulin, may not be stimulated to develop normally. Another way of looking at this is to see fetal life as a practice run that sets up pathways for metabolic functions. If survival requires that the developing body live on fewer calories, that body learns to use those calories very efficiently, to store them whenever possible, and to reclaim them from fat stores at a slower rate.

Barker hypothesized that undernourished babies develop a thrifty phenotype, one with a thrifty metabolism adapted to starvation. Such a thrifty metabolism is somewhat resistant to insulin and also less able to make more insulin if obesity develops. A thrifty metabolism is well adapted to food shortages. But if food becomes plentiful later in the person's life, the thrifty metabolism means a predisposition to diabesity. For those with both thrifty genes and a thrifty metabolism, the risk of obesity and diabetes is greatest.

When I first read about this research, I realized that Grandma

Sadie probably got diabetes in part because she was starved in the womb. I don't know how much she weighed at birth—my grand-mother wasn't even sure of the date or year of her birth. But she used to tell me that when she was born, she was so small that she was put in a box to sleep. Sadie was born in Russia in the last years of the nineteenth century. Her mother had been subsisting on insufficient calories for years and through multiple pregnancies. Because Sadie received inadequate nutrition before and after she was born, she had to develop a degree of insulin resistance in order to survive. During her childhood in Russia, her thrifty metabolism served her well. One of her brothers starved to death and her mother died, probably from malnutrition, when Sadie was still a young child. But my grandmother was able to survive her terrible circumstances.

When Sadie was a teenager, her father, my great-grandfather, sent her to the United States so that she could have a better life. Sadie's diet changed considerably in America, where she was ex-posed to abundance for the first time. But her body's metabolism had been formed in infancy. Those early years of deprivation set her up to get diabetes sixty years later when food was abundant and Sadie could indulge in my mother's chocolate cake.

I often think of Sadie as a tiny infant sleeping in a box when I walk through the newborn nursery in my hospital. No babies are born at Childrens Hospital Los Angeles. The infants in the nursery have been sent here from other hospitals for specialized care. Our nursery cares for some of the sickest babies on the planet. Some of them are here because they were born with deformities or suffered a catastrophe during birth; others were born too early. And some of the babies are sent to us because they were born too small.

Many of the tiny infants who were born small for gestational age stay in the nursery for weeks or even months, until they can gain enough weight to go home. The neonatal nurses wrap them in re-ceiving blankets—swaddling soothes them, because they're used to the restrictive environment of the womb. They look like little foot-balls, with their arms held at their sides, their legs straightened and secured, heads covered with little knit bonnets made by hospital vol-unteers. We must feed them sparingly and carefully, because their stomachs are so small. Looking at these tiny infants, it's difficult to imagine that one day—as a result of their struggles now—they may tip the scales in the opposite direction.

Thrifty genes and a thrifty metabolism are advantageous to the littlest babies in the nursery as they adjust to life outside the womb, just as they were an advantage to Grandma Sadie as an infant battling to survive. These same genes helped our long-ago ancestors cope with the challenges of their environment. Now all of us must learn how to live with our genetic heritage, despite the blessings of abundant food and modern technology.

NINE

The Land of Plenty

I grew up in Oak Park, Illinois, not far from the first McDonald's opened by Ray Kroc, the empire's founder. My father, who was well known in our community, was invited to become an early investor in McDonald's. One Sunday in 1957, he announced, "We're going to try a new kind of restaurant for lunch." Grandma Sadie wasn't interested. But the rest of us—my two older brothers, my parents, and I—got into our Chevrolet station wagon and headed to McDonald's.

My brothers and I were excited. Our family didn't eat out often. My mother was skeptical about restaurants. "Unless I've seen the food being cooked, I can't be sure it's safe," she'd say. But once a month we went to Big Al's, a hamburger joint in nearby Maywood, the town where my father grew up. This was a real treat. Each of us kids would get a burger and a malt; my father usually bought a Polish sausage sandwich. My mother got a burger, too, but she hardly ate any of it. "Who knows what Al puts in this?" she would say every month. My parents also bought one order of fries for the whole family to share, which worked out to about ten fries apiece. "That's plenty," said my mother. Her preference for fresh food, her dislike of anything greasy, and her firm ideas about proper portion size probably explain why my mother was slim her whole life.

Big Al's burgers were cooked on a grill. They were thick and juicy, with lettuce and slices of fresh tomato and onion tucked into the bun. Since Big Al's was a drive-in, we'd eat in our station wagon, trying to keep the juice from running down our arms. The new restaurant, McDonald's, was not a drive-in. We all went inside, very curious. My father ordered one burger and one glass of milk for each of us, and he ordered the usual single portion of fries for the family. I remember that the burgers cost fifteen cents each.

Even I could tell that the McDonald's burgers couldn't compare to Big Al's. But I liked the fries. They were thin and crisp; they tasted sweet and salty. Big Al's fries were fatter and soggier. You had to add salt to them, because they weren't salted. My brothers, as usual, eagerly ate everything. I didn't finish my burger. My mother, after scrutinizing hers, refused even to taste it. My father bit into his hamburger. He frowned as he chewed. He opened the bun and poked at the thin, dry patty. Then he shook his head and delivered his verdict: "No one is going to eat this crap."

My father—as we never let him forget—was wrong. Every family in America was about to eat differently, and my family was to be no exception. By the 1950s, Americans had already begun a dietary shift. But many more significant changes were to come. These changes would increase our average daily caloric consumption. What's more, our lives would shift in other ways that would significantly affect how many calories we burned. As caloric intake pulled ahead of caloric expenditure for most Americans, the inevitable result was an epidemic of obesity.

EXPANDING AMERICA

When I was a child, every pharmacy had a scale. You could step on the scale, put in a penny, and learn your weight. Sometimes you got your fortune, too. On top of the scale were printed normal weights for men and women of different heights. The numbers were based on standards established by the Metropolitan Life Insurance Company. These days, height-and-weight tables are no longer used to determine normal weight. Instead, we use the Body Mass Index (BMI), in which a single number can help us tell if a person's weight is appropriate for their height.

The Body Mass Index is sometimes called the Quetelet Index after Adolphe Quetelet, a nineteenth-century Belgian astronomer and statistician. Quetelet searched for statistical patterns in human size. For raw numbers, he used military data. Armies needed to take measurements of thousands of young men so that they could fit soldiers for uniforms. He discovered that these numbers—whether the chest circumference of Scottish soldiers or the heights of French conscripts—tended to follow a bell-shaped curve: there were relatively few soldiers who were much smaller or larger than average; most were clustered in the middle. Also following a bell-shaped distribution was the index he devised, now called the Body Mass Index, based on body weight and height.

The BMI is a person's weight in kilograms divided by his or her height in meters squared: kg/m^2. A more complicated formula is used to compute BMI for weight in pounds and height in inches. Many Web sites will perform the calculation instantly if you enter your height and weight; you can find them with Google or another search engine.

A normal BMI is between 18.5 and 24.9. That's true for adult men and women, and it's true for adults of any height and shape. Women may be slender or curvy; men may be slight or muscular. But if their BMI is between 18.5 and 24.9, their weight is normal. This simplicity is the advantage of using BMI rather than the old height-weight tables. For example, for a women of average height, 5 feet 4 inches, a normal BMI corresponds to a weight of 108 to 144 pounds; for the average man, 5 feet 9 inches tall, the normal range is between 125 and 168 pounds.

At a BMI between 25 and 29.9, an adult is considered overweight; anything higher is termed obese. The higher the BMI, the higher the proportion of fat a person's body is likely to have. But there are exceptions. Some very muscular individuals may have BMIs in the above-normal range even though their bodies contain no excess fat. An example is Arnold Schwarzenegger. According to published reports, he is 6 feet 2 inches tall and weighs 257 pounds. Though that makes his BMI 33, he's neither obese nor overweight. He's heavier than average because he has more muscle. Nevertheless, BMI represents a useful yardstick for most adults. For the average woman who's 5 feet 4 inches, overweight means a weight between 145 and 174 pounds; obesity starts at 175 pounds. A man who is 5 feet 9 inches would be considered overweight at 169 to 202 pounds and obese at 203 pounds or more.

BMI is used for children, too. However, different standards are used to interpret them. A youngster's BMI is calculated by the same formula. But then the BMI is compared to standard childhood growth charts that were developed by the Centers for Disease Control and Prevention (CDC). Because the CDC wished to avoid stigmatizing heavy kids, they don't use the term "obesity." If a child's BMI is in the top 15 percent for gender and age—in other words, if the child is at or above the 85th percentile on standard growth charts—the youngster is considered "at risk for overweight" by CDC standards. Those in the top 5 percent (at or above the 95th percentile) are labeled "overweight."

The 1999–2000 National Health and Nutrition Examination Survey found that an astonishing 64 percent of American adults are either overweight or obese. The number was approximately 8 percent higher than a decade earlier and continues to climb. Even more alarming is that nearly one-third of American adults—31 percent—are obese. That's double the rate of obesity of the late 1970s.

Rates of overweight in American children have increased similarly over time. In the 1960s, 5 percent of children age six to nineteen were overweight. By 2000, the proportion of overweight youngsters had leaped to 15 percent, a threefold increase over four decades. For African American and Hispanic children, the rate of overweight is over 30 percent. And remember, the term "overweight" applied to children corresponds closely to "obese" in adults.

I've seen this trend in my medical practice. Each year, more and more children are referred to me because they weigh too much. And each year I notice that the parents of my patients have gotten heavier and heavier, too. How did this happen? Why have so many

Americans become obese? It's not hard to understand when we think about our thrifty Paleolithic genes and how our world has changed over the past fifty years.

THE EVOLUTION OF SADIE'S KITCHEN

Grandma Sadie left Russia in 1906, when she was about sixteen. She settled in Chicago because her father, my great-grandfather Joseph, had a cousin who knew someone who had promised to help my grandmother get settled in her new world. Sadie's mother had died years earlier; her father stayed behind in Russia, and Sadie never saw him again. Within a year of arriving in America, a marriage was arranged for her. She met my grandfather Harry for the first time on the day of their wedding. Over the next twenty-two years she gave birth to five children; my father was the next-to-youngest.

After her food-deprived childhood, Sadie was determined to feed her family well. To her, food was a sign of love. She became an excellent cook, famous among friends and relatives for her generous portions. In her early years of marriage and motherhood, Sadie shopped for food nearly every day. Everything she bought to feed her family was fresh: meat and poultry from the butcher, fish from the fishmonger, fruits and vegetables from the market. She used to tell me how she would go to the butcher and pick out the best chickens, the ones with plump breasts. She would discard the heads, pluck each feather, and cut off the feet to simmer in soup. "Fisel," she called the feet. "Such a delicacy."

Sadie bought carrots when they still had the green tops. She put carrots in the bottom of the pan when she roasted chickens; she added them to soups, along with the tops; she peeled them so her family could eat them raw. Sadie kept a supply of juicy apples for snacks. My father told me he would often sneak an extra apple out of the house to give to his teacher.

Every night, when my grandfather came home from his job driving a delivery truck, the entire family would sit down in the small parlor and eat dinner together. All the food was made from scratch, including the bread and cake. Sadie dished out everything with care. Because her sons were more active than her daughters and would one day be bigger, she knew intuitively that they should eat a little more. Any leftovers found their way into the next meal in another form. Friday night was the best of all. My grandfather's parents, Max and Anna, joined the family for dinner. Sadie's mother-in-law, my great-grandmother Anna, arrived early to help Sadie prepare soup and twisted challah bread. They roasted two chickens, cooking potatoes in the pan; they made a tsimmes, a casserole of carrots with prunes and brown sugar. Wine was poured, prayers were said, and the family was nourished and nurtured together on the Sabbath.

In 1920, when Sadie was about thirty years old, she opened a candy store to help support the family. It was called Sadie's Confectionery Shop, and she made every piece of candy herself. I have a cherished picture of my grandparents, Sadie and Harry, standing outside the candy shop on the day it opened in Maywood, Illinois. Sadie is wearing a long white dress with a high lace collar. You can just see her lace-up boots sticking out beneath the hem. Harry is wearing a suit and tie, with his white collar standing up underneath his suit coat. A large cigar hangs between his lips. His expression is stern, but Sadie's smile is radiant. By 1920, Sadie had already given birth to four of her five children. Yet she was slender in that picture—you could have wrapped your hands around her waist. When I look at that photo, I'm always struck by the sharp contrast to the Sadie I knew more than thirty years later. That Sadie was heavy.

Despite the thrifty metabolism that resulted from Sadie's early malnutrition, she remained slim in her first three decades of adulthood. The candy prepared for the store was made to sell; she and the family ate very few pieces. And like the Pima Indians of Mexico, Sadie led a life that included sufficient physical activity to burn the calories she consumed. She was up at dawn to tend to her family, run to the market for supplies, and prepare the day's inventory of candy for the shop. The confectionery opened at ten in the morning. She was on her feet every minute until closing time; then she came home and made dinner. With help from her mother-in-law, she somehow managed to get everything done—and also gave birth to her fifth and last child in 1928, two years before she turned forty.

In 1932, when Sadie was in her early forties, she sold the candy store to a younger woman and retired. Without the store, and with her older kids grown, she could relax a little for the first time in her life. She would sip a cup of tea in the parlor and finally enjoy a piece of candy that she hadn't slaved to make.

During Sadie's early years as a housewife, she didn't serve store-bought bread or soup from a can. She feared that processed or canned foods might be contaminated; she doubted they would taste as good as what she cooked. But gradually, like most American housewives, Sadie started to try them. She bought Heinz vegetarian beans; she bought Wonder Bread, which promised to "build strong bodies eight ways." My grandmother once told me about the first time she tried canned corned beef hash: "I opened the can and looked inside. Vas it cooked already? I didn't know. So I cooked it, just to be safe."

I have another old photo of Sadie, the one my father took with him as a young soldier serving in the Army Medical Corps in World War II. In this picture, Sadie is heavy. She still stood 5 feet 4 inches tall. But she probably weighed 175 to 180 pounds, about 40 pounds more than on the day the candy store opened. Twelve years of increased food consumption and decreased physical activity had transformed my grandmother from slim to obese.

FROM THE FIFTIES TO FAST FOOD

When I was growing up, my nourishment came almost exclusively from food eaten at home and prepared by my health-conscious mother. I remember the first time I ate a TV dinner. I was ten years old and was spending the day at a friend's house. As dinnertime approached, I could smell food cooking, and I expected that any minute we'd be called into the kitchen or dining room. Instead, my friend and her younger brother pulled several folding chairs from behind the living room sofa and set them up in a row, facing the TV. Then they lifted little tables that had been stacked in a corner and put one table in front of each chair. I was mystified, but I didn't want to ask questions and reveal my ignorance.

My friend and her brother each took a seat, so I did, too. Her father came into the living room and turned on the TV. We sat silently for a few minutes, watching *Lassie*. Then my friend's mother entered carrying knives, forks, napkins, and five small tinfoil trays on a large platter. She distributed the cutlery and placed one tinfoil tray on each of the little tables.

I'd noticed Swanson's TV dinners in the freezer compartment at the grocery store. The package looked like a television screen, with knobs on both sides that were supposed to represent the knobs on a TV. But I'd never seen what was inside the box. At first, I wasn't sure what I was supposed to do. When everyone else began eating from the tinfoil tray, I started, too. The tray was divided into four compartments. The largest held slices of turkey in oily, salty gravy; the other three contained stuffing, peas, and chunks of sweet potato. I thought it was fantastic—watching TV and eating greasy, salty food from a tinfoil container.

At home later that night, my mother asked me what I'd had for dinner. When I told her, she seemed startled. My father said provocatively, "That sounds like fun." My mother poked him in the ribs. It was clear that our family wouldn't be eating TV dinners any time soon.

Once I became a teenager, I began to eat more meals with my friends. We'd go to White Castle for burgers and fries; we drank sodas and shakes. In college, late-night pizzas, greasy burgers, chips, and candy bars were my common fare. I avoided weight gain only because I was physically active.

My diet changed considerably after I started medical school. I was fascinated by biochemistry—it explained what we're made of and how we metabolize food and nourish our bodies. This theoretical knowledge suddenly became real on the day when we reached a part of the medical curriculum I'd dreaded, the part that involved dissecting a human body. Four of us would be assigned one cadaver, a body that had been willed to the medical school by the deceased person or donated by his or her family. The cadavers were stored in embalming solution in the anatomy laboratory of the medical school. We would work with our particular cadaver for almost an entire year.

Our assignment on the first day was to learn to feel comfortable with our cadaver. It wasn't easy. The body belonged to a middle-aged woman who had died of a gunshot wound. When I first looked at her and realized what I had to do, I wanted to run out of the room. It was difficult just to sit next to her, to think that once someone had been her friend or her lover. She became so real to me that I had the irrational thought she might suddenly sit up.

Meanwhile, my lab partners, all men, were busy examining her. I tried not to show my fear and disgust. After about fifteen minutes, I got hold of myself. I slowly moved my hand and touched her arm and then her hand. I stared at her face. All of a sudden, I felt profoundly grateful to her. She was going to reveal to me the mysteries of anatomy, physiology, and medicine. She was going to be my guide to understanding the human body. Somehow, on that first day, I learned to feel comfortable with her. When I came home, I realized that my hands were numb and that they smelled from the embalming fluid. I soaked in a tub filled with sweet-smelling soap and bubbles.

Over the months that I studied my cadaver, I came to admire her. She had little body fat; her muscles were well developed; her bones were sturdy; her organs were healthy. Before she was shot down, she must have gotten plenty of exercise. Everything she'd ingested and imbibed had been made into her skin, her hair, her muscles, and her organs—and she had made them well. It dawned on me that everything I ate and drank became part of my body, too. Medical school didn't include nutrition courses back then; even now, they're not always part of the curriculum. But I knew that if I were to have a healthy body, with strong bones and muscles and little fat, I'd need to think about what entered my mouth and found its way to my stomach. I found myself preferring fresh food and avoiding grease and sweets, just like my mother. These feelings were magnified once I became a pediatrician and a parent.

When our children were young, my husband, Neal, and I tried to protect them from fast food and junk food. We sent them to a preschool where sugar, soda, and candy were forbidden. At this school, snack time meant chunks of cheese, sticks of red pepper, raisins, and apple slices. Parents were required to send a "wholesome" lunch from home. I once arrived at the school carrying a doughnut hole and a Styrofoam cup filled with coffee. I hadn't eaten anything since six-thirty in the morning, and that's all I could grab as I dashed out of the hospital to pick up my boys in the late afternoon. Jonah's preschool teacher, shocked as much by the Styrofoam as by the pastry, stopped me before I could enter the classroom and set a bad example.

Neal and I allowed the children's babysitters to take our kids to fast food restaurants occasionally. But we insisted that they follow certain rules: one order of fries for all three of them—my family tradition—and no sodas ever. The sitters also were required to remove any toys that might entice the children to demand frequent return visits. Until Adam was six years old and joined a T-ball league at the local park, neither he nor Jonah, then age four, knew what they were missing.

After the second T-ball game, when the kids finally hit the ball off the tee and ran around the bases in the right direction, one of the fathers presented a McDonald's Happy Meal to each child and each sibling. My children's eyes widened when they saw the brightly colored boxes, and they laughed with delight when they looked inside. So many fries! A Coke! They couldn't believe they got a tiny toy circus car, too. That was the end of fast food innocence for our children and for us. Other parents bought Happy Meals for their children and my sons. When they joined friends' families at the movies, candy bars and buckets of greasy popcorn were part of the excursion.

Neal and I resisted and resisted. We were both pediatricians, and both of us were strongly committed to healthy eating as individuals, as doctors, and as parents. We didn't want fast food to be part of our family's diet. But one day when Adam was seven and Jonah was five and we were on a family skiing vacation in Utah, we found ourselves driving through a snowstorm on unfamiliar slippery roads, all of us hungry. As we came to yet another cluster of fast food eateries, Neal said, "We'll stop as soon as I find a real restaurant."

Adam responded, "McDonald's is real, Dad."

"Look!" cried Jonah. "Here's one right now."

Neal and I looked at each other, feeling the force of social change as well as the pressure of the storm and our hunger—and we capitulated. That was the first time, but not the last. The following year, when Jonah turned six, we yielded to his urgent pleas and scheduled his birthday party at Chuck E. Cheese's. Nevertheless, we made sure that these exceptions did not become the rule.

The trends I've seen in my own family echo the experiences of most Americans. The home-cooked family meal has not disappeared. About three-quarters of the meals we eat—including breakfast and lunch, as well as dinner—are prepared and eaten at home, according to statistics from the NPD Group, a company that tracks consumer behavior for its business clients. However, "prepared at home" doesn't necessarily mean homemade in the traditional sense. Family meals have evolved considerably since Grandma Sadie served chicken soup in her parlor. In 2002, the most recent year for which numbers are available, only 35 percent of main meals were prepared from scratch, down from 41 percent a decade earlier. Most of us are using processed foods or take-out food in the meals we serve at home. We're also eating more meals at restaurants, especially fast food restaurants. On a given day, over half of Americans eat meals and snacks away from home. That's a much higher proportion than in the past.

Some days I feel surrounded by fast food. One of the first things you see when you enter my hospital is a McDonald's restaurant. McDonald's, Wendy's, and other fast food restaurants are not rare inside children's hospitals. It's unfortunate, but understandable. Hospitals are open around the clock; doctors, nurses, and other staff members work all day and all night and need to eat. Hospital administrators look for food services that will be cheap, quick, and familiar to their patients and staff.

In my clinic, families often arrive in the waiting room carrying bags of fast food take-out. Sometimes when I walk into the examining room to meet with parents and their children, I'm overwhelmed by the smell of hamburgers and fries. Or I overhear a parent telling a child, "I'll take you to Jack in the Box later if you behave." Many of these youngsters are coming to see me because of weight problems. Often their parents are overweight, too. I can understand why they buy inexpensive fast food. Many are impoverished; nearly all of them are juggling jobs and family responsibilities. They've rushed from work, dashed to pick up their kids at school or child care, and have just made it through Los Angeles traffic to get to their appointment at the clinic. The inducements of taste, ease, and low cost make fast food hard to resist.

Fast food restaurants have changed what we eat and how much we eat, as well as where we eat. Soda has replaced milk; ketchup and fries have replaced fruits and vegetables. Fast food typically contains more saturated fat, more sugar or other sweeteners, and more salt than food prepared at home. These ingredients add taste appeal; sometimes they make foods easier or cheaper to produce. But extra fat and sugar pile on the calories.

Consider, for example, the McDonald's Mighty Meals, which are marketed to preteens. One version includes a double cheeseburger, french fries, and a 16-ounce soda. It contains a total of 860 calories, which is 43 percent of the 2,000 calories that a ten-year-old should be eating for the day. This single meal packs more than half of the fat recommended for a child of ten (37 grams out of a daily suggested maximum of 65) and more than half of the maximum amount of sodium a youngster should consume in an entire day (1,420 milligrams out of a maximum of 2,500). It also supplies an excess of refined sugar: 47 grams, the equivalent of about 9 teaspoons. A Mighty Meal is mighty on calories, fat, salt, and sugar, but it's puny on nutrition. Growing children need fruits and vegetables for their vitamins, minerals, and fiber. But they get none from a Mighty Meal—unless you consider ketchup a vegetable.

Portion distortion is another alarming trend exacerbated by fast food. There's more on our plates and in our cups, so we're consuming more. When I was growing up, my father would take me and my brother, Gary, who was three years older, to Blue Bell on North Avenue as a special treat on weekend afternoons. John, five years my senior, was off with his friends. Blue Bell had it all. Blue Bell was heaven. In front were a pharmacy and a mini grocery store. In back was our destination: the soda fountain. I learned how to ride a two-wheel bike on those ten-block trips to Blue Bell, my father steadying me the whole way there. When we arrived, he bought me a Coca-Cola. The soda came in a 6-ounce glass with a straw. My older brother, who had been riding circles around me, got a root beer float: a scoop of vanilla ice cream in a glass of root beer. My father had a cup of coffee. I savored that 6-ounce Coke. It must have taken me an hour to drink it. I wanted it to last forever. I spun around on my red vinyl seat at the soda fountain. My father talked to me about being a doctor, and my brother slurped every last molecule of his root beer float from the sides of his glass.

Soda now comes in quantities that make my 6-ounce Blue Bell treat look like a mere sip. The smallest bottle of Coca-Cola sold today is 12 ounces. At Wendy's a "small" soft drink contains 16 ounces; "medium" refers to a 20-ounce cup; and a "biggie" holds 32 ounces, one full quart. Other fast food chains offer similar super-sizes. But the 7-Eleven convenience store chain outdoes them all, with the X-treme Gulp, a mug that contains 52 ounces of soda. That's more than three pints in a single serving.

Supersizing isn't limited to soda. As health journalist Greg Critser documented in his fascinating book *Fat Land: How Americans Became the Fattest People in the World*, McDonald's discovered in the 1970s that offering much larger portions at only slightly higher prices boosted sales. Doubling the size of a cup of soda or a bag of fries added just pennies to the cost. The labor, overhead, marketing, and other fixed costs were the same, no matter what the portion size. Customers swallowed the bait of these large-size "bargains." So profits soared.

The price doesn't increase in proportion to the size, but calories do. Coke contains about 12 calories per ounce, so my 6-ounce Blue Bell serving was a modest 72 calories, approximately the same as one and a half Oreo cookies. An X-treme Gulp portion of cola—52 ounces—is a whopping 624 calories. A man who quenched his thirst with an X-treme Gulp would have consumed 28 percent of his daily calories; a woman would have consumed 35 percent.

Traditional sit-down restaurants have also increased portion size, using the same more-for-your-money lure that worked so well for the fast food industry. Supermarkets and warehouse stores offer supersize "bargains," too, like chocolate chips in gallon bags and bricks of cheese big enough to build a house. All of us learned to pile food on our plates and overflow our bowls. From 1971 to 2000, average consumption by men in the United States increased by 168 calories per day; for women, it jumped by 335 calories per day.

SLOWING DOWN

While the input side of the caloric equation was going up, the expenditure side—how many calories we burn—has been going down. In current surveys, 40 percent of American adults report that they are completely sedentary. Of the remaining 60 percent, seven in ten are somewhat active but fail to meet the minimum recommended standard of engaging in thirty minutes of moderate or strenuous physical activity five or more days a week. One recent study found that Americans spend nine times as many minutes on TV and movies as they do on all leisure-time physical activities combined.

When I was in elementary school, I rode my bike to and from school nearly every day in the fall and spring. Walter, the crossing guard, made me and all my friends get off our bikes to cross the busy road, Division Street, where he was on duty. When I arrived at school, I would play in the playground until the bell rang. And every day, I had physical education, which we called PE. Mr. Schultz, the PE teacher at my grade school, was tall and stern. During PE, he would blow his whistle to keep us moving. At the end of the period, we'd be hot and flushed from playing so hard.

After school, our mothers directed my friends and me to "go outside and play." And we did. We rode our bikes to the forest preserve at the edge of town. It was a long ride. Once there, we ran around, played hide-and-seek, and climbed trees. Back in the fifties and early sixties, parents didn't worry when their children played unsupervised, because parks and neighborhoods were considered safe to explore. In the afternoons, America's children were outside playing. We watched much less TV than today's kids do. There were no home computers and no video games. So most of our play was active.

All this had changed by the time my own children were born, Adam in 1978 and Jonah in 1980. They were driven to school not only because we lived many miles away, out of biking range, but also because stories of children being abducted or hit by cars dominated our lives. And as a pediatrician, I'd cared for too many children who were the victims of accidents or hurt by adults. So I could not have conceived of allowing my children to go off with other youngsters to explore a forest preserve. All of their outdoor activities were supervised. Lance was great at taking them to parks and playgrounds, teaching them karate and keeping them active. But none of that was as easy as it was when I was growing up.

According to government transportation surveys, walking and bicycling by children age five to fifteen dropped 40 percent between 1977 and 1995. Physical education, which was once a required part of the school curriculum, has been drastically cut back in many communities. Only 17 percent of middle and junior high schools—and a mere 2 percent of senior high schools—now require students to engage in physical activity every day.

As opportunities to be physically active became more limited, sedentary indoor distractions proliferated. Though television was a major part of American life by the 1950s, until the 1970s children watched no more than an hour of TV per day, on average. But by 1990, kids spent an average of three hours daily in front of the tube, and today it's close to four hours. Children's programming has expanded, from Saturday morning cartoons to afternoon soap operas and sitcoms, adventure programs, and reality shows every night. On top of TV-viewing time, hours are spent on the equally sedentary pursuits of Nintendo, Game Boy, computer games, the Internet, and instant messaging.

These days, when kids are asked about their physical activity, only about half of American youth between twelve and twenty-one say that they regularly participate in any kind of vigorous physical exercise. About one-fourth acknowledge that they get just about no exercise at all.

TIPPING THE BALANCE

Looking at the changes in our lives over the past several decades, it's not difficult to understand why America faces an obesity epidemic.

We're eating more—more than we need and more than we can expend in physical activity. And we're moving less. That's all it takes to tip the balance to obesity. Surprisingly small changes in what we eat or do can make a big difference.

Mark, a former colleague of mine, is a good example. I first met Mark when he was a resident at Childrens Hospital Los Angeles. We stayed in touch after he joined a nearby pediatric practice. Mark was funny and smart. He was slim, with dark curly hair. When he laughed, a dimple formed in his right cheek. About five years ago— after Mark took a job with an insurance company and stopped practicing medicine—we lost track of each other.

In the years when Mark was a practicing physician, his office was on the third floor of his medical building. He got into the habit of using the stairs to get there. Lunch was another habit: every day he went to the coffee shop in the lobby of his building and ordered a roasted turkey sandwich with lettuce and tomato on a whole-grain roll. After a while, the coffee shop owner had the sandwich waiting for him when he came downstairs at noon. Mark ate well at home; his wife was a nutritionist and she watched the family diet very carefully. On the weekends, they took their two young children to the park or to the pool.

I'd missed our occasional get-togethers over the past five years, so I was delighted when Mark telephoned recently to invite me to give a lecture on diabesity at a community meeting sponsored by his company. We agreed to meet for coffee before the lecture. I was shocked to see that he'd gained about 50 pounds. "You look the same," he said when he greeted me. Then he added, "Not like me." He chuckled as he patted his protuberant belly. I noticed that he no longer had a dimple when he smiled—his cheeks were too puffy.

Over coffee, Mark brought me up to date on his life. Shortly after he began working for the insurance company, he learned that his wife was having an affair with her tennis instructor, and their marriage ended. Since he wasn't interested in cooking, he'd begun picking up drive-through dinners at the KFC he passed on the way home from work. His children, who spent every other weekend with him, begged for fast food. "Their mother won't let them eat junk, so I indulge them," he said. "Makes the visit more fun." At the insurance company, his office was on the twenty-third floor, so he never took the stairs. His children preferred going to the movies to more active recreation on their weekend visits. Mark had become almost completely sedentary.

On the way home, I thought about how all these changes in Mark's life had added up to a 50-pound weight gain in five years. A pound of fat represents about 3,500 calories. If you change your life in some small way that consistently causes a 10-calorie-per-day excess—either you consume 10 extra calories or burn 10 fewer calories in physical activity—over the 365 days of the year, you'd gain about a pound of fat. And if you make changes that amount to an excess 100 calories per day (a latte with whole milk instead of skim would do it), you could be up 10 pounds in a year, just like Mark. When he was practicing medicine, he burned about 15 calories each time he walked up the three flights of stairs to his office, something he did twice a day for a total of about 30 calories. It wasn't hard to imagine that his new fast food habit—the difference between roasted turkey and fried chicken—could account for at least 70 additional calories per day.

Our margin of error is very small. Just a few extra calories every day, coupled with a sedentary lifestyle, can cause extra pounds to accumulate. As individuals with free will, we can choose to grab a bag of chips, plop ourselves down in front of the TV, and slurp an extra-large soda. Or we can down a glass of water, get on our bikes, and go. As individuals, we can make the better choices no matter where we live. But our environment helps shape these decisions, by making good choices easy or difficult. As America has changed in ways that nudge us in undesirable directions, the balance has tipped to diabesity. And as our lifestyle has spread throughout the world, the obesity and type 2 diabetes seen in this country have become a global epidemic.

TEN

Diabesity Around the World

In 2002 I attended the World Health Organization's Fifty-fifth Assembly in Geneva, Switzerland, as a member of the United States delegation, which was led by Secretary of Health and Human Services Tommy G. Thompson. The assembly floor looked like the United Nations, with people of every color and shape, many in traditional garb, talking in over a hundred languages. Speakers from undeveloped nations described the major health challenges they faced: starvation, HIV/AIDS, the terrible injuries created by horrific wars. Others, from the so-called "advanced" nations, described their major problem: diabesity. Some of the world's countries suffered from an inadequate food supply and others from an obscene overabundance. And a growing number of developing nations were coping with both problems simultaneously.

In 2000, 151 million adults worldwide had diabetes. Experts predict that by 2010 there will be 200 million people on the planet with diabetes, and the figure may reach 300 million a decade later. Although too many of the world's peoples are still threatened by malnutrition or outright starvation, diabetes is escalating in every continent and in every country.

Because type 2 diabetes is exploding in the populous countries of China and India, by 2010 more than half of the people in the world with diabetes will be Asians. In Latin America, diabetes is expected to increase by 44 percent, in Africa by 50 percent, in Europe by 24 percent, and in Australia by 33 percent. No place is immune.

What's causing this worldwide explosion of diabetes is the increasing number of people across the globe who have become obese—a phenomenon now referred to as "globesity." According to the International Obesity Task Force, which is composed of world experts in the field, an estimated 300 million people are obese and 750 million more are overweight. Each year 34 million people die from obesity-related causes, including not only diabetes but also heart disease, stroke, and certain types of cancer. That's about 60 percent of annual disease-related deaths worldwide. Obesity has doubled in Japan since 1982. The prevalence of obesity has increased by 10 to 40 percent in most European countries in the last decade. In the United Kingdom and the United States, it has doubled in the past two decades.

Many think that obesity is a problem only in industrialized nations. But that's not true; it has infiltrated the developing world as well. In Egypt, Chile, Peru, Mexico, and Tonga, about a quarter of children are overweight or obese. According to the International Obesity Task Force, 0.7 percent of children in Africa suffer from insufficient nutrition—but 3 percent are overweight or obese. Where we have obesity today, we will have type 2 diabetes tomorrow.

Diabetes is an enormous challenge for any country's healthcare system. To cope, there must be diabetes-trained doctors, diabetes educators, nutritionists, psychologists, and people able to transport emergency cases to healthcare facilities. Countries must have the ability to care for all the complications of diabetes, including heart disease, kidney failure, and retinopathy, as well as the consequences of gestational diabetes. To do that, there must be hospitals, intensive care units, operating rooms, clinics, dialysis machines, and facilities for childbirth and for the care of high-risk newborns.

People with diabetes often require medication to control blood sugar. Some inject insulin; others take pills. Both insulin and pills come in different forms, all of which must be available. Insulin users need syringes, which must be sterile to be safe. They need access to refrigeration, since insulin must be refrigerated. To optimize blood sugar control, patients must have glucose meters to test their blood several times a day; they also need the strips upon which the blood is placed, and batteries to run the meters.

I've had the privilege of traveling around the world to teach about diabetes and to observe a variety of healthcare systems first-hand. I've met with physicians, scientists, nurses, nutritionists, and care providers; I've talked with patients. I have seen and touched diabetes in China, Japan, Taiwan, Mongolia, Ecuador, Mexico, Kenya, Slovenia, Lithuania, Australia, and most of the countries of Western Europe. Diabetes is devastating in every one of them, but some countries are managing more successfully than others.

Many developed countries are able to provide excellent care for people with diabetes. The United States, Canada, New Zealand, Australia, Japan, and most of the countries of Western Europe are in that category. Some developed countries—including many of the Western European and Scandinavian countries, but not the United States—have national diabetes databases that track patients and their outcomes, thereby coordinating care for the patient's lifetime. So far, the developed countries have been able to cope with the increased prevalence of diabetes. Yet to be seen is whether they can continue to meet the demands that the diabesity epidemic will place on them in the future. Most developed nations, in contrast to the United States, provide health care for all citizens. In the U.S., where 43.6 million people are without health insurance, many people with diabetes do not have access to any medical care, and certainly not to the best care the nation offers. Those who are uninsured or under-insured must sometimes manage without adequate medications or supplies, just as people in impoverished countries do.

Diabesity is a particular challenge for developing nations, such as India, China, the Pacific Island nations, and Latin American countries. With increased prosperity and adoption of Western ways—including fast food and sedentary leisure activities—comes obesity. People with economic resources can afford to eat too much. Manual labor is no longer part of their lives. Once they can purchase a car or motorcycle, they don't need to expend calories on walking or pedaling a bicycle. As the middle-class population gains weight, their incidence of diabetes inevitably increases.

In 2003, when my son Adam was working and studying in Monterrey, Mexico—the country's third largest city—I lectured on type 2 diabetes and obesity at a local private hospital, Hospital de San José. After my talk, doctors crowded around me to ask questions. Everyone moved aside to permit a distinguished-looking elderly man to come to the front. I later learned he was the retired head of the department of medicine at the medical school in Monterrey. His question was hardest of all. "Doctora," he said, continuing in perfect English but with a thick Mexican accent, "in Monterrey we have many poor people. They can only get emergency medical services and services from the public health department. My country can barely care for them now. What do you think will happen in the next decades as these people live longer, labor less, and eat more?" I had no answers. Both of us knew that the Mexican healthcare system, and Mexico itself, could sink under the weight of the diabesity epidemic. And I thought of other nations I'd visited—India, China, and Ecuador. All of them were struggling now. And all face far more difficult challenges in the future.

INDIA: A SYSTEM THAT WORKS FOR SOME

I traveled to India in 2002 as part of a group teaching a postgraduate medical course hosted by the American Diabetes Association and the Madras Diabetes Research Foundation. Type 2 diabetes was uncommon in India until about a decade ago. Now there's an emerging epidemic. Almost 6 percent of the Indian population between ages twenty and seventy-nine have type 2 diabetes. So far the disease in India is almost exclusively confined to the urban areas. That's where the population has become less active: they drive cars, watch TV, and play computer games. Urban dwellers also have more food in general and more non-Indian food in particular.

The postgraduate course was held in the M.V. Diabetes Specialities Centre, a clinic located in Chennai, a city in the south of India that was once called Madras. The Diabetes Centre is run by Dr. V. Mohan and his wife, Dr. Rema Mohan. They follow 75,000 people with diabetes. Our clinic in Los Angeles follows about 2,000 people, and we feel overwhelmed almost all the time. So it was mind-boggling to imagine how any medical facility could care for such a large number of potentially complicated patients. But this clinic in India did.

When our delegation arrived at the clinic's reception desk, a line of about fifty people snaked through the lobby. There were two long rows of sturdy wooden chairs on one side. Every seat was taken, with two or three children squeezed together in some seats. Along the edge of the room, men and women squatted against the walls, some with children in their laps. People stood or squatted along every corridor and in every stairwell. The clinic was overcrowded by any criterion, but there was no sense of chaos. Everyone waited quietly and patiently. The day was hot. Intermixed with the scent of perspiration, a suggestion of curry wafted through the air. I later learned that there was a kitchen in the clinic. It was used to teach people how to eat and cook, and to prepare meals for patients who were staying overnight.

After brief introductions and a cup of British-style tea in his office, Dr. Mohan gave our group a tour of the clinic and introduced us to many of his staff. At my request, a nurse asked one of the patients in the clinic's intake area if he'd speak to me. He agreed and introduced himself as Vijay. I spent the next two hours following him through the clinic, observing his care, and learning about his life.

Vijay was forty-five years old. He had dark hair, a ready smile, and twinkling black eyes. His arms and legs were skinny, but he carried excess weight around his middle. That meant he had visceral fat, the kind inside his abdominal cavity that's associated with health risks. Two months earlier he had been diagnosed with type 2 diabetes.

He'd been slim as a young man, Vijay told me; now he was about 30 pounds overweight, with a BMI (Body Mass Index) of 29, close to obese. In the previous year alone he'd put on 15 pounds, and almost all of it had gone to his midsection. "It used to be that when I entered a room, my big nose was the first part of my body across the threshold," he told me with a wry laugh. "Now it's my belly."

Vijay worked as a manager for a private computer chip company. His wife was not employed outside the home; she cared for their two teenage boys, Vijay, and Vijay's mother. Over the past ten years, as Vijay advanced at work, the family income had increased. Hearing how his lifestyle had changed as a result, it was easy to understand why he'd gained weight.

When Vijay and his wife were first married, they had traveled around Chennai on foot or by bicycle. But when they had enough money, they bought a car and gave away their bicycles. Vijay equipped the house with an air conditioner; he bought a big TV and a VCR. During the sweltering Indian summer, no one in the family wanted to go outside. Relative affluence altered their diet, too. Though they still ate traditional Indian food, they could afford extras, such as sweetened soda, candy, and ice cream.

The more weight Vijay put on, the more rundown he felt. He began awakening in the middle of the night to urinate, and there were a few sores on his legs that weren't healing. A few months before I met him, he had mentioned these problems to a friend at work. The friend urged him to go to the Diabetes Centre.

He'd filled out forms, met with a nurse, and told her his symptoms. The nurse immediately sent him to the blood-drawing area, where another nurse took a vial of blood from a vein in his arm and pricked his finger. A drop of blood was placed on a special paper strip and inserted into a glucose meter. Vijay's blood sugar was 287 mg/dl. The nurse told him he had diabetes; the laboratory would test the venous blood to confirm the diagnosis. I asked Vijay how he felt when he heard those words. He looked down and said, "I felt ashamed. I knew I had indulged myself by eating too much, and this was the result."

On his first visit to the clinic Vijay had spent the whole day. It took that long to attend the classes given by the diabetes educators and nutritionists. They explained what was happening in his body now that he had diabetes; they provided dietary instructions and advice about exercise. Vijay learned how diabetes medications work and what side effects they might cause. He was shown how to use a glucose meter and how to keep a log of his sugar levels. At the end of the day he received a bottle of pills—an insulin sensitizer—to take two times a day. From his description, I thought that he'd received excellent instruction and care, equivalent to what we offer patients at our clinic.

Now it was two months later, and Vijay was returning for his first follow-up appointment. I could tell he was proud of himself and his diabetes management. He told me he'd started to lose weight. His blood glucose levels were returning to the normal range, and he felt better. As I followed Vijay over the next few hours, I was impressed by the efficiency with which he was poked, scanned, measured, treated, and evaluated by clinic staff members, each of whom wrote their findings in the chart Vijay carried. It was almost like an assembly line, but an assembly line with a heart. Members of the staff directed him from one area to another. They seemed to be looking out for the patients, ensuring they received their full evaluation.

Vijay went first to the nutritionist, a young woman wearing a sari. She reviewed his nutrition plan, cautioned him about salt, and wrote a few things in his chart. She seemed pleased with his progress, and so did he. Their encounter took about ten minutes. After the nutritionist, Vijay had a similarly brief visit with a nurse educator who checked his log, nodding approvingly at his improved blood sugar readings. She ascertained that Vijay was having no problems or side effects from his medications, made notations in his chart, and sent him to his next appointment, a cardiovascular assessment.

To show me he was committed to exercising, Vijay suggested that we take the stairs. The stairwell was filled with people waiting to be seen. As we trekked up the two flights, dodging other clinic patients, Vijay quickly became out of breath. "I'm not quite there yet," he admitted, panting slightly.

Inside another small room was an ultrasound machine that can assess cardiovascular risk noninvasively, by evaluating the major blood vessels. The technician, a friendly young man in a white coat, told Vijay to take off his jacket, sit in a chair, and place his arm, palm up, on an armrest. The technician held a device over his radial artery (the artery at his wrist, below the thumb), sending sound waves into his blood vessels and receiving the echoes as they bounced back. For several minutes the technician was transfixed by a computer screen, which showed waves that looked like the bleeps and sweeps on a radar screen. These waves represented the flow of blood in Vijay's arm. The technician explained that the test results would take a few days to analyze. Then he added with a smile, "But it looks good. You must keep it that way."

In yet another office, Vijay was weighed and the number recorded in the chart he carried. He had lost 3.1 kilograms (about 7 pounds) in two months. At the news, Vijay smiled and bowed to the scale. I bowed to him. Though Vijay's waist wasn't measured, I knew from his "apple" shape that he had too much fat around his liver and in his abdomen. Fat distribution is in part genetically determined. Indian men and women tend to have more abdominal fat than Caucasians. Vijay had about 20 percent more fat in his abdominal cavity than a similarly overweight Caucasian man with the same BMI, which meant that he was at elevated risk for both diabetes and cardiovascular disease. This probably explained something that had struck me when I looked at the patients in the Chennai clinic: although most were overweight, Indians with diabetes were not as heavy as typical patients with type 2 diabetes in the United States.

After his weigh-in, Vijay excused himself to use the bathroom. He needed to provide a urine sample so that his kidneys could be checked. He left the little jar at the clinic's clean but sparse laboratory. A doctor would telephone him later if a kidney problem were detected.

We made our way to the ophthalmologic department, which had two examination chairs with all the ophthalmology equipment I have at my hospital. About thirty patients were waiting to be seen. Some already had trouble with their vision and required the help of family members to navigate the room. A nurse dilated Vijay's eyes with drops, and he received a full ophthalmologic examination from a doctor.

Vijay's final appointment was with one of Dr. Mohan's associates, who examined his chart and reviewed the morning's findings with him. I waited outside, eager to hear the results. When Vijay emerged from the doctor's small office, he looked triumphant. "The doctor says I'm doing very well," he announced. "There's no evidence of any diabetes complications." As a smile crossed his face, I felt one appear on mine.

Vijay's last stop before leaving the clinic was at the pharmacy. He needed to purchase more glucose strips and more pills. About twenty people stood on line in front of the pharmacy window. Behind the pharmacist, I could see a huge room with row upon row of shelves filled with bottles of pills and boxes of supplies. While we waited, I asked Vijay how he paid for his health care and how much everything cost.

Vijay did not have health insurance; he worked for a small computer company that was unable to offer him coverage. There's a public health system in India for those with no insurance and no financial resources. But Vijay told me he wouldn't want to use the public health clinics, because they are overcrowded, overwhelmed, and unable to provide first-rate medical care. So Vijay paid for everything himself. Looking around this clinic, where waiting people lined every hall and stairwell, I couldn't imagine how crowded the public health clinics must be.

Medical bills had already consumed some of Vijay's savings. This morning's comprehensive evaluation had cost almost 3,500 rupees, nearly one month's wages. Though his glucose meter and its supplies were also relatively expensive, his diabetes pills—manufactured by an Indian drug company—were not. The same medication would have cost about ten times as much in the United States.

To afford his treatments, Vijay had sold his big TV and VCR. He'd spent some of the money to buy a smaller television of lesser quality, and put the rest in the bank. I asked him how this made him feel. "Good and sad," he told me. "Good because I'm doing something positive for my health. But sad because my children no longer have the biggest TV."

"Well, perhaps your family will become more physically active," I said, trying to sound encouraging. Vijay told me with a smile that the new television is so small, no one watches it for very long.

Vijay had received a thorough evaluation. But less than 5 percent of the population in this part of India could afford such comprehensive medical care. Each of the health professionals with whom he met had provided individualized, competent—and caring—service very efficiently. The Diabetes Specialities Centre's "assembly line with a heart" approach could teach those of us in developed countries how to provide care to greater numbers of patients. But when I thought about the crowds of people, I wondered how this clinic and others in India could possibly meet the increased demand for their services that the country's diabesity epidemic would soon create.

CHINA: A BLEND OF EAST AND WEST

Childrens Hospital Los Angeles has a sister hospital in Guangzhou (formerly Canton), China: Guangzhou Children's Hospital. In 1994, a group of our physicians was invited to Guangzhou to teach and exchange ideas with our counterparts there. I was particularly excited about the trip when I learned that my husband, Neal, and our two sons—then ages fourteen and sixteen—would be able to join me. China was emerging from an isolated past and was at long last opening its doors for interchange, including medical interchange.

For the month before the trip, I spent every spare moment in preparation. I created slides to show how diabetes develops. I added pictures of common complications: eyes displaying signs of retinopathy, feet with gangrenous sores. My presentation included equipment used by patients: glucose meters, different insulin preparations, and syringes. I copied our educational manuals. I called pharmaceutical companies and asked them to donate pamphlets and samples for us to distribute. I also bought breakfast bars, cups of soups, and boxes of nuts and raisins in case my children found Chinese food too exotic. These supplies filled a large suitcase.

Our group was welcomed not only by leaders of the medical community and our hosts from Guangzhou Children's Hospital but also by Guangzhou's Communist officials. We were housed at the best hotel in the city and treated to an elaborate welcoming banquet. While Neal and I met with our Chinese colleagues, a tour guide entertained our sons.

Each morning members of our group were driven through the streets of Guangzhou to the hospital. We were in cars, but cars were not the dominant mode of transportation in the city. The overcrowded streets were filled with men and women walking quickly to their destinations, as well as people pulling rickshaws or pedaling bicycles, some transporting a second person sitting side-saddle at their back. Everyone I saw was dressed in drab colors. The weather was extremely hot, and they wore loose-fitting shirts and shorts that came to mid-thigh. Almost everyone looked thin. Obesity, which was soaring in America, was not a problem in Guangzhou.

Guangzhou Children's Hospital was huge. The building was drab and gray. Though the halls were overflowing with people, the rooms and floors were spotlessly clean. We were taken to a big lecture hall—there must have been close to a hundred doctors and nurses in attendance—and our lectures began.

Neal was one of the first speakers. A translator stood next to him. Neal's talk was about middle-ear infections, a common problem in the United States. At the end he asked the Chinese doctors in the audience, "How often do you find middle-ear infections?" The translator repeated the question. No one answered. Finally the chief pediatrician of Guangzhou Children's Hospital explained to Neal that their doctors did not actually examine the ear during routine examinations, because only specialists had otoscopes, a viewing instrument that allows doctors to see the eardrum. In the United States, consumer versions of otoscopes are sold in some drugstores for less than $50. But in Guangzhou, a child with a suspected ear infection needed to visit an ear specialist for diagnosis.

My turn came next. I explained the importance of blood glucose control. I described the techniques and tools we use to help patients achieve good control: multiple medications, frequent blood testing, and careful balancing of food and activity. Between slides, I waited for the translator. But after Neal's experience, I realized that my Chinese counterparts probably didn't have the equipment I was describing.

My hosts had arranged for me to spend the rest of my day with Dr. Shu, the one and only pediatric endocrinologist in Guangzhou. She was thirty-eight and had trained in both Russia and Hong Kong, I'd been told. I could not have guessed her age by looking at her. Her back was bent; her hands were rough and cracked. These features made her look ancient. But the skin around her dark eyes was devoid of lines, and the short black hair that bobbed around her face made her look like a teenager. Her eyes suggested she was all business. Looking in her eyes, I surmised that she had laughed very few times in her thirty-eight years. She spoke English. But I had to concentrate to understand her, because her voice was quiet and her Chinese accent was strong.

After our formal greetings, Dr. Shu took me to one of the hospital's wards. A total of about thirty beds were lined up on both sides of a long hall. There were no curtains between the beds. Attending each child was a parent, a grandparent, or both. Some youngsters were being bathed; some were being fed; some were being fanned in the sweltering heat. Others were being coaxed to sit up or to stand and walk. I looked up and down the long ward but didn't see any nurses. Relatives were tending to all the caretaking tasks that nurses would have performed at my hospital in Los Angeles.

Dr. Shu stopped to point out two girls in adjacent beds on the ward, one age seven and the other fifteen. The youngsters had type 1 diabetes, which is rare in Asians. They had come to the hospital with very high blood sugar levels, suffering from dehydration. "We give many insulin shots," Dr. Shu said. "Better now." Both children were so thin that they seemed to disappear in their beds.

"How long have they been in the hospital?" I asked. In the United States, children who arrived in similar condition typically spend two or at the most three days in the hospital.

"Two weeks this one," she replied, pointing to the fifteen-year-old. "And three and half weeks that one," she continued, indicating the seven-year-old.

I blurted out, "Why, that's forever! Why do they need to be here?"

Dr. Shu explained that their families couldn't afford glucose meters, batteries, or glucose strips. But if the children stayed in the hospital, she could give them the frequent tests they needed to bring their blood sugar under control. She was right: if I faced the same choice, I'd keep my patients in the hospital, too.

We left the ward and went downstairs to the second floor. On one side of the hall, behind glass doors, was the Western pharmacy; on the other side, behind two giant wooden doors, was the traditional or Eastern pharmacy. Dr. Shu led me into the Western pharmacy. It reminded me of drugstores from my childhood in the 1950s. Large bottles and jars were on display in neat rows, with balances to weigh medications.

The hospital stocked many of the newest drugs: third-generation antibiotics, cutting-edge medications for pediatric cardiac disease, and cancer drugs. But there were significant gaps. Only animal insulin was available in China. In the United States and Europe, animal insulin had been phased out rapidly since 1994 in favor of bio-engineered insulin, which is not only cheaper to manufacture but also safer, since animal insulin can trigger allergies.

We left the Western pharmacy, and I followed Dr. Shu through the two giant wooden doors into the Eastern pharmacy. We entered a vast room lined with wooden medicine chests, each with many small, narrow drawers. Some of the drawers were open, and I could see roots and plants and insects in them. A pharmacist was using a mortar and pestle to grind up something that looked like the wings of a big moth. Dr. Shu tried to tell me what it was, but all I could comprehend was that some patient was going to brew this into a tea and drink it.

Dr. Shu showed me a whitish powder that could have been powdered sugar, baking powder, or cocaine. "Good for muscles," she told me, and noted that she gave this powder to children with diabetes. I nodded, wondering if I was looking at something revolutionary and helpful or something potentially disastrous and lethal. She showed me a clear liquid: reptile venom. They added this liquid to the IVs of children who had cardiac surgery to prevent clotting. I knew that the venom of some poisonous snakes has anticoagulant properties, which is how those snakes kill people. I was eager to see more, but Dr. Shu's three-hour clinic session was about to begin. She said, "Must go now. Many patients waiting." I looked back as I followed her out the wooden doors, thinking that somewhere in one of those drawers might be a magical cure for something.

The clinic looked like a long hall. It was stark and crowded. At the far end were two examination rooms; between them was a desk. There were a few chairs against the walls, but most of the people—children and teenagers with their parents or grandparents—were standing in line, waiting to see Dr. Shu. There were at least fifty youngsters in the line. Dr. Shu walked to the end of the room and took a seat at the desk; I sat down next to her. Dr. Shu's assistant, a young woman with thick glasses and dark black hair tied in a ponytail, stood at her side. She was not a nurse but a clerk, who was there primarily to help with paperwork and to promote efficient patient flow. I couldn't imagine how all these children could be moved through two examining rooms in three hours, with only one doctor to care for them. But I soon saw how: Dr. Shu didn't examine most of the patients. She spoke with them and with their families, made diagnoses, gave advice, and dispensed Eastern and Western medications. But only a few children were asked to step into the examining rooms.

Patients streamed by. Dr. Shu talked with the mother of a six-year-old boy with rickets; he was doing well on an Eastern medication that consisted of powdered bone. Another patient was a twelve-year-old boy who was the size of a six-year-old. Dr. Shu told me that she would have liked to treat his severe growth problem with growth hormone. But it was impossible to get that expensive medication in Guangzhou. All she could do was reassure his family that apart from his size he was healthy.

Ten patients had diabetes. The assistant checked their blood sugar levels, which were elevated in all cases. Dr. Shu adjusted their insulin doses accordingly. But I wondered how it was possible for patients and doctors to achieve good control without follow-up monitoring of blood sugar levels at home.

One of the older teenage girls with diabetes looked exhausted. Her face was flushed, and I thought she might be feverish. Dr. Shu brought her to one of the examining rooms. She took out a stethoscope—it was the first time I'd seen her use it—and listened to her lungs. The young woman had pneumonia. Dr. Shu prescribed an antibiotic and an Eastern herb and told her to come back in two days. I would have arranged an X-ray for a patient with diabetes who had pneumonia, and might have admitted her to the hospital. But Dr. Shu told me she could order an X-ray only if there was a life-threatening problem, and said, "Her parents take care of her at home with prescribed medicines."

During the three hours of the clinic, Dr. Shu saw more than fifty patients. It was arduous work. I see four, at the most five, patients an hour during my Tuesday clinic at Childrens Hospital Los Angeles, and I'm always exhausted at the end of the long day. I have the support of nurses, nutritionists, social workers, psychologists, fellows, residents, and medical students. But Dr. Shu did almost everything herself, and it seemed to me she accomplished what she did with her hands tied and her eyes blindfolded.

I worked for one week at Dr. Shu's side. I watched her struggle without staff support; I watched her mix East and West with the medicines she gave; I watched her hide her emotions. I shared with her what I knew and told her how we did things in my clinic. In our brief free time together—during lunch, walking from the clinic to the ward—I questioned her about her private life. She told me that she had a nine-year-old son. He lived with her parents in a province to the north. Her husband, a computer specialist, worked and lived in yet another province. She saw her child only twice a year and her husband not much more often. She seemed resigned, not bitter. That was the way they did things in China, she told me. No one expected anything different. After all, she wouldn't have time to care for her own child when she was so busy working—so busy caring for other people's children.

On my last night in Guangzhou I asked Dr. Shu to join our group for our final banquet. When she arrived at the hotel, I almost didn't recognize her. Instead of her white lab coat, she wore a traditional Chinese dress, red and embroidered in gold. Her hair was combed back from her face, and I thought she might have put rouge on her cheeks. As she walked through the luxurious lobby of the hotel, she looked radiant. She had brought me a gift in a small gold box. I opened it. Inside was a statue of a cricket, carved from a green stone. She explained that it was a symbol of good luck. I bowed in appreciation, feeling lucky to have worked at her side and to have shared her world, if only for a week.

On our way back to Los Angeles, we spent two days in Beijing, the capital of China, which is almost 1,200 miles north of Guangzhou. On the streets of Beijing I saw many more cars and fewer bikes—and many of those bikes were motorized. As we drove through the city, I spotted a huge McDonald's and signs advertising Coca-Cola. And for the first time since I'd been in China, I saw a few Chinese people who were obese.

I returned to China three years later, in 1997. This time I was in Beijing, so I did not see Dr. Shu. The hospitals still blended East and West. But we saw more books, more equipment for clinical care, and even a few otoscopes. Outside the hospitals, however, China looked very different. The streets were now completely filled with cars. Wherever I looked, I saw Western goods and products, including McDonald's and other fast food chains, and 7-Elevens selling candies and enormous sodas. This time, when I visited a pediatric clinic, I saw obese Chinese children. In the halls of the hospital and in the streets, it was obvious that globesity had arrived. Diabetes was exploding. I thought of Dr. Shu at Guangzhou Children's Hospital and wondered how long the lines had become at her clinic. I could only hope that she had more help now than she'd had in 1994.

ECUADOR: HEALTH CARE ON THE EDGE

In 1999 I spent one week at a diabetes camp in Quito, Ecuador. The camp had been organized several years earlier by two remarkable teenagers from Washington, D.C., Jesse Fuchs-Simon and Nick Cuttriss. Back in 1994, the year Jesse and Nick entered high school, Ecuadorian friends of Jesse's family had brought their eleven-year-old son, José, to the United States so he could be treated for diabetes. Both of José's parents were physicians and could afford to buy insulin for their son. Yet they lacked the practical information they needed to use it properly—information about blood tests, diet, and exercise. José's life was saved by the education and treatment he received in the United States.

During the family's visit, Jesse and Nick learned that in Ecuador most youngsters with type 1 diabetes die before age thirty. With help from their parents and adults in the U.S. diabetes community, the two boys decided to do what they could to teach Ecuadorian youth and their families how better to care for their diabetes. They founded an international nonprofit organization called AYUDA, which stands for American Youth Understanding Diabetes Abroad; also, "ayuda" means "help" in Spanish. Each year AYUDA sends dozens of young volunteers to help develop and implement diabetes programs in Ecuador and other Latin American countries.

I first heard about Nick and Jesse from my son Adam, who met them when they were all in college together at the University of Pennsylvania. My children had also experienced diabetes, working with me at diabetes camp and living with Lance. The next time I visited Adam at school, he introduced us. Jesse and Nick looked like typical college students, dressed in jeans and T-shirts. But their dreams and their visions were anything but ordinary. They talked rapidly, intensely. When they told me about their work and asked if I would come to Quito that summer to help teach Ecuadorian children and their families, I couldn't resist. Since Jesse and Nick needed all the assistance they could get, Neal and my sons came, too.

We arrived in Quito with insulin, glucose meters, batteries, strips, instruction sheets, pamphlets in Spanish—everything I could think of that might be useful. Jesse and Nick, working with Ecuador's Diabetes Association, had arranged for the camp to be held at an inactive military base. The buildings were old and barely functional. For our meetings, there was a central building made of wood and sheet metal. It was essentially a shell, with paint peeling from the ceilings and walls. The only furnishings were old tables and wooden chairs, which reminded me of the ones I'd sat on during grade school. In another building was our mess hall, with a rusty refrigerator, two ancient gas stoves, and a deep porcelain sink that was badly rusted. Rows of metal tables, with the same wooden chairs, had been set up to create a makeshift dining room.

The camp had eight American staff members—Jesse, Nick, my two sons, two other college kids, Neal, and me—as well as more than a dozen Ecuadorians: three nurses, one nutritionist, a cook, and a few other nonmedical assistants, plus eight parents, including José's parents, who were both physicians, though not diabetes specialists. On the first night, we met to plan the camp's activities. We decided to check blood sugars before bedtime to be sure no one was hypoglycemic, because I didn't want to face middle-of-the-night seizures in Quito, Ecuador. We would teach everyone how to manage diabetes with two blood tests a day, since that was all that would be practical for the majority of campers once they returned home.

About twenty adults and fifty kids had signed up for camp. Some wore traditional Ecuadorian ponchos and blankets; others wore jeans. Most of the youngsters had type 1 diabetes; two teenagers and five of the parents had type 2. They stayed in barrack-like huts, each of which held about twelve people. We assigned at least two adults to each hut, along with both American and Ecuadorian staff members. Neal and I stayed in a bleak little cabin. Once camp started, the primitive living conditions no longer mattered. We were inspired by the enthusiastic young people—both the staff, who were devoting a week of their summer vacation to helping others, and the campers, who had to struggle to stay alive. Many of the children and their families had traveled long distances, by multiple buses, to spend this week at camp.

Alejandro, age fourteen, who'd had diabetes since he was six, had journeyed for three days on five buses. He lived in a small village; there was no running water and no electricity in his home. He had never attended school. Regional health workers, not physicians, provided his medical care. If Alejandro had been my patient in Los Angeles, I would have prescribed thirty to forty units of insulin per day for him. But insulin was in low supply in Ecuador, and Alejandro couldn't afford a glucose meter to check his blood sugar at home. So he could take no more than ten to twenty insulin units a day. This meant that his blood sugar was chronically high and his cells did not receive enough nutrients. As a result, his health was compromised and his growth was stunted. Though he was fourteen, he was the size of an eight-year-old. At camp, he received insulin and other medications that would last him almost six months. Twice during the year, he and his mother traveled to the regional health center and received supplies for another three months. Because the family had no refrigerator, the insulin was stored in a box that was kept submerged in a nearby creek.

Each day at camp in Quito everyone came to the central building to learn how to manage diabetes. With help from a translator, I lectured to the parents. The American teenagers, all Spanish-speaking, met with the kids. We explained how to balance diet and exercise. A healthy lifestyle would reduce their insulin requirements. This is helpful for anyone with diabetes but is particularly important for people in a country where insulin supplies are limited.

Neal met with the parents; I held a daily question-and-answer session for parents and another for kids. We used a mini-curriculum similar to what we use at Childrens Hospital Los Angeles, but made practical for the realities of Ecuador. Since they couldn't check their blood sugar four times a day, we taught them to manage on two tests by varying the testing times. For example, they might check blood sugar first thing in the morning and before the evening meal on one day, then check before lunch and before bedtime on the next. Occasionally they'd test themselves in the middle of the night or after exercise. And they'd perform extra tests if they were ill.

We learned that Ecuadorian parents usually gave injections to their children, even after the children were in their teens. That meant the youngsters were not learning to take responsibility for their diabetes. All of us encouraged campers to take their own shots. One youngster shyly admitted that he felt embarrassed about the injections. Others nodded. At this, Jesse rolled up his sleeve and put an empty needle into his skin. Nick did the same. In fluent Spanish, Nick asked, "Why should I be embarrassed by this if it saves my life?" Jesse said, "I would be glad that I could do it, and proud that I knew how." I could tell from the expressions on the children's faces that the two young men had made an impression.

Ecuador and its people are dealing with pressing issues—political, economic, and social. Diabetes is barely able to make the list. Because most people are poor, excess food is not a problem in many parts of Ecuador. Physical labor is still common. So far, diabetes is confined mainly to children and young adults with type 1; type 2 diabetes is still rare. But this is changing. According to the International Obesity Task Force, obesity is on the rise in Ecuador. A 1999 study found that 19 percent of schoolchildren in Quito were obese. And data on pregnant women from the Ecuadorian Ministry of Public Health suggest that obesity is increasing among adults, too. I read these numbers with dread. The limited healthcare systems of Ecuador and other developing nations, which can barely cope with type 1 diabetes, couldn't possibly handle a type 2 epidemic.

LITHUANIA: WHICH PATH WILL IT FOLLOW?

In the fall of 2003, I went to Vilnius, Lithuania, to speak at the Third Oskar Minkowski Advanced Postgraduate Course for Eastern Europe, sponsored by the European Association for the Study of Diabetes. The course brought together a faculty of twenty experts on diabetes and obesity from around the world; our audience was several hundred Eastern European doctors. I lectured under the picture of Oskar Minkowski, the man whose seminal work revealed that insulin is made in the pancreas. Diabesity had not yet arrived in the economically emerging country of Lithuania. But the nation's doctors were trying to prepare for it.

After the first day of lecturing, I went for a walk through the streets of Vilnius. Grandma Sadie had come from Russia, from someplace near and similar to Vilnius. I wanted to get a feel for the place where she'd lived and the streets she'd walked down. And I wanted to see what the people were like now, as they turned from their Communist past and prepared to join the European Union.

As I walked, I saw an incredible mix of old and new. There were old dilapidated buildings and old church spires dotting the horizon, with new and renovated buildings sprinkled between them. Walking down the streets were elderly women dressed in black, with hats and scarves covering their heads. Past them brushed jeans-clad teenagers with purple stripes coursing through their hair. I'd worn a shawl, because it was September and the air was turning cool. I wrapped myself in my shawl and envisioned Grandma Sadie, with a similar shawl around her head and shoulders, walking out of Russia. Sadie had been dead for over two decades, but I felt close to her in Lithuania. I walked through an open-air market. Breads, fruits, and vegetables were on sale in the stalls but in scant amounts, not like the abundance in the markets I frequent in Los Angeles. I saw cakes and cookies, none topped with frosting or chocolate. People didn't appear to be buying very much. I looked at them. They were closer to ideal body weight than one could ever imagine finding on the streets of America. A few of the older people looked overweight, but most were not. Only rarely did I see anyone who was obese. Young mothers pushed strollers with bundled babies. Teenagers clustered near the clothing stands, laughing and joking with each other. All of them were slim and seemed physically fit. Suddenly it struck me that not one person I'd seen in the market was eating. They were not holding sodas, bags of chips, or ice-cream cones.

At the end of my trip, a young Lithuanian physician drove me to the airport. She was tall and slender with curly blond hair; she wore blue eye makeup and bright red lipstick. "Do you think diabetes will come to Lithuania?" she asked.

"I don't know," I responded. "It all depends on how much you become like America."

"But that is our goal," she said. "That's what I hope for."

As we said goodbye at the airport, I wondered if she really understood the risks. And I wondered if there were any way for Lithuania, or any other emerging country, to reap the advantages of development without also reaping diabesity.

PART 3

Engines of Change

ELEVEN

The New Normal

When I first met fourteen-year-old Cami, she was lying on a bed in the emergency room of my hospital. She'd been assigned to one of the cubicles in the ER's observation area. Cami wore a cardiac monitor, and both of her arms were hooked up to IVs. She clutched a small stuffed dog with one hand and her mother's hands with the other. I related to her instantly, knowing what a difficult place she inhabited—that baffling territory between growing up and still being totally dependent on a parent.

I could see that Cami was about 50 pounds overweight. She'd been crying: her eyes were red and slightly swollen; her skin was blotchy, with scattered acne lesions. She wore three earrings in her right earlobe and two in the left. Her brown hair was cut short. The top was streaked blond and spiked up with gel. Despite the trappings of adolescent rebellion, she was appealing. Here was a spirit trying to express itself. Cami's mother, Barbara, was sitting very close to her daughter, holding Cami's hand in both of hers. Barbara was well dressed and attractive, with carefully coifed brown hair. Like her daughter, she was obese.

I knew from the ER resident that Cami and Barbara had been following a low-carbohydrate diet for three weeks—and Cami had tried to take shortcuts. For the past two weeks, without telling her mother, she had taken Lasix, a potent diuretic. This was more evidence of her emerging independence mixed with rebellion. She'd found the pills, an old prescription of Barbara's, in the medicine cabinet. Each night she awakened two to three times to use the bathroom, and she'd vomited nearly every night as well. All this fluid loss—in large part induced by the diuretics—plus her diet had caused an alarming drop in her blood potassium level. Now my ER colleagues were trying to replenish her body with this essential mineral.

Most of us get sufficient potassium from the fruits and vegetables we eat, but Cami's overly restrictive diet had not included adequate amounts of these fresh foods. Potassium, along with sodium, helps regulate water balance in the body, and it plays a critical role in transmitting electrical impulses to the heart and muscles. People with abnormally low potassium levels may experience an irregular heartbeat or even cardiac arrest. Fortunately, that hadn't happened to Cami, though some of the waves on her electrocardiogram (EKG) had flattened. These flattened waves meant that electrical conduction was impaired within her heart. If the situation deteriorated enough, the chambers of her heart might not be able to pump sufficient blood. Not surprisingly, Cami complained of muscle pain and generalized weakness throughout her body; these are neuromuscular consequences of low potassium. I introduced myself as I entered the cubicle. "How do you feel?" I asked Cami. "Are you still weak?"

"I guess so," she said.

"Is it a big effort to lift your arms?" I asked.

"Yeah," she said, sounding miserable. "And now my arms are killing me."

"That's because you're getting potassium," I explained. "Potassium hurts when it is infused into the veins. We could never give you what you need through one IV line. It would be too painful and could injure your veins. That's why you have to have two IVs, so we can spread it out. You'll feel better in about three hours," I promised, then added: "After we fix your potassium, we'll talk about a healthier way for you to lose weight and keep it off."

Over the next few hours in the emergency room, Cami's blood potassium level normalized. The pain and weakness in her face, hands, and feet went away, and her electrocardiogram became normal. Her IVs were disconnected, instantly relieving the pain in her arms that had been caused by the potassium infusions. Cami smiled with relief. She had a wonderful smile, with glistening white teeth.

We offered Cami and Barbara something to eat. "Give us carbs!" Barbara said. Cami asked for toast; Barbara wanted a bagel. They devoured the snacks. "This is the best thing I've ever eaten," Cami said. Before they went home, they promised to make an appointment to see me.

Two weeks later Cami and Barbara came to my office, and I learned more about them. At Cami's fourteen-year-old checkup with her pediatrician, four weeks before she wound up in the emergency room, she weighed 184 pounds. Since she was 5 feet 4 inches tall, her BMI was 32. That's greater than the 95th percentile for a girl of her age on the growth charts developed by the Centers for Disease Control and Prevention (CDC). A normal weight for a fourteen-year-old girl of her height is between 120 and 135 pounds. An adult of Cami's size would have been considered obese, but the CDC prefers not to use that term for children.

The adverse health consequences had been obvious to her physician. Cami had borderline high blood pressure, and her periods, which had started when she was twelve, had stopped the following year. The doctor told Cami and Barbara that the cause was polycystic ovarian syndrome, a hormone disorder that can cause menstrual irregularity, infertility, and other symptoms such as excessive body hair growth. Because of Cami's excess weight, her cells had become insulin-resistant. In response, her body was producing more insulin. High insulin levels had caused her ovaries to overproduce androgens, male hormones. A woman's ovaries normally produce some androgens, but when there's overproduction, the signals between the ovaries and the pituitary gland are interrupted. Those are the signals that trigger the ovaries to release an egg every month.

"Cami, you probably won't have regular periods until you lose weight," the pediatrician had said. He'd turned to Barbara and asked: "Do you want your daughter to be fat like you?" Remembering this question, Barbara's eyes filled with tears. She told me she'd been struggling with her own weight since she was Cami's age, gaining and losing—and then regaining—"hundreds of pounds." She was now thirty-nine years old and had reached her highest weight, 230 pounds, just before they started the low-carbohydrate diet. Since she was 5 feet 5 inches tall, her BMI had been 38.

Cami's pediatrician gave them handouts on dieting and exercise. But Barbara had read dozens of handouts like these and none had ever helped. So she decided they'd try something different, a diet her friends talked about, a diet she'd read articles about in women's magazines. She decided to try carbohydrate restriction.

I asked Cami what she'd been eating before they began the diet, starting with breakfast. "I don't have time for breakfast. That alarm goes off, and I don't hear it. Mom has to come in and get me," she said, with a glance at Barbara. I could see this was part of Cami's routine, a cryptic way to show her mother she still needed her. "By the time she drags me out of bed and I do my hair—"

"Oh, I can see that might take some time," I interrupted, looking at Cami's blond spikes. She ran her fingers over the tips of her hair and smiled a wide, toothy smile. Her hair was her signature, and she seemed proud that I had noticed.

"So I go to school," Cami continued, "and by my first break, I'm starved. I get a candy bar and a soda from the vending machines. Later, me and my friends buy something on the snack line, like juice, fries, and maybe a cookie. Usually we go to Ben and Jerry's for ice cream after school. Then I have dinner at home with my mom."

Barbara looked embarrassed. "Our eating habits are terrible," she admitted. Since her divorce ten years earlier, dinner was mostly take-out from fast food restaurants. "After work, I'm too tired to cook," she said. "I pick up two meals at McDonald's and something at Taco Bell, so Cami has plenty of choice. But then we eat it all." Barbara and Cami acknowledged that they got little exercise beyond walking from the car to school or work, or pushing a cart through the convenience store as they shopped for groceries that all too often included lots of candy and chips. Most evenings, after Cami finished her homework, they sat and watched television together.

We talked about diet and exercise, and I could see that Barbara and Cami felt strongly motivated. They swore off fast food take-out and sweetened sodas; they vowed to take walks instead of turning on the TV. They were scheduled to see a nutritionist after their appointment with me. As they left, Cami said, "Thank you so much, Dr. Kaufman. This is really going to work." I was delighted to hear the determination in her voice. But I wondered if she really understood the immense challenge that lay ahead.

Anyone can go on a diet, change behavior temporarily, and lose weight. Cami and Barbara had done this many times. But then they'd returned to their normal lives. In her normal life, Cami wanted to fix her hair in the morning, so she didn't have time for breakfast. For Barbara, normal life meant being too tired after work to cook dinner or get some exercise. Their normal lives inevitably led them back to candy bars, fast food, and TV. And just as inevitably, the weight they'd lost returned. What Cami and Barbara needed was not merely a new diet but a new normal—a new way of life in which wholesome eating and daily exercise could become their comfortable, natural routine.

THE BALANCE AND THE SEESAW: HOW WE GAIN AND HOW WE LOSE

The laws of thermodynamics apply to us all: for our weight to stay stable, our energy input—the calories we consume—must equal our energy expenditure. If we eat more food than our body burns, we gain weight. Each pound of fat represents an excess of about 3,500 calories. To lose that pound of fat, we must create a caloric deficit. In other words, we must burn 3,500 calories more than we eat.

We expend energy every minute that we're alive, even when we're sleeping. In adults, resting energy expenditure—known as our basal metabolic rate (BMR)—accounts for approximately 10 to 12 calories per pound of body weight per day. Though BMR varies from individual to individual, it works out to about 1,400 calories a day for an average person, just to keep our body running—our heart beating, our lungs breathing, our nerves transmitting, and our gastrointestinal system digesting. On top of that, we burn calories every time we get up and move. Add it all together, and the average adult man has a total daily energy expenditure of about 2,300 calories; the average woman expends only 1,800 to 2,000 calories.

Physically active people burn considerably more. If we add sustained strenuous activity to our lives—the kind of exertion that makes us huff and puff—we might need 3,000 calories or even more in a day. All this energy comes from the food we eat.

Since we don't eat constantly, we rely on stored energy to meet our needs between meals. Our first backup energy source is the glycogen in our liver and muscles. Each of us carries approximately 2 pounds of glycogen, which amounts to 4,000 calories. For each pound of glycogen, the body also stockpiles approximately 2 pounds of water. As our glycogen stores are used up, the associated water is excreted via our urine. This process is accelerated on carbohydrate-restricted diets because the body can't readily replenish its glycogen stores without available carbohydrate. That's why most people see a dramatic drop in weight when they begin a low-carb diet. But they're shedding mostly water and glycogen.

When a person doesn't consume enough calories to match caloric expenditure, and stored glycogen doesn't suffice to make up the difference, the body turns to its fat. As fat is broken down, it releases free fatty acids and compounds that can be made into ketones, which can be used for energy by the nervous system, including the brain. Excess ketones may be expelled in the urine and in the breath, which is why people on calorie-restricted low-carbohydrate diets sometimes develop a fruity smell to their breath. Ketones usually aren't dangerous in a healthy person, though they may decrease appetite and produce fatigue and weakness. However, if a person with type 1 diabetes is untreated or doesn't take sufficient insulin and becomes dehydrated, excess ketones in the blood can produce diabetic ketoacidosis (DKA), a potentially deadly condition.

Insulin plays a key role in regulating our energy stores. After a meal, our insulin levels increase in response to the rise in our blood sugar. The presence of insulin enables our muscles to use this glucose for immediate energy. Any excess is moved into the liver, where it becomes a building block to replenish our glycogen stores. If there's still more glucose beyond what we need to store as glycogen, it's turned into fat. After a meal, the presence of insulin stops the breakdown of fat; thus the body meets its immediate energy needs with the food just eaten.

Insulin also affects the hormones that regulate our appetite, encouraging us to stop eating when we've had enough. Later, when the insulin has been used to move sugar out of the bloodstream, regulatory hormones prompt us to feel hungry again. The human body is equipped with multiple mechanisms designed to keep food intake in balance with our needs. We're supposed to become hungry when we need fuel; our appetite should subside after we've eaten. However, as soaring obesity rates testify, these mechanisms aren't always effective in today's world. For example, it takes at least thirty minutes for the satiety signals to kick in. But a grab-and-go fast food meal lets us overeat before we've given our bodies time to register that we've had enough. Moreover, when food is abundant and tempting, we're spurred to eat beyond our true hunger. This urge is probably built into our Paleolithic genes, since our ancestors needed to take advantage of bountiful food supplies when they were available.

Our body is genetically programmed to reach a set point: once we establish a weight, our body strives to keep it. So when we try to reduce food consumption, various built-in systems thwart us. For example, when we cut caloric intake in the hope of burning stored fat, the hormones that help metabolize the fat also signal a general metabolic slowdown. This protects us from starving to death, which was helpful in our Paleolithic past when the food supply was sometimes poor. But it also makes weight loss more difficult.

DEVOURED BY DIETING

A myriad of dietary plans have been proposed over the decades. Barbara told me she'd tried dozens of them. For example, two years earlier she and Cami had gone on the cabbage soup diet, which permits little food other than a vegetable soup made mostly from cabbage. After a week, each of them had lost about 3 pounds. But they were fed up with cabbage and resumed their previous eating patterns.

"We gained back the 3 pounds we'd lost, plus another 3 pounds," Barbara said. "That was so discouraging."

"The soup was gross," chimed in Cami. "I told you it was a stupid idea, Mom."

After Cami's visit to the pediatrician, Barbara had bought *Dr. Atkins' New Diet Revolution.* According to the book, they'd be able to eat plenty of meat, eggs, chicken, and cheese, so they wouldn't feel deprived. Barbara had explained the diet to Cami. "You can have lots of protein and fat, as long as you don't eat cookies, cakes, candies, breads, pasta, potatoes, or anything else with carbohydrate. I'll get rid of everything we can't have, so it will be easy. We're also supposed to drink at least eight glasses of water and take a multivitamin pill every day."

Cami asked, "What about ice cream?"

"Not on the diet," Barbara answered.

"What about fruit?" Cami wanted to know.

"Not on the diet," Barbara told her.

"Butter?"

"You can cook with it if you want," Barbara replied.

Cami agreed to try the Atkins diet. They decided to start the next day. That evening they devoured everything in the kitchen that contained carbohydrates.

For their breakfast on the first day, Barbara scrambled five eggs for the two of them. She also packed two lunches. Each contained a large chicken breast, two chunks of string cheese, and a hard-boiled egg. To keep everything cold, she added a bottle of water that had been frozen the night before. After Barbara finished packing the lunches, she took a vitamin and mineral pill and left the bottle on the table so that Cami could do the same. But she didn't notice that Cami never took her pill.

That night Barbara served large portions of ham for dinner, along with a small salad of lettuce, raw celery, and cucumbers. They topped the salad with liberal amounts of ranch dressing, which was allowed because it was almost all fat. In the evening Barbara made a meat loaf and roasted a turkey breast so the refrigerator would be filled with cooked meats for meals and snacks. As soon as the meat loaf was done, they each ate a slice.

By bedtime Cami felt slightly nauseated and more tired than usual. Barbara tried to encourage her. "That's probably from the ketones. It must be a sign that you're breaking down fat," she said. For the rest of the week, Barbara continued to cook plenty of meat and poultry. They helped themselves to large portions and snacked on the leftovers through the evening. Barbara took a multivitamin every day, but Cami never did. She didn't remember that was part of the program, and Barbara didn't notice the omission.

Cami always felt nauseated by the end of the day; sometimes her head hurt, too. Both of them were constipated. They felt irritable and slightly lightheaded. Because they'd been drinking so much water, they had to get up in the middle of the night to urinate, which left them tired during the day. At the end of the week, they weighed themselves. Cami had lost only 2½ pounds, and Barbara had lost 3½. Both of them had expected to lose much more. They felt discouraged, though they shouldn't have. Successful dieting is usually slow—1 or 2 pounds per week. Diets that induce rapid weight loss often cannot be sustained. "It's probably water weight because we're drinking so much," Barbara told Cami, trying to make her feel better.

A few hours after the weigh-in, Cami's head began to hurt. She went to the medicine cabinet to get a painkiller. There she found a bottle that Barbara had marked "water pills." In the past, Barbara had tried to augment her weight loss with diuretics, but they'd made her feel sick. Cami was worried about failing and didn't want to disappoint her mother. It occurred to her that the pills might help her lose "water weight" really fast. Without telling Barbara, she decided to take one pill each evening.

After she began taking the diuretic, Cami felt even more nauseated. A couple of times she vomited before going to bed. But in the morning she felt well enough to go to school. Barbara wasn't alarmed by these symptoms; she thought Cami must be breaking down fat and forming ketones. By now, both of them were tired of the limited food selection, so they were eating less. After the second week, they weighed themselves again. Cami had lost 4 more pounds,

Barbara 5 more. Though Cami felt terrible, both of them were encouraged.

During the third week, Cami vomited every night. She hadn't
had a bowel movement in days. Then she began to experience muscle cramps—particularly in her hands and feet—and weakness. She
didn't mention these new problems to Barbara. At the end of week
three, Cami had lost a total of 9 pounds and Barbara had lost 12. But
the morning after their weigh-in, Cami felt so weak that she
couldn't get out of bed. She felt numb around her mouth; her lips
felt like plastic. The cramps and pains in her hands and feet felt like
electric shocks.

Cami was terrified; she thought she was going to die. Finally she
told Barbara about the water pills and about her symptoms. Frantic,
Barbara called Cami's pediatrician, who was appalled. He realized
that Cami's alarming symptoms were probably the result of a dangerously low potassium level, and he told Barbara to take Cami immediately to the nearest emergency room—which is where I met
them.

CARBOHYDRATES COUNT

Cami's experience by itself can't be taken as an indictment of low-
carbohydrate diets. She might have avoided this crisis if she hadn't
decided to use a diuretic and if she'd taken the daily vitamin and
mineral pill suggested in the Atkins book. But is a low-carbohydrate
diet, followed correctly, really more effective than a balanced low-
calorie diet?

Advocates of low-carbohydrate diets say that they work by decreasing the amount of insulin secreted into the bloodstream. The
idea is that with lower insulin levels, there should be less insulin resistance, less fat storage, less glycogen storage, less hunger, and easier weight loss. But opponents argue insulin secretion can be
diminished by any diet that is low enough in calories so that more
energy is burned than is consumed. This is an area of much contro-
versy, with consumers, physicians, and scientists taking sides. I've

read a plethora of articles, listened to this debate among colleagues, and debated with myself. The conclusion that makes the most sense to me is that we don't yet have sufficient scientific evidence to know for sure.

We know that it's important for people with diabetes to account for carbohydrate intake. Since the 1990s, carbohydrate counting has been the key element of nutrition counseling for people with diabetes. They've been told to count how many grams of carbohydrates they consume and to keep track of how it affects their blood sugar; those using insulin adjust their dose according to their carbohydrate consumption. Usually they're also told that it doesn't matter whether these grams come from sugar, pasta, or fruit.

However, some nutritional counselors have argued that carbohydrates are not all the same, because some raise blood sugar more than others. They've turned for guidance to an index, called the glycemic index, that indicates how much a particular food elevates blood sugar. The glycemic index was invented by Dr. David Jenkins and his colleagues at the University of Toronto—the same university where insulin was discovered in 1921. Foods are compared to some standard, usually pure glucose or a slice of white bread. Those foods with a high glycemic index break down quickly and cause blood sugar to rise; those with a low glycemic index break down more slowly and have less effect on blood sugar elevation.

While you might think that it makes sense to avoid foods that score high on the index, it turns out that things aren't quite that simple. First, what are being compared are not normal servings of these foods, but the amounts that yield 50 grams of carbohydrates. This can lead to distortions. For example, carrots have a relatively high glycemic index, but you'd have to eat many servings to consume 50 grams of carbohydrates. Not only is there no harm in eating a normal portion of carrots, there are important nutritional benefits from its fiber and vitamin content.

The glycemic index is determined in the laboratory following a procedure similar to the oral glucose tolerance test I described earlier, which is used to diagnose diabetes. Volunteers fast overnight, then eat a fixed amount of the food being indexed. Their blood is drawn at intervals to track the rise of blood sugar. But few of us eat single foods; most of us eat foods in combination. How quickly blood sugar rises after we eat a particular food depends on what else we've eaten at the same time. If a meal contains more fat and fiber, all of the food will be digested more slowly, and blood sugar will rise more slowly, too.

In most studies done so far, the benefit of carbohydrate restriction seems to be that people consume fewer calories overall. That was certainly the case for Cami and Barbara. During the second week of their diet they lost more weight because they'd become bored with the food and consequently ate less. But with the current proliferation of low-carb treats—everything from muffins to cookies to ice cream—I'm not sure the boredom factor will continue to operate.

The true test of a diet's effectiveness is not whether it works quickly but whether it can be followed successfully in the long term. Highly restrictive fad diets can produce short-term weight loss. But they rarely solve the problem permanently, because people can't stick to them. They begin to crave what they're denied; if restrictions are too severe, they may even suffer adverse effects from loss of important nutrients.

Careful studies of low-carbohydrate diets suggest that they initially achieve more rapid results than conventional low-calorie diets but that this advantage is short-lived. In one such study, reported in the *New England Journal of Medicine* in 2003, doctors at the University of Pennsylvania followed sixty-three obese dieters for a year. Participants were assigned at random to follow either a low-carbohydrate diet or a conventional low-calorie food plan. At the end of six months, volunteers on the low-carbohydrate diet had lost significantly more weight. However, the difference had disappeared by the end of the year.

Many nutritionists and doctors had feared that low-carbohydrate diets would increase cardiovascular risk, because these diets are usually high in fat. However, research suggests that this is not the case. People following these diets do not show increases in blood cholesterol or triglyceride levels; in fact, these risk factors typically are reduced. That's because weight loss—even if it's induced by increasing fat intake—decreases insulin resistance and all of its adverse effects on fat metabolism. If weight loss can be maintained, these benefits are likely to persist. However, if weight gain occurs later on, then cardiovascular risk will likely return.

Humans have been eating fat, protein, and carbohydrate—all three of them—for eons. Carbohydrate is the essential fuel of our bodies. Fiber, one form of carbohydrate, is required for normal digestion. Lack of fiber explains why Cami and Barbara became constipated on their version of the Atkins diet. Fat is essential for cellular function. Protein is the building block of our bodies, which allows us to maintain and rebuild our cells. Our problem is not that we eat all three of these macronutrients, but that we eat too much of all of them.

LOOKING FOR ANSWERS

When patients ask me how to lose weight, they look at me expectantly. Sometimes I think they're hoping I can give them some magical prescription or secret. But all I can offer is the same advice that most of them have heard many times before: to follow a food plan with healthy variety, to eat appropriate portions, and to get physically active. As I recite this familiar formula, I see the disappointment in their faces. They don't want to believe that I have no magic to offer. But the truth is that this familiar advice, unexciting as it might seem, really does work.

If you want to learn about successful weight loss, a good place to start is to ask those who have managed to take weight off and keep it off. That's exactly what Rena Wing at the University of Pittsburgh and James Hill at the University of Colorado did when they set up the National Weight Control Registry. This database includes more than 4,000 people who have maintained a weight loss of at least 30 pounds for at least one year. A study of their participants—who had lost an average of 66 pounds and maintained at least 30 pounds of that loss for an average of five years—found that nearly all of them were successful with a combination of a low-calorie, low-fat diet and physical exercise. Not rocket science, not magic, just the plain and simple truth.

Nevertheless, medical science has long sought a cure for obesity—or at least ways to make weight loss less difficult. The current diabesity epidemic has intensified the search. Though our understanding has increased in the process, the problem has so far eluded safe and effective medical solutions. I've learned to be skeptical when new "breakthroughs" are announced.

For example, in 1994 scientists were excited by the discovery of a hormone they thought would be the holy grail of obesity. This hormone was called leptin, and it is released by fat cells after a meal. Leptin signals the hypothalamus, the part of the brain that controls appetite, that it's time to stop eating. Mice lacking the gene that controls production of leptin become obese. When investigators gave these same mice injections of leptin, their appetites became normal and they lost weight.

This dramatic effect in mice raised hopes of a cure for human obesity. But it turned out that obese people, unlike these obese mice, produce plenty of leptin; the problem is that they're resistant to it. We are not sure why this resistance occurs. Perhaps it was an advantage in ancient times so that when our ancestors had the opportunity to gorge, they would not be inhibited. But that gorging was infrequent and advantageous, since it enabled them to store food to protect themselves from famine. Today, our daily gorging—uninhibited by the leptin signal—is killing us.

Despite the leptin disappointment, pharmaceutical companies continue to search for drugs that can promote weight loss and that can be used for years with a minimum of side effects. But I doubt there's a magic bullet for obesity. The body has so many regulatory pathways that affect weight—pathways that control appetite, metabolism, and gastrointestinal absorption—that it's difficult to imagine how a single drug could have much effect. And if drugs are used in combination, the risk of side effects is increased.

Many drugs are under investigation as potential agents in the weight loss armamentarium, including some medications currently used to treat depression and epilepsy. However, only two prescription drugs are currently approved for weight loss treatment in the United States: sibutramine (trade name Meridia) and orlistat (trade name Xenical). They approach the problem in different ways. Sibutramine is an appetite suppressant that affects chemicals in the brain; orlistat works by reducing the body's ability to absorb dietary fat.

These medications produce only a modest, temporary benefit. On average, they cause a weight loss of 5 to 20 pounds in about six months. After that, weight tends to plateau or to increase again, probably because people develop a tolerance to the drug. Side effects of sibutramine include high blood pressure and irregular heart rate. Orlistat may interfere with the absorption of certain vitamins and can induce unpleasant gastrointestinal side effects, including oily rectal spotting and excess gas.

Yet another medical approach to weight loss—one that's even more drastic than medication—involves gastrointestinal surgery. Operations for obesity were first developed in the 1950s. Doctors had noticed that people lost weight after surgical treatment for cancer or severe ulcers that involved having part of their stomach or intestines removed. Surgeons reasoned that similar procedures could induce weight loss on purpose. These operations came to be called bariatric surgery, because "baros" means "heavy" in Greek.

Some versions of bariatric surgery reduce stomach size; this greatly limits the amount of food that can be eaten at once and may also reduce hunger by altering the stomach's signals to the brain. Other techniques bypass portions of the digestive tract where nutrients are absorbed. These days, most such operations are performed through tiny incisions with the aid of a viewing instrument called a laparoscope. This change and other refinements in surgical techniques have made bariatric surgery safer. Nevertheless, it remains a serious undertaking.

The benefits include significant weight loss—and improved blood sugar control for those with diabetes. But the risks are enormous. Surgery of any kind involves risk, but the dangers are even greater for the obese. An estimated 10 to 20 percent of those who undergo bariatric surgery subsequently require additional surgery to correct problems, such as abdominal hernias. Many patients develop gallstones, a common consequence of rapid weight loss.

Thirty percent become anemic; others suffer from loss of bone mass, setting them up for osteoporosis, or they develop other nutritional deficiencies. Fatal complications are reported at between 0.1 and 2.0 percent.

Despite the risks, there's been a dramatic rise in bariatric surgery performed in the United States over the past decade. In 1991 the National Institutes of Health issued a consensus statement indicating that surgery was an acceptable treatment for obesity in carefully selected patients. At the time about 16,000 procedures were performed each year. In 2003 there were 103,000.

Bariatric surgery costs approximately $20,000 to $50,000; the procedure is sometimes covered by health insurance. Because of the risks as well as the expense, surgery is advised only for people who are severely obese or who suffer serious obesity-related health problems. For the most part, it's restricted to those with a BMI above 40—in other words, those about 100 pounds overweight for men or 80 pounds overweight for women. This degree of excess weight is termed "morbid obesity," because it's almost always associated with medical problems. Surgery is also considered for people with a BMI above 35 if they suffer from significant health difficulties (including diabetes) because of their weight.

UNDER THE KNIFE

We don't yet know if bariatric surgery is a long-term solution for morbid obesity. The National Institutes of Health has established a study group to answer key questions about the risks and benefits. But their results won't be available until 2008, and many potential patients don't want to wait that long. Among them are Hank and his daughter Judi.

I first met Judi—along with her mother, Kathleen, and her father, Hank—when she developed type 2 diabetes at age fourteen. She was 5 feet 6 inches tall and weighed 283 pounds. Her BMI was 45, in the range termed morbid obesity for an adult. Kathleen was overweight, too, but only slightly. However, Hank was even more obese than his daughter. He was one of the largest parents I'd encountered in my practice. I noticed that before he sat down in my office, he surveyed the available chairs and selected one without arms, so that he would fit.

Judi was dressed in jeans and a loose-fitting black sweatshirt, probably chosen to conceal her body. She slouched and her facial expression was sullen; she didn't make eye contact. I could tell she was suffering. Judi told me she hated school, that other kids whispered comments to each other as she walked by. Her diabetes had been discovered after she got sick with the flu. A routine blood test revealed that her blood sugar was 266 mg/dl. To lower it, I prescribed metformin, a medication that increases sensitivity to insulin, and arranged for her to consult a nutritionist about diet and exercise.

A month later, the family returned for a follow-up appointment. Judi had responded well to medication and to the nutritionist's advice about changing her eating habits. She'd lost 5 pounds, and her fasting blood sugar was now 122 mg/dl, which is within the acceptable range for a child with diabetes. I read the results aloud and said, "That's great. Congratulations!" Judi blushed but didn't smile; Hank and Kathleen beamed. Judi was scheduled to see the nutritionist again. As she and her mother rose to leave, Hank asked if he could speak with me for a minute.

"Doc," he began as soon as we were alone, "what can you tell me about bariatric surgery?"

"I've had very little experience with it," I told him. "It's rarely done in children and adolescents."

"I'm not asking for Judi. It's for me. I'm thinking pretty seriously about having the surgery," he told me. "I've tried every diet known to mankind. I've tried all the diet pills. Nothing works, and I don't know what else to do. I want to live to see Judi grow up."

Hank told me that he weighed 350 pounds, nearly 200 pounds above the normal weight for his height of 5 feet 9 inches. His BMI was 51. He'd always been heavy. Eight years earlier, at age thirty-four, he'd developed type 2 diabetes; two years after that, he was diagnosed with congestive heart failure, a condition in which the heart's ability to pump blood is impaired. I wasn't surprised to hear this, since I'd noticed that even the slight exertion of walking from the waiting room to my office left him breathless. It was a struggle for his heart to supply his body with adequate oxygen. His doctor had placed him on a medically supervised fast after his heart failure diagnosis, and he'd lost over 100 pounds. But he quickly regained the weight once he began eating again. Hank struggled to control his blood sugar, but it was nearly always too high and he knew he was at risk for developing additional complications of diabetes.

"You'll need to consider this very carefully," I told him. "There are risks. But being extremely overweight is risky, too."

The next time I saw Judi, three months later, she'd lost another 6 pounds and her fasting blood sugar was down to 116 mg/dl, even better than before. She informed me that her father was in the hospital getting ready to have his gastric bypass. Judi seemed excited. "My dad will be brand-new after his surgery," she said.

"I hope so, but it might take some time," I warned. And it did. During her checkups over the next year Judi kept me informed about Hank's progress. Right after the surgery, Hank lost nearly 25 pounds. Six months later he was down 41 pounds; at nine months it was a total of 60 pounds. That was a lot, but Hank still weighed 290 pounds. His blood sugar was still too high, and he still became breathless with even slight exertion. Meanwhile, Judi continued to lose about 2 pounds per month. She was eating well but was still sedentary. Every time I praised her, she'd say, "My dad's doing a lot better than I am."

About ten months after his operation, Hank had to return to the hospital to fix some of the sutures inside his abdomen. At the end of a year, he'd lost 87 pounds altogether. Finally he could see significant improvements in his diabetes. But walking still left him breathless. Judi, over that same period, had lost a total of 26 pounds, and her diabetes was under excellent control. "I wish I could have that operation," she said. "But my parents say it's not for kids."

A year later, Hank accompanied Judi on one of her appointments with me. While Judi went to the prep room to be weighed and then to the lab to have a blood sample drawn, Hank gave me an update. "The surgery helped, but not enough," he told me. He'd lost weight much more slowly during the second year after his operation, reaching 240 pounds, which was his lowest weight since college. Then, as sometimes happens with bariatric surgery, he stopped losing. His BMI was 35, which was still far from optimal. Though his stomach could hold only a few ounces at a time, Hank confessed that he ate frequently throughout the day. That's why he was unable to lose more weight.

When Judi came back from the lab, she asked to see me alone. Now age seventeen, she was down to 237 pounds, still obese but 46 pounds lighter than she'd been at age fourteen. She had grown another inch, so her BMI was down to 37. I started to say something encouraging, but Judi interrupted me. "Look, this isn't working," she said. "I've lost 46 pounds. Big deal. My dad's lost 110. We're almost the same weight. I really want to have this operation. Everyone asks me when I'm going to do it, but my parents say no way. Could you please, *please* talk to them?"

I felt moved by the despair in her voice, but I could also understand why Hank and Kathleen didn't want her to risk surgery. I tried to explain: "Judi, teenagers are not the same as adults. They're still growing or have just completed the growth process. Their sexual maturation may not be complete, and their hormone levels are different from adults'. We don't know how this operation might affect their development. You have a lifetime ahead of you. We have no data to tell us what gastric surgery might do to your health twenty, forty, or sixty years down the line."

Judi brushed off these concerns. No surprise. Even as I spoke, I knew that a teenager doesn't worry about her seventy-eight-year-old self. I told her about the NIH research that will be finished in 2008. "I'm not going to wait forever!" she wailed.

We continued talking. She sounded more interested when I mentioned that investigators are exploring less invasive surgical approaches, such as a gastric pacemaker that reduces appetite by stimulating receptors in the stomach that signal fullness. Judi was also receptive when I told her that a fitness center in her neighborhood had started a program for overweight teenagers. This was the first time she'd been interested in exercise. She said she'd think about calling the fitness center. We agreed to talk again at her next checkup.

After my appointment with Judi, I went back to my office feeling as if I had just won a skirmish but not the war. I ran into a colleague and told her what had transpired. My colleague—a pediatric gastroenterologist—was adamant about avoiding surgery. She showed me an article from a 2004 issue of *Pediatrics*, in which a group of experts had suggested criteria for performing the surgery in adolescents. "Your patient doesn't meet any of the criteria," she said. "The BMI cutoff is 40, so her BMI is too low. She's lost weight, her diabetes is managed, and she doesn't have any other obesity-related conditions. There's no way she should have this operation." My colleague was right, but it didn't erase from my mind the look of disappointment on Judi's face.

MAINTAINING A HEALTHY WEIGHT

One of the challenges doctors face is figuring out what to tell patients and families about a healthy lifestyle. We need to provide specific recommendations that are relevant to their lives, advice they can actually put into practice. And these suggestions must be simple enough to explain during a brief medical visit, because healthcare providers still need to perform a physical examination, assess mental health, discuss issues such as smoking cessation, consider giving immunizations, and talk about other health issues.

Blue Cross/Blue Shield of Massachusetts came up with a supersimple message that I repeat constantly: 5-2-1 Jump Up and Go. The 5 means "Eat five fruits and vegetables a day." The 2 is shorthand for "Reduce screen time—television, videos, video games, and computers—to no more than two hours a day." And the 1 is a reminder to do one hour or more of moderate-to-vigorous exercise every day.

5-2-1 Jump Up and Go is great advice, but most families struggling with weight problems need more. Even a series of nutrition classes didn't help Randy, an eleven-year-old boy who was referred to me by his pediatrician in 1998 because he was about 80 pounds overweight. Some heavy children enter puberty as early as eleven, but not Randy. He was cherubic, with fair skin and blond curls. He looked like a baby somehow expanded into a bigger body. Randy's intelligence was normal, but he had a learning disability. For a month he and his mother, Vivian, attended weekly nutrition lectures offered by my staff; they took home pamphlets and information sheets. But at Randy's next checkup, a month after his first visit, he hadn't lost any weight.

While I was examining Randy, I asked him how things were going. "Okay," he replied with a sweet smile.

Vivian, who looked like a slim female version of her son, erupted with complaints: "I send him off to school with a healthy lunch. Then I find out from his teacher that he trades it for doughnuts! He won't stop eating. There's no junk in the house anymore, but he overeats on the good foods. He polished off a whole box of cereal the other day—a whole box, all by himself! I tell him over and over what he's supposed to eat, but he just doesn't listen. And forget about exercise!" Randy's smile disappeared. I felt bad for both of them.

Several months earlier, members of my staff at Childrens Hospital and I had realized that we needed to do more to help overweight kids and their parents. We were receiving referrals for weight reduction counseling from the entire L.A. metropolitan area. Our nutritionists and endocrinologists simply didn't have the clinic time for everyone who needed us. And as Randy's experience suggested, our standard classes had dismayingly little impact on those who needed our help most.

"We should have a program, not an appointment," said Marsha Mackenzie, a nutritionist, at one of our staff meetings. She had researched the medical literature to learn about successful weight loss programs for children elsewhere, and she reported her findings: "The programs that work involve the whole family. Most meet weekly for an intensive phase that lasts at least two months, then there's a maintenance phase that meets less often. The most effective programs are hands-on. Activities such as making healthy snacks or playing games seem to be the most engaging and fun."

Over the next few weeks we began to plan a practical program for kids and their families. Our previous classes had taught nutrition basics. In our new program we'd also show them how to navigate grocery stores and read food labels. We wouldn't simply urge them to increase physical activity—we'd get them moving in our weekly sessions to show them that being active was fun. As we talked, the name for the program became obvious to us all: KidsNFitness.

I told Vivian and Randy about KidsNFitness and invited them to join our first session, which was about to begin. Randy was enthusiastic; his mother was skeptical, but she agreed to participate. A total of fourteen children ages eight to seventeen registered. Among them were African Americans, Hispanics, and Caucasians. Half of the parents spoke only Spanish. We weighed each youngster privately before the program began. One boy weighed more than 300 pounds. The lightest was 171 pounds, and he was nine years old.

Our first meeting started with a hands-on nutrition lesson. Marsha had brought about a hundred food models, plastic representations of spaghetti, pizza, hamburgers, fries, mashed potatoes, tacos, fruits, vegetables, butter, milk, cheese, meats, ice cream, and just about every other kind of food you could think of. Nutritionists use these models routinely to teach proper portion size, but most of the youngsters had never seen them before and were fascinated. Marsha led a simple game that required them to identify good food choices. The kids were running around, throwing and catching food models, and chattering away. "Look!" Randy said excitedly, tossing a plastic apple toward the ceiling. "A good food choice!"

Next, Barry Conrad, another staff member, brought the kids downstairs to the biggest conference room in the hospital. The parents remained behind to meet with Sharon Braun, a staff nutritionist, and Mary Halvorson, a Spanish-speaking nurse educator who was also our lead research person. I stood to the side of the room, watching the parents. To my dismay, one mother pulled a bag of fries from Wendy's out of a tote bag. I wasn't sure what to do. In the front of the room, Sharon was explaining principles of nutrition. As she listed which foods to buy and which to start eliminating in their homes, the mother took a fry right out of her mouth, threw it in the bag, crushed the bag in her hands, and dropped it into her tote. Mary and Sharon shared pointers on encouraging children to watch less TV and become more physically active. The best motivator, Mary said, is a parent's good example.

I slipped out of the room and went downstairs, where Barry led the children in warm-up exercises and dances. Everyone participated, laughed, and had fun. These youngsters had never met each other before. But they shared a bond and an understanding. In a world where obesity is stigmatized, it must have been comforting to be in a room where everyone else was of similar size. Half an hour later, drenched with sweat, they rejoined their parents.

The following week, Marsha focused on portion size. This time she'd brought real food, plus a small scale and a plastic bowl for each youngster. "Who likes Cheerios?" she asked.

There was a chorus of "I do!" and "Me!"

Marsha passed around boxes of cereal and asked the kids to read the nutrition label. "Okay," she said after everyone had checked the label, "put one portion of Cheerios into your bowl." Staff members helped the youngsters pour cereal into their bowls. "Now weigh your portion," said Marsha.

There were shouts of astonishment. "Hey, this is four portions!" cried one of the girls. "One portion is *nothing*!"

After the second session, Randy came up to me and said, "A portion is what fits in my palm." I was so excited, I kissed his head and ran my hand through the curly locks surrounding his angelic face.

By the fourth session, Randy had lost a total of 6 pounds. He could actually read a nutrition label, and he was able to keep a food diary. Vivian stood with an arm around her son, smiling proudly. "He packs his own lunch," she said, "and that's what he eats at school. He's been riding his bike more, and every evening he takes the dogs for a walk," she told me.

Since that first group, hundreds of children and teens have gone through the KidsNFitness program at Childrens Hospital. We've had a waiting list since the start. Two hundred and sixty kids were in the initial KidsNFitness program that lasted eight weeks. Based on this experience, we improved the curriculum and lengthened the program to twelve weeks. One hundred and nine kids have participated in the new version, and it seems even more effective. In addition to the sessions at the hospital, we've led KidsNFitness programs in schools in the Los Angeles Unified School District and in our outreach clinics. We've also created specialized sessions for children with diabetes, for youngsters with other medical or genetic conditions that predispose them to obesity, and for those who have already experienced obesity-related illness. Our kids have been filmed for national and local TV shows, and the program has been covered in magazines and newspapers not only in the United States but also around the world.

KidsNFitness is a research program, too. We've gathered reams of data; we've written papers and developed ancillary studies. In 2000, at the annual American Diabetes Association meeting in San Antonio, Texas, we presented our initial analysis of KidsNFitness, based on the first eighty-three participants. Before joining the program, all were overweight and gaining, on average, nearly 3 pounds per month. During the eight weeks of the study, plus the following half year when they attended monthly maintenance sessions, their average weight gain dropped to only ounces per month. Since the children were still growing, that meant that they achieved a lower BMI, an important step in the right direction. Parents and children also increased fruit and vegetable consumption while cutting back on high-fat foods. In 2004 we reported at the annual ADA meeting in Orlando, Florida, that the first group of thirty-five youths who attended our new twelve-week KidsNFitness program had a decrease in BMI and blood pressure and improvement in cholesterol and insulin levels. Our next step is to learn if these benefits can be maintained over the long run.

KidsNFitness worked for Cami and her mother, Barbara. They joined the program a few weeks after Cami's low-potassium symptoms brought her to the Childrens Hospital Los Angeles emergency room. By the time they started, each of them had gained back 2 of the pounds they'd lost on their carbohydrate-restricted diet. After eight weeks in KidsNFitness, Cami lost 10 pounds and Barbara lost 12. Cami lost weight without nausea, fatigue, tingling, and numbness. Both of them felt healthy, energetic, and raring to go.

We're delighted with the results of KidsNFitness, but it's by no means a panacea. The families who participate in this program live in a toxic environment that undermines everything we teach them. The children attend schools that sell unhealthy snacks. They live in neighborhoods where fast food is abundant but fresh fruits and vegetables are difficult to find or prohibitively expensive. In their communities, parks and streets often are not safe places for them to be physically active. When we ask them to make fundamental changes in their lifestyle—to adopt a healthy new normal—we're asking them to swim against the tide of the old normal. Some can make that heroic effort, but it's simply not realistic for most people.

To stop the diabesity epidemic, the new normal must become not just an individual but a societal choice. I think of the world my grandmother Sadie lived in when she was a young mother. In that world, it was normal for people to walk; it was normal to eat fresh homemade food. We can't go back to Sadie's world. In the last three generations, we've changed the landscape of our lives. But we can—and we must—create new ways of living in our world. We need a new normal that will encourage the appropriate food choices and physical activity our bodies need to remain healthy. The new normal must be supported by our schools, our workplaces, our communities, our healthcare system, and our government. The changes won't be easy, but they're within our power. In the next four chapters I'll describe successful programs that are already making a difference.

TWELVE

Who's Responsible?

Erendira was one of the first teens in my practice with type 2 diabetes. I liked her right off the bat; she was one of those wonderful patients with whom it was easy to bond. She had a round face, brown skin, black eyes, and a wide smile. She'd been born in El Salvador to an impoverished young couple. Shortly after her birth, her mother had left El Salvador and come alone to the United States in search of a better life for her family. She'd worked as a housekeeper and babysitter, sending money back to El Salvador every month. Not until twelve years later, when Erendira was thirteen, were they finally able to save enough so that the family could be reunited in Los Angeles. Over the next three years, Erendira's parents had two more children.

Erendira's father found occasional manual labor in wealthy sections of Los Angeles, but his income was unreliable and money was tight. After school Erendira watched her two younger siblings while her mother cleaned other people's houses and babysat other people's children. I related to this: someone else had to watch my children when they were younger because I was caring for other people's children, too.

Erendira's life was difficult, but she was always cheerful, always ready to laugh. She looked as if she were still living in her small village in El Salvador. She wore traditional white blouses with colorful embroidery around the slightly scooped necks, full skirts made of woven fabric, and flat leather sandals. Even in the summer, she covered herself with a poncho. Her long black hair was always twisted in two braids right behind her ears. Silver earrings dangled from both earlobes. Tied around her right wrist—from the first day I met her—was a bracelet of red threads. These threads were to ward off *mal de ojo*, the evil eye.

When I first met Erendira, she was sixteen years old and weighed 180 pounds, far too much for her height of 5 feet 3 inches. She told me that she'd started to gain weight right after she and her father came to this country. Though she'd continued to wear the garments of her village, she no longer ate the healthy staples—fish, beans, fresh vegetables and fruits—of a traditional Central American diet. Her family, despite their poverty, did not go hungry. However, they were nutrition-insecure: the foods they could afford were laden with sugar and fat; fresh fruits and vegetables, lean meats, and fish were out of their reach. Erendira's diet featured cheap Mexican-style fast food, loaded with greasy ground beef and cheese, and leftovers brought home from her mother's housecleaning job, mostly day-old breads and cakes.

Because Erendira had diabetes, she was eligible for California Children's Services (CCS), a medical entitlement program that didn't bother to determine who was born in the United States and who was not. I have been thankful for CCS throughout my career because it has enabled me to care for every child who has diabetes and who is in need. CCS even pays for counseling and nutrition services. After our first meeting, Erendira saw a nutritionist and therapist at Childrens Hospital. They helped her manage her diabetes and her weight, adjust to life in this country, and deal with twelve years of being separated from her mother.

Erendira remained in counseling for one year, and it helped a little. She seemed to gain a better understanding of her family dynamics. But she could never get her diabetes or her weight under optimal control. Erendira faced too many other pressures to be able to do that. She had to help her family survive.

Over the years, Erendira graduated from high school and became a part-time student at Los Angeles City College. She continued to live with her parents. When she wasn't in school, she was caring for her two younger brothers or helping her mother clean and babysit in the fancy houses in Beverly Hills. She outgrew her CCS but was covered by another California entitlement program, MediCal, thanks to the fact she was from war-torn Central America. MediCal enabled me to continue to see her at my hospital. That was good, because neither of us was ready to end our doctor–patient relationship. This is not unusual for me and many of my pediatrician colleagues. We find it difficult to send our patients to an internist or family practitioner after watching them grow up. And many of our patients don't want to be sent away. Erendira was not offended when the receptionist assumed she was a patient's mother rather than the patient herself; she didn't mind sitting in a waiting room with screaming babies and toddlers. I was glad to continue to help her and curious to see first-hand the long-term course of type 2 diabetes that first appeared at an early age.

At age twenty-two Erendira weighed 182 pounds, which was about what she'd weighed at sixteen. But her test results concerned me. Her blood pressure had crept up to 132/88—higher than it had been when she was sixteen, and well above 120/80, which would have been normal for a woman her age. Because her blood sugar control had always been less than optimal, she was at risk for developing diabetes complications. So I was particularly alarmed that her urine test revealed excess protein, an early sign of kidney damage. I explained the findings and said: "Erendira, you must lose weight and get physically active. Your blood pressure and kidney tests aren't normal. I have to repeat these—and if they are still abnormal, I will have to give you pills to lower your blood pressure and protect your kidneys."

"I try," she'd said. "I like to walk, so I've been taking a bus to Griffith Park on the weekends."

"That's excellent," I said. "But it's not enough. You should be walking every day, not just on the weekend."

Erendira sighed. "I don't have time to go to the park during the week. And it's difficult to walk where I live," she said. I knew Erendira lived in a rundown section of downtown L.A., but I thought she was making excuses. Trying to conceal my annoyance, I told her, "Exercise is essential for your health. Once the kidneys fail, they don't recover."

"I could try walking in my neighborhood," she replied hesitantly. "The problem is, it's dangerous and I'm scared. But I guess that if I stick to busy streets, where they have patrol cars, it should be okay." She described a route that would take her past a school and a strip mall.

A month later, I saw Erendira again. She'd been walking every day. As a result, she'd lost 5 pounds. Her blood pressure had improved and her kidney test was now normal. "I feel better, like there's more muscle in my body," she told me as I examined her. "Sometimes I take my little brothers with me. But man, are they slow—they stop like puppies to look at everything. I like it better by myself. I can listen to music and move."

"How have your blood sugars been?" I asked her.

"A lot better," she replied. "I haven't had sugars so close to normal since I first got diabetes. I'm pretty amazed at what this walking has done." I told her that if she kept it up, she wouldn't need blood pressure or kidney medication and that eventually she might even be able to do without one of her diabetes drugs. She left my clinic with a quick and confident stride.

The following week, my name rang out over the hospital loudspeaker: "Dr. Kaufman—ER—stat!" I'm seldom paged that way. "Stat" means "immediately." Stat means catastrophe. I ran down four flights of stairs to the emergency room, my heart pounding. I didn't know what I was running to, but I knew it was going to be terrible. I flew through the ER doors, my mind racing. Which of my hundreds of patients was nearly dead? I found my answer when I looked at the gurney and saw Erendira. Her face was barely recognizable behind a breathing mask. But I immediately recognized the red threads she wore tied around her right wrist to ward off the evil eye.

"My God!" I cried. "What happened?"

"She was shot," the ER resident explained. "Two bullets to the abdomen. She was out walking or something and got caught between two gangs. In broad daylight."

One of the paramedics was pressing hard on her abdomen, trying to control her internal bleeding. He was covered in blood. Two intravenous lines had been placed in Erendira's arms to give her the lifesaving fluids necessary to keep her circulation going; an endotracheal tube was installed in her throat, and a pediatric resident was using the tube to deliver oxygen to her lungs. A MAST suit—a special garment to decrease blood flow to non-vital body parts—had been inflated around her lower legs and abdomen. This would maintain her circulation to the extent possible despite her loss of blood. I had imagined a disaster as I ran down the stairs, but nothing like this: as a result of exercising in her community, Erendira had been shot. Because she'd been walking in her neighborhood to lose weight and stay healthy, Erendira might die.

Four surgeons appeared. Half a dozen nurses ran in and out of the room. A respiratory therapist hovered over Erendira, adjusting the settings of her oxygen tank and assisted-breathing apparatus. More and more equipment was brought in. Bags of blood were hung on the two intravenous lines. I checked Erendira's blood sugar and discovered it was high: 412 mg/dl. One of the nurses helped me prepare an insulin infusion to go into yet another intravenous line. I calculated the infusion rate and projected it would take less than one hour to bring Erendira's blood sugar down to an acceptable level.

I'd made my contribution, but that was all I could do. As I watched my colleagues, all of them working furiously to save Erendira's life, I felt helpless—and I felt guilty. Intellectually, I knew that what had happened wasn't my fault. But I still felt guilty, because I'd encouraged her to exercise, and she'd been shot doing what I'd suggested.

Within minutes, Erendira was on her way to surgery. I checked her blood sugar again as we ran to the operating room. When we arrived, I put on the gown and mask that would allow me admission to the operating theater, and I scrubbed my hands. I kept imagining Erendira walking briskly down the street straight into two bullets. The next minutes would determine whether she would live or die.

They would determine if taking a walk in Erendira's neighborhood was a mortally dangerous activity.

The surgeon opened her up and scanned her abdominal cavity. Carefully he pulled her intestines this way and that to look for puncture wounds and lacerations. "She's lucky," he commented. "I won't need to remove any of her bowel." As I looked at Erendira lying unconscious and bloody on the operating table, I had trouble thinking that she was lucky, even though I knew she was. Lucky meant that she wouldn't lose part of her intestines or stomach, that she wouldn't need to be fed through a gastrostomy tube, or wear a colostomy bag for the rest of her life.

Erendira made it through surgery and through the tenuous postoperative hours. Her injuries were severe and progress was slow. She stayed in the intensive care unit for two weeks and then spent another two months on one of the hospital wards. She couldn't eat for six weeks. During the entire time, Erendira's mother sat by her side, crying and fussing over her and caring for her in the way that only a mother can.

Before Erendira left the hospital, I wanted to apologize to her for being so adamant about the need for her to exercise every day. I sat on the side of her bed, looked her straight in the eyes, and said: "Erendira, I'm so sorry. I still can't believe what you went through, and I feel so badly that it happened because you were trying to get fit and healthy."

"Look at the bright side," she said.

"What bright side?"

"I lost 22 pounds," she said with a chuckle. Her braids, now loose behind her ears, wiggled from side to side. That little laugh made her wince in pain, and she pressed one of her pillows into her abdomen for support. "My walking program worked," she said. "And so did my red threads."

I thought of Erendira recently when I gave a talk for a program called Beyond the Bell, which is run by the Los Angeles Unified School District. I stood on a podium at the Foshay Learning Center, a school in South L.A. that goes from kindergarten to twelfth grade, and talked to fifty or sixty concerned parents and community members about the importance of physical activity and good nutrition.

My message was the usual 5-2-1: Jump Up and Go. Parents need to give their children five fruits and vegetables each day, limit young-sters to two hours per day in front of a screen, and see to it that their children get one hour of moderate to vigorous physical activity daily.

A hand went up. The hand belonged to an articulate African American woman who said, "Doctor, you're up there telling us what we need to do. I'm down here telling you we can't do it. We want to, but we can't. I can't afford to buy fresh vegetables. They cost too much and they rot too soon. I can't go for a walk with my kids if it's after four p.m. It's too dangerous. And those fancy gyms? There just aren't any here."

I felt despair, because she was right. Many of our urban areas present similar problems. A Los Angeles County Health Survey conducted in 1999 and 2000 revealed that 25 percent of all parents with children under age five did not have easy access to a safe park or playground. The figure was even higher for parents living at or below the federal poverty level: 33 percent of those mothers and fa-thers reported that they lived out of range of a safe play area for their children. The same neighborhoods that lack resources for physical activity often don't have supermarkets that sell affordable fresh food. When I sit in my office and tell the parents of one of my patients that they need to help their child lose weight, I may be making recommendations they're unable to follow no matter how hard they try.

AN UNEVEN PLAYING FIELD

Americans are ambivalent about the role society and government should play in fighting obesity, according to a national poll con-ducted in 2003 on behalf of Harvard University's Interfaculty Pro-gram for Health Systems Improvement. About half of the respondents to the Harvard survey said that obesity was a private matter that people needed to deal with on their own. The other half viewed it as a public health problem that society should help solve. Though a majority supported government-funded efforts involving education about how to lose weight, most wanted to leave it at that. Only 35 percent felt that the government should play a major role in fighting obesity; less than half (41 percent) endorsed the idea of placing a special tax on junk food. Interestingly, those surveyed were more willing to accept government intervention on behalf of children, particularly efforts focused on schools, such as requiring healthier school lunches or more physical education.

Governor Mike Huckabee of Arkansas—who lost 105 pounds after being diagnosed with type 2 diabetes—has begun a far-reaching crusade to turn his state, currently one of the unhealthiest in the nation, into one of the healthiest. The campaign, called Healthy Arkansas, is as attentive to the realities of politics as it is to those of public health. Much of the effort is focused on children. For example, the state is weighing and measuring all of its public school students, from kindergarten to twelfth grade. A pilot program is sending a Child Health Report to parents, warning them if their son or daughter is overweight and offering suggestions to improve the situation. To head off concerns about the government intruding into the private lifestyle choices of individuals, Healthy Arkansas emphasizes voluntary efforts. For example, they offer incentives to employers who adopt initiatives such as providing educational programs to their workers. And rather than regulating restaurants, they've proposed a "Healthy Arkansas restaurant" designation that could be displayed by establishments that offer healthy foods on their menus, are smoke-free, and have passed existing state and local sanitation inspections.

Federal, state, and local government agencies struggle to convey information about good health. In 2003 the National Cancer Institute's 5-a-Day program, which encourages Americans to eat five fruits and vegetables every day, had a $1.1 million annual budget. Meanwhile, the food industry spends approximately $25 *billion* a year on advertising to deliver their messages. According to Marion Nestle, author of *Food Politics* and chair of the Department of Nutrition and Food Studies at New York University, $13 billion of that— more than half—is spent in marketing to America's children.

Why so much emphasis on children? It turns out that kids are extremely susceptible to advertising and they have tremendous influence over what foods their parents buy. Instead of spending money trying to persuade skeptical adults, the food industry reaches parents via their naive children. In the process, parental influence is diminished. Moreover, industry experts believe brand loyalty begins as early as age two. If youngsters can be "branded" by a company, their lifetime loyalty is worth many thousands of dollars.

As Nestle points out, advertising presents food as entertainment and fun, making immediate pleasure more important than nutrition and long-term health. Four out of five food ads aimed at children are for sugary cereals, snack foods, candy, soft drinks, and fast food. Only 2 percent of food advertising promotes fruits and vegetables.

Advertising is not limited to TV commercials. Children's toys and books are linked to beverage and food products. For example, Coca-Cola Barbie wears a hat and apron with the Coca-Cola logo; she carries a tray with burgers and Cokes. A McDonald's Food Cart, for children ages three and up, comes with play food items, including burgers, fries, chicken nuggets, and pie. Numerous learn-to-count books aimed at preschoolers feature junk food, among them *Kellogg's Froot Loops! Counting Fun Book* and *The M&M's Brand Counting Book*. For older children, there's *Skittles Riddles Math* and *The Hershey's Milk Chocolate Bar Fractions Book*.

The European Union has developed specific guidelines about TV advertising to children. Sweden has banned all advertising to children under age twelve. In Greece, commercials that could influence children can't be shown until after 10:00 p.m. Companies in these countries are able to make healthy profits nevertheless. It's a disgrace that Americans place such a low value on the health of our children that we allow direct marketing of foods to vulnerable youngsters.

NOBODY NEEDS TO SMOKE; EVERYONE MUST EAT

When I was a teenager, I became convinced—from watching TV commercials and movies with women lighting up cigarettes—that smoking could make you seductive and attractive. I tried cigarettes in high school, but it wasn't until college that I got hooked. Smoke filled the air in my college dorm, and most of my friends smoked. We smoked to look sophisticated; we smoked to relax; we smoked because we thought we'd gain weight if we quit.

I continued smoking when I started medical school. I remember having a cigarette after anatomy lab. Spending time with my cadaver left me feeling tense, so I would light up. And I wasn't alone. Back then, doctors smoked in the doctors' lounge, in the doctors' dining room, and in the changing rooms off the obstetrical suites. The stench of smoke permeated the labor wards. Women in labor inhaled secondhand smoke as they panted with each contraction. Patients and visitors were permitted to smoke in hospitals; cigarettes were on sale in hospital gift shops and vending machines.

In the mid-1970s, when the anti-smoking campaign took off, I stopped smoking, and so did most of my colleagues. These days it's rare to encounter an American doctor who smokes, though it's common in Europe and Asia, where anti-tobacco efforts have been less strenuous. Smoking and tobacco products have been banished from hospitals and from an increasing number of other workplaces and public facilities. All this didn't happen overnight. The battle against tobacco has lasted over thirty years.

Although there are many similarities between the anti-tobacco and anti-diabesity campaigns, there are fundamental differences as well. The most obvious is that no one needs to smoke. Tobacco is the only legal product whose accepted use has no benefits and only liabilities. Therefore, it's easy to ban its use in public spaces, to vilify it, and to portray it as poison. But food is a necessity for all life. It cannot be banned or vilified. Still, we must apply the lessons learned from the successes of the anti-tobacco effort to the prevention of diabesity.

Perhaps the most important strategy used to reduce smoking has been educational efforts making people aware of the ill effects on smokers and on those exposed to passive smoke. We must educate the populace more effectively about the consequences of poor eating and poor fitness. This must be done through multiple venues, such as schools, communities, work sites, and the healthcare system.

All of us eat, and many of us read about nutrition. Nevertheless,

I'm amazed at the information gaps I discover when I speak with the parents of my patients or present public seminars. For example, many people don't really know how to read a food label. Like youngsters in the KidsNFitness program, they usually assume—often incorrectly—that the portion referred to on the label is the same as the portion they've dished or poured out. They don't know how to translate information on calories or grams of sugar into practical guidelines for what they should consume during the day. As a result, they don't comprehend how much sugar they drink. Nor do they realize what they're doing to themselves when they drink a sweetened beverage. They don't know that they're stimulating an insulin spike; they don't understand the connection between all this and insulin resistance and type 2 diabetes.

At my lectures, people are astonished when I show a slide with different sizes of soda and connect the dots. Twelve ounces of sweetened soda equals 150 calories and 37 grams of sugar; 20 ounces equals 250 calories and 62 grams of sugar; 32 ounces equals 400 calories and 100 grams of sugar. This slide bears little resemblance to a Pepsi or Coke ad, showing attractive people having fun with their friends, bonding between generations, and finding romance. But as my audience absorbs the information, they begin to understand what they need to do to improve their health.

We can also use the mass media for education. In his movie *Super Size Me*, Morgan Spurlock—producer, director, and guinea pig—dramatically made points about the health hazards of fast food by documenting changes in his own body over a month in which he consumed nothing but food purchased from McDonald's. Even his doctors were surprised by the disastrous consequences: a weight gain of nearly 30 pounds, elevated blood pressure and blood lipids, loss of energy and sexual potency.

The anti-tobacco campaign changed social norms about the acceptability of smoking. We were exposed to negative images of people who smoke: they were unattractive and wrinkled. Obesity is already stigmatized. Rather than trying to create unappealing images for the couch potato, the junk food consumer, and the soda guzzler, we can create positive messages celebrating the new normal—a lifestyle that includes exercise and healthy eating and drinking. With cigarettes, you can only say no. But with fitness and good nutrition, there's so much you can say yes to.

We've cleaned up the environment concerning cigarettes by tightly regulating cigarette advertising, banning smoking in an increasing number of public spaces, getting rid of convenient cigarette vending machines, and making it difficult for juveniles to buy cigarettes by enforcing age restrictions. In the same way, we must improve our food environment. That means developing junk-food- and soda-free zones in schools and healthcare facilities (something I'll discuss in later chapters) and placing constraints on advertising and marketing.

Taxation made cigarettes more expensive, placing them out of the financial reach of many teens. In many cases these taxes were used to fund anti-smoking efforts and treatment of tobacco-related illnesses. Similarly, we can support programs to combat the diabesity epidemic by taxing products that contribute to it. Currently Arkansas, Missouri, Rhode Island, Tennessee, Virginia, Washington, West Virginia, and the city of Chicago have specific taxes applied to carbonated beverages. Arkansas has the highest tax, with a surcharge of 21 cents per gallon of liquid soft drink and $2 per gallon of soft drink syrup. Revenues from these taxes generate over $40 million per year to support the state's Medicaid health insurance program.

Legislators elsewhere are attempting to introduce similar laws, but it's been an uphill battle. For example, in 1992 California voters passed Proposition 163, which forbids taxation of candy, gum, and other snack foods. This proposition, heavily supported by the food industry and not completely understood by the electorate, was also put on the ballot at a time when most people were unaware of the looming obesity and diabetes epidemics. But a decade later, Proposition 163 thwarted California state senator Deborah Ortiz when she authored a bill that would have imposed a 2-cent surcharge on every can and bottle of soda sold in California. And it denied the citizens of California an estimated $512 million that could have supported programs to promote fitness and good nutrition.

Other legislative efforts throughout the country and in the United States Congress have aimed at increasing healthy food choices and physical activity. Most of these bills focus on reducing childhood obesity by modifying the school environment or by regulating marketing to children, as I pointed out earlier. While it's encouraging to see that state and federal legislative bodies are interested in preventing diabesity in children, that's only part of the solution to this epidemic. The full positive impact of government intervention won't be felt until our legislators realize that adults need similar measures to improve their health.

TAKING FAST FOOD TO COURT

Litigation against the tobacco industry went a long way toward changing tobacco use in this country. Today, veterans of the tobacco wars are retooling their weapons to go into battle against "big food."

In 2002 two obese teenage girls in New York made headlines worldwide by suing McDonald's. Ashley Pelman, age fourteen and 4 feet 10 inches tall, weighed 170 pounds; Jazlyn Bradley, age nineteen and 5 feet 6 inches tall, weighed 270. In the complaint filed by their attorney, Ashley and Jazlyn blamed McDonald's for their excess weight and elevated risk for associated ills, including diabetes, coronary heart disease, and high blood pressure. Ashley had been consuming Happy Meals and Big Macs three to four times a week since age five. Jazlyn was an even more devoted customer. She often started the day with a McDonald's breakfast and returned during school lunch breaks or after school. Typically, she ordered whole meals: a Big Mac, Chicken McNuggets, or a fried fish sandwich, along with fries and a soda or shake. Sometimes she added apple pie or another dessert. Both girls collected the prizes McDonald's advertised to draw children to their restaurants, such as Beanie Babies and Walt Disney glasses.

The lawsuit was widely denounced and ridiculed. The girls and their parents were criticized for poor judgment and lack of self-control. One editorial cartoon showed a fat man on a scale; dismayed by his weight, he was planning to call a lawyer. McDonald's fought back vigorously. Their attorneys argued: "Every responsible person understands what is in products such as hamburgers and fries, as well as the consequence to one's waistline, and potentially to one's health, of excessively eating those foods over a prolonged period of time."

The judge agreed, at least in part. He wrote:

> If a person knows or should know that eating copious orders of supersized McDonald's products is unhealthy and may result in weight gain (and its concomitant problems) because of the high levels of cholesterol, fat, salt and sugar, it is not the place of the law to protect them from their own excesses. Nobody is forced to eat at McDonald's. (Except, perhaps, parents of small children who desire McDonald's food, toy promotions or playgrounds and demand their parents' accompaniment.)

Although the judge dismissed the case early in 2003, his ruling suggested arguments the plaintiffs might make for a more successful outcome and gave them thirty days to amend the lawsuit. Perhaps, he said, the dangers of McDonald's products are not commonly known. If so, the company would have an obligation to warn customers. As an example, he cited Chicken McNuggets, which he described as "a McFrankenstein creation of various elements not utilized by the home cook."

Attorneys for Ashley and Jazlyn filed an amended complaint. Among other additions, it included the chemical-laden ingredients list for Chicken McNuggets and revealed that one serving contained three times as much fat as a hamburger. The amended complaint also documented that comprehensive nutritional information about McDonald's products was not readily available to consumers at their stores. Unfortunately, this complaint was dismissed, too.

Despite the failure of this lawsuit—not only in the court of law but also in the court of public opinion—I believe it delivered an important message: the food industry is potentially culpable for the kinds of foods they sell and how they market their products, especially to our children. We hold the tobacco industry responsible for knowingly manufacturing and promoting a harmful, addictive substance. Why shouldn't we do the same for the food industry? After all, they entice our taste buds by adding unnecessary fat, sugar, and

salt to our food without regard for our health and without adequately informing most consumers. They try to capture our children from an early age with advertisements on children's television
programs, with the toys they package with their meals, and with the
playgrounds available at their stores. And they don't think about nutrition if it interferes with profits.

The parallels don't end here. High-calorie, high-fat foods may
in fact be addictive for some people. Certain foods that are high in
fat and carbohydrate, such as chocolate, appear to trigger the creation of opioids in our brain. These opioids make a person feel calm
or happy; they also produce a desire to overeat. One study found
that blocking the effects of opioids decreased food intake by 21 percent in people of normal weight and by 33 percent in those who
were overweight. Conversely, the same study found that eating
high-fat, high-calorie foods increases food intake.

The food industry recognizes that litigation is a major threat. In
2003 their lobbyists and political supporters persuaded members of
the United States Congress to introduce legislation to protect them.
The bill, H.R. 339, bars consumers from bringing obesity-related
lawsuits against restaurants and food manufacturers. At this writing,
it has passed the House of Representatives and is headed for the
Senate. The bill is called the Personal Responsibility in Food Consumption Act. The name was designed to distract us from the fact
that it makes the food industry immune from litigation and culpability. Passage of this bill would deprive all of us of an effective way
to press for positive change to combat diabesity.

Apparently in response to Ashley and Jazlyn's lawsuit, as well as
to increasing public concern about obesity, McDonald's and other
fast food chains have made changes in their menus. These are very
small steps, but at least they're in the right direction. McDonald's is
phasing out supersize fries and sodas, though they haven't yet revealed how small their serving sizes will go. Unless there's a significant reduction, the elimination of just one excessively large size is an
empty gesture. At the moment, a 21-ounce sweetened soda, containing over 200 empty calories, is termed "medium" at McDonald's.

In one constructive 2004 promotion, McDonald's sold adult
Happy Meals consisting of a salad, a bottle of water, and a pedome-

ter with an instruction booklet encouraging walking. A new Happy Meal for kids presents the options of apple juice or low-fat milk (plain or chocolate) instead of soda, and includes apple slices instead of fries. But the apple slices come with a caramel dipping sauce.

Burger King, Carl's Jr., McDonald's, and other fast food restaurants now offer sandwiches without the bun. But the fat and its calories are still there because the same fillings—many high in saturated fat—are placed on lettuce instead of a bun. Nutritional information is becoming easier to find for customers interested in ordering meals that are lower in fat, calories, and carbohydrates. Though these improvements are welcome, much more is needed.

Yes, individuals and families must change their behavior if we are to turn around the diabesity epidemic. But they cannot do it on their own. Reversing the trends of physical inactivity and unhealthy eating will require coordinated efforts from local, state, and national governments, public and private industry, community and religious organizations, schools, and the healthcare system. We must provide information; we must change social norms. Most of all, we must create an environment that supports healthy lifestyles. In this environment, Erendira will be able to take a safe walk outside her front door; employers will expect workers to take exercise breaks; school and workplace cafeterias will ban junk food and serve wholesome meals and snacks; if kids turn on the TV, they will be bombarded by messages to eat fruits, vegetables, and whole grains. Only when all of us have this kind of support will we truly have the freedom to make the right choices.

Reading, Writing, and Diabesity

About ten years ago, sixteen-year-old Lewis, a husky teenager who lived in my neighborhood, mentioned that he drank a six-pack of Mountain Dew every day. I was concerned to hear this. Not only was he consuming many empty calories, he was also creating a pattern that might lead to drinking a six-pack of beer every day. And I was puzzled, too. I knew that Lewis, who was on his high school's junior varsity football team, arrived at school early in the morning; he left late in the afternoon, after practice. How did he manage to drink six cans of soda in the remaining hours of the day?

I was so curious that I asked him. His answer floored me: Lewis consumed most of that soda at school. Until then, it had never occurred to me that a child would drink soda during school. But Lewis purchased five cans of Mountain Dew from school vending machines every day. He bought soda before his first class, after second period, and just before lunch. Before football practice he downed a fourth can, and he topped it off with a fifth soda when practice was over. That left one for home.

By now I'm no longer surprised by what children buy at school, though I'm just as dismayed. When I take dietary histories from youngsters with weight problems, I often learn that they've made poor food choices throughout the day. But it's especially discouraging that some of the really bad choices involve foods sold to them by their schools.

When I went to school, in the 1950s and 1960s, food and beverages were not allowed anywhere but in the lunchroom at lunchtime. Until two or three decades ago, schoolchildren ate either a homemade lunch or a lunch prepared by food service workers under the National School Lunch Program (NSLP) of the United States Department of Agriculture (USDA). Lunch was fresh and healthy, appropriate in size, and washed down with milk. Daily physical activity was part of the curriculum, and it was safe to ride a bike or walk to school. But that's no longer true.

To understand how schools contribute to the rising rates of obesity and type 2 diabetes, visit elementary, middle, and secondary schools in any city across the country. To appreciate the real impact, go to schools in impoverished neighborhoods—the areas where diabesity has struck hardest. If you believe that one of schools' educational roles is to model and promote healthy behavior, you'll be astonished and disappointed by what you see.

In theory, youngsters should be able to eat healthy meals at school. But in practice, too much food is available—and a great deal of it is anything but wholesome and appropriate. Under NSLP and the Department of Agriculture's breakfast program, youngsters can still buy a breakfast and lunch that follow federal nutrition guidelines. However, schools also sell foods that don't meet these standards. "Competitive foods"—so called because they compete with USDA meals—are sold on the snack line of the cafeteria, by the school store, and in vending machines. Under USDA regulations, the sale of competitive foods with minimal nutritional value (basically, candy and soda) is prohibited in the food service areas during the school meal periods. But not all schools comply with this rule; moreover, candy and soda usually are available in nearby vending machines. Efforts to change the situation often meet with resistance, because our schools profit from sales of the unhealthy foods and beverages they're dishing out to students.

The nation's schools are facing budget crises and overcrowding; they're struggling to address the fundamental needs of at-risk children—all the while straining to improve academic tests scores as outlined in the No Child Left Behind Act of 2001. At a time when physical education programs and other enrichment programs are being cut for lack of money, food sales have become an important source of revenue. In the School Health Policies and Programs Study 2000, conducted by the Centers for Disease Control and Prevention (CDC), 82 percent of schools reported that clubs, sports teams, or the PTA sold food to augment the program budget. School administrators and school boards have been forced to make compromises. They've compromised on nutrition; they've compromised on physical activity and physical education. But to fight the childhood diabesity epidemic, schools must stop compromising in these areas.

THE NATIONAL SCHOOL LUNCH PROGRAM, THEN AND NOW

The National School Lunch Program is one of the federal government's great triumphs. World War II revealed that malnutrition was widespread in the United States; many men were rejected for military service because they were underweight. After the war, in 1946, President Truman started the NSLP to combat the problem. Advocates for the poor had long urged that schools provide food for needy students. Hungry youngsters couldn't learn properly, they argued. As a result, school lunch programs were already in place in many cities and states. But under NSLP they proliferated. In 1946, when the program was established, 7.1 million schoolchildren participated. During the 2002–2003 school year more than 27.8 million children received meals.

The NSLP provides public and nonprofit schools with donated commodities from the USDA as well as cash subsidies for each meal they serve. These meals must meet certain requirements: they must provide one-third of the recommended dietary allowances of calories, protein, iron, calcium, and vitamins A and C. Caloric requirements for lunch are 517 calories for preschool children, 664 calories for youngsters in kindergarten through sixth grade, and 825 calories for middle and high school students. No more than 30 percent of those calories may come from fat, and less than 10 percent may come from saturated fat. Any child may purchase the lunch. But children from poor families receive their lunch free or at a reduced price, depending on need.

Over the years, the NSLP expanded to add breakfast. The breakfast program, called the School Breakfast Program (SBP), is smaller because many schools lack the personnel needed to prepare the meal, serve it, supervise the youngsters, and clean up afterward. But on a typical day during the 2002–2003 school year, 8.2 million children in more than 76,000 schools and institutions participated in the SBP. Of these children, 79 percent received free or reduced-price breakfasts.

Unfortunately, the positive role of the NSLP has been compromised by all the other food that schools now make available to students. According to the CDC's School Health Policies and Program Study 2000, 43 percent of elementary schools, 74 percent of middle and junior high schools, and 98 percent of senior high schools sell food and beverages via snack lines, vending machines, and the school store. Typically these offer less-than-optimal food choices.

The snack line is usually placed in the school cafeteria. It provides easy-to-grab items that allow students to move rapidly through the lunch area. This is particularly helpful in crowded schools, where students may have as little as twenty minutes for lunch. A typical snack line menu includes chips, fries, sandwiches, hot dogs, pizza, cookies, and cakes. Candy and sodas aren't supposed to be sold during meals, but they often are; they're also available at other times during the day. According to the CDC, 20 percent of schools offer brand-name fast food items from chains such as Pizza Hut, Taco Bell, and KFC. Profits from the snack line usually remain with the school's food service department.

Vending machines offer beverages—sweetened sodas, juices, sports drinks, milk, and water—as well as chips, cookies, and candies. The machines also promote: nearly all of them carry large and colorful advertisements for the junk food they sell. Schools share in vending machine profits, and they receive bonus payments when vending contracts are signed. As I'll explain shortly, these revenues can be substantial.

Few of the snacks dispensed by vending machines meet federal nutritional guidelines, and many of them are poor food choices for youth. For instance, a typical cookie offering is a 2-ounce package of Oreos containing six cookies—what Nabisco describes as a single serving—with a total of 270 calories and 12 percent saturated fat; 40 percent of the weight of the cookies is sugar. For the average middle school student, who is thirteen years old and who should consume an average of 2,300 calories a day, this is about 12 percent of the daily calorie allotment with very little nutritive value. If a youngster presses the button for a bag of chips or a candy bar instead, the empty calorie count may be even higher. Similar snack foods and drinks are sold in school stores, along with notebooks and pencils. These stores are often under the purview of the student council or a parent organization such as the PTA, which uses the profits for school programs or to support itself.

There's no doubt in my mind that these readily available unhealthy choices are displacing the healthy ones and contributing to the diabesity epidemic. In one telling study, investigators from Baylor College of Medicine in Houston, Texas, recruited nearly 600 fourth and fifth graders to complete lunch food records over a two-year period. During the first year, the fourth graders were in elementary school, where snack lines were not available. But in the second year, these same students graduated to middle school, where they had access to a snack bar. The change had a significant effect on what they ate for lunch. Once they entered middle school, their consumption of fruit and non-fried vegetables dropped, and they drank less milk. Instead, they ate 68 percent more fried vegetables (usually potatoes), and their consumption of sweetened beverages increased by 62 percent. Many states are trying to regain control by instituting standards for the sale of competitive foods. One example is the California Pupil Nutrition, Health and Achievement Act of 2001, locally known as Senate Bill 19. This legislation, authored by state senator Marta Escutia, was designed to ban high-sugar, high-fat snack foods altogether in elementary schools and to limit student access to these products until after the lunch period in middle schools. Fearing that the schools themselves might resist the ban because of lost sales revenue, the state of California offered to offset these losses by increasing the state subsidy of meals served in public schools by 10 cents per meal.

The problem of competitive foods is one of quantity as well as quality. Because food is now so abundant at school, often available throughout the day in multiple locations, youngsters can easily consume many more calories during the school day than they did in the past—and many more than they need. As a result, the caloric guidelines established by the USDA, which once made sense, now contribute to excess consumption.

For Henry, a twelve-year-old in the KidsNFitness program at my hospital, an SBP breakfast plus an NSLP lunch added up to too much food. Henry was referred to our program by his pediatrician because of his weight. He was 5 feet 1 inch tall and weighed 230 pounds, giving him a BMI of 44. Henry's father was African American; his mother was Caucasian. Both were heavy. Henry had mocha-colored skin and curly black hair; his eyes were hazel, with a hint of green. Henry came to the weekly KidsNFitness sessions with his maternal grandmother, who lived with Henry's family. She was spry, opinionated, and loving—and the only slim person in Henry's household.

Before we could work with Henry and his grandmother on principles of nutrition, we needed a dietary history to find out what he was currently eating. Henry laughed when we asked him about the details of his meals and snacks. "Why would you want to be knowin' all that?" he asked.

We learned that he drank a tall glass of whole milk shortly after he woke up (200 calories). He ate breakfast at school (250 calories). Since he became hungry in the middle of the morning, he brought a snack from home, usually a bag of Cheetos or potato chips (240 calories). Henry ate the NSLP lunch (664 calories). When he came home from school, he had a big snack—an amount that would have been a large lunch for most twelve-year-olds. His after-school snacks varied, but his favorite was a can of Chef Boyardee over-stuffed beef ravioli (560 calories) and a glass of orange juice (120

calories). Dinner was usually fast food take-out, including soda
(likely adding up to over 600 calories in food plus 200 in sweetened
soda). His typical bedtime snack was two pieces of toast with butter
and a generous amount of grape jelly (about 300 calories). Including
occasional candy bars and other snacks, we estimated that Henry
was consuming nearly 3,000 calories a day. An active boy of twelve
should have been eating about 2,200 calories—and Henry, who was
out of shape as well as overweight, wasn't very active.

We presented the numbers to Henry and his grandmother.
"Henry," I began, "when we add up all the calories you eat in a day,
it comes to eight hundred more than you need. That's the equivalent of a whole dinner."

"Goodness gracious!" said his grandmother, clearly surprised
and distressed.

"Henry, what do you think about that?" I asked. I wanted to involve him in problem solving.

"I guess that's a real lot," he answered slowly. Out of the corner
of my eye I saw his grandmother preparing to comment, but I sig-
naled her to be quiet and let Henry continue.

"What do you think would be the best way to start cutting
back?" I asked, looking directly at Henry and smiling to encourage
him.

"The candy and soda?" he said.

"Hey, you're some smart guy," I said. "You picked exactly the
best things to start with. So how do you think you can do that?" I
wanted him to be concrete.

"I'll stop drinking soda at home. And I could have candy—just
one piece—only on the weekend."

With that, we had the beginning of a plan.

During the first week, Henry made excellent progress. He gave
up soda and brought a bottle of water to school; he had only one
bite-size Hershey's chocolate on the weekend. Each week during
the KidsNFitness program, Henry set more goals, and the following
week he returned with his food log and reported that he'd met his
goals. KidsNFitness taught Henry and his grandmother about
proper portion size. Henry learned to stop himself and look at the
clock if he wanted seconds; if he still wanted more after half an hour,

he took another small portion. But to Henry's surprise, he often wasn't hungry then or he simply forgot about it.

By the fifth session he had made major alterations. For his morning snack, he substituted baked chips for fried ones. As his afternoon snack, instead of ravioli, he ate a turkey sandwich on one piece of bread. Henry's parents—at the insistence of his grandmother—began buying healthier take-out, such as rotisserie chicken and salad. As a result of all these changes, Henry had lost 4 pounds. This was acceptable as far as we were concerned, but Henry was disappointed and so was his grandmother. "I thought you said I could lose 2 pounds a week," Henry told me.

"Well, if you cut out your midmorning snack, you'd lose more quickly," I said.

Henry shook his head. "I'd get hungry if I did that. Everyone else has a snack then."

Together with Barry Conrad, the nutritionist in my center, we went through Henry's food diary. His school breakfast and lunch added up to over 900 calories each day. These meals included french fries, fried chicken strips, hot dogs, cookies, cupcakes, fried eggs, bacon, and biscuits. Henry thought the school meals were great. "There's soooo much food," he said with a big smile on his face. "I'm so stuffed after lunch, I can hardly move."

Barry suggested that Henry split each item on his breakfast and lunch trays into three parts. He was to eat only two-thirds and put one-third in the garbage can. His grandmother said, "Now that's a shame, that's a real shame. Someone who's hungry would like that food."

Henry wasn't enthusiastic, either. But he agreed to try it for a week. For one week Henry threw a third of the federally subsidized breakfast and lunch into the garbage bin at school. He did that even though he would have liked to eat the whole portion. At the next KidsNFitness meeting, he'd lost 2 pounds. We were delighted, and Henry was triumphant. "I'm king of the thirds!" he told Barry. He now knew what was an appropriate portion size for breakfast and lunch—and that was what he ate, even if it meant he had to throw good food away.

The NSLP provides a potentially sound foundation for healthy nutrition in schools. But the program needs improvement at both the federal and school levels. Although a small percentage of children still suffer from hunger, there are many more children who get sufficient—and in many cases too many—calories but insufficient nutrition. Their calories come from sugar and fat and processed foods, not from fresh foods replete in vitamins, minerals, and fiber. And as Henry's case illustrates, the required calorie counts of the NSLP meals are now too high in light of other foods typically eaten at school, as well as the epidemic of childhood obesity.

The NSLP nutritional guidelines currently apply to all the meals served over a week, rather than to individual menus or specific items. Most of the calories, sodium, and fat come from the entrées; some popular entrées, such as pizza and burritos, are particularly high in all three. These entrées are allowed on the menu because they're balanced by other low-calorie, low-fat items such as a salad or vegetable. But many youngsters simply discard the salad and vegetable, and wind up eating a high-fat meal that consists of an entrée, beverage, and dessert. When the food service assesses its compliance with federal guidelines, it considers only what's offered. But what really counts is what children actually eat.

Food service workers want to offer healthy meals, and they want the kids to eat their meals. But as they can tell you, children often choose the less healthy items. If the food service takes them off the menu altogether, they won't be able to balance their budgets because sales will drop. And more kids will eat from the snack line or vending machines, where the options are even worse. For nutritious items to win favor, children need to learn about good food choices and adults have to model healthy behavior. Also, competitive foods must become healthier.

School services receive compensation from the USDA for each meal they serve; they also get full or partial payment from students not entitled to a free lunch. Nevertheless, to balance their budgets, they count upon foods purchased and donated by the USDA. The most popular USDA-donated foods are cuts of beef, pork, chicken, and turkey that are often high in fat. Despite the USDA's recommendation that schools "ensure financial decisions do not undermine nutrition goals," school cafeterias generally must rely on these subsidized high-fat foods. Fruit, which is not generally subsidized, is offered for only 58 percent of meals in the NSLP.

Change is also needed at the school level. Children who receive free or reduced-price lunches in the NSLP are often stigmatized and teased by their peers. Though federal law requires that children receiving subsidies should not be differentiated, some schools violate these laws and have separate lines for those receiving free lunch. I have seen teachers, food service workers, and school administrators point to the NSLP line and say, "That's for the poor kids." It's easy to understand that students might be embarrassed to stand on such a line. But when children don't buy the NSLP lunch, all that's left—unless they bring lunch from home—are the relatively unhealthy options from the snack line, vending machines, and school store.

Another problem is that schools often serve lunch at inappropriate times. Because of overcrowding, over a quarter of schools begin serving lunch before 11:00 a.m.—and nearly 5 percent start before 10:30 a.m. In about 13 percent of schools, a child may not get to eat lunch until 1:00 p.m., and more than 2 percent keep stomachs growling until after 1:30 p.m. Youngsters expected to eat lunch too soon after breakfast may opt for a snack instead, which means they'll probably hit the vending machines or snack lines later. Children forced to wait until they're extremely hungry will have a tendency to overeat, or they'll grab a quick snack before lunch.

SELLING SODA TO STUDENTS

Our Paleolithic genes never conceived that one day we would consume large quantities of sodas—beverages that contain water plus sugar, caffeine, salt, and chemicals. Other than the water, sodas offer nothing healthy. Sodas ruin kids' teeth and interfere with bone mineral deposition. Particularly if they're caffeinated, sodas affect children's behavior and their ability to pay attention in class. And sodas help make kids fat. There's absolutely no reason to push sodas on kids during the school day or at any other time. Yet sodas are not merely sold on school campuses, they're promoted. Banners with the brand names appear on the walls in school hallways and on the athletic field scoreboard. Schools bind themselves to beverage companies with exclusive contracts.

In an influential report titled *Liquid Candy*, the Center for Science in the Public Interest (CSPI) documented the increasing consumption of soda by America's children. Youngsters start drinking soda at a remarkably young age. One-fifth of one- and two-year-old children consume soft drinks. These soda-drinking toddlers swallow an average of 7 ounces—nearly a full cup—per day. Almost half of all children between ages six and eleven drink soda daily, with the average drinker consuming 15 ounces per day. In part because soda is now available in middle school and high school, consumption increases through young adulthood. Teenagers drink much more soda now than in the past. From 1977 to 1996, soda consumption by teens jumped by 75 percent for boys and 40 percent for girls. Sixty-five percent of adolescent girls and 74 percent of adolescent boys consume sodas daily. One-third of teenage boys drink three or more cans of soda every day. Teens now drink twice as much soda as milk.

Sodas are the leading source of added sugars in children's diets. Teenage girls consume an average of 36.2 grams of sugar per day from soft drinks—about 140 empty calories a day. Teenage boys consume 57.7 grams on average, which amounts to 223 calories. That's nearly one can of soda per day for girls and one and a half cans for boys. The extra calories are sufficient to cause weight gain—and mounting research evidence suggests that soda consumption is indeed a factor in childhood obesity.

A 2001 study of sixth- and seventh-grade children in Boston, published in *The Lancet*, found that the odds of becoming obese increased by 60 percent for each 12-ounce can of sweetened soda consumed daily. In a 2004 report in the *British Medical Journal*, another team of investigators documented the benefits of a school-based "ditch the fizz" campaign. Fifteen classes in six English primary schools participated in a four-session program designed to reduce soda consumption. They received nutrition instruction and engaged in related motivational activities, such as songwriting and observing a tooth dissolve when it was immersed in cola. Youngsters in fourteen other classes simply followed the usual curriculum, serving as a control group. The results: a year later, soda consumption had decreased in youngsters exposed to the "ditch the fizz" curriculum, and their incidence of overweight and obesity had decreased as well. But soda consumption, along with obesity and overweight, increased in the control group.

Soft drink companies are eager to sell their products in schools. They receive much more than the profits from current sales; they also "brand" our children and make them customers for life. Because these sales and advertising opportunities are so valuable, companies dangle large financial incentives before school boards and administrators. In exchange for the exclusive right to sell drinks at a school or in a school system, they offer substantial up-front payments, commissions, and other inducements such as scholarship funds. The money may go directly to the school, or it can go to a school district, which distributes it to the schools according to some predetermined formula. Specific amounts depend upon the size of the school or school system and their negotiating skills. But here's just one example, from an article in *Beverage World*, a trade publication for the U.S. beverage industry: the second largest public school system in Virginia, Virginia Beach, signed a five-year $7 million contract with Pepsi in 2001. That $7 million doesn't include commissions. In the 2002–2003 academic year, vending machine commissions brought another $786,000 to the Virginia Beach schools.

The money is particularly tempting for schools and districts facing budget crises. Because their budgets may become dependent on soda sales, schools can turn into accomplices in encouraging soda consumption during the school day and at after-school activities. They may fail to comply with federal restrictions designed to limit soda consumption. Or they may be slow to fix their antiquated, non-functioning water fountains.

What do the revenues from soda sales support? In a 2001 survey by the National Association of Secondary School Principals, 90 percent of the principals reported that they need business partnerships to supplement their budgets. The survey showed that 66 percent of schools used the money to purchase sports and physical education equipment, with lesser amounts going to other student activities such as arts programs and computers.

THE BAN HEARD ROUND THE WORLD

I'd been appalled for years that schools were making it possible for children to drink large quantities of sugar- and chemical-laden colored water. So in 2002 I was delighted to join a coalition working to ban the sale of soda in the Los Angeles Unified School District (LAUSD). The group, led by Harold Goldstein of the California Center for Public Health Advocacy, included health educators, concerned students, the American Diabetes Association, the Los Angeles County Department of Health Services Nutrition Program, and nearly a dozen other advocacy organizations. We also had a champion on the LAUSD school board, Marlene Canter. Together, we decided the time was ripe for a ban of soda sales in the Los Angeles public schools. Many people had become worried about the diabesity epidemic in our youth, and sweetened soda was implicated as a major contributing factor.

Marlene crafted the Healthy Beverage Resolution and enlisted the support of two other school board members as co-sponsors. The resolution began:

> Whereas, the Los Angeles Unified School District has a strong interest and obligation in promoting the health of children, which leads to better attendance, improved behavior, lower incidence of illness, and increased attention, creativity and academic achievement,

and cited alarming statistics about the increase in obesity. Our proposed law followed:

> Resolved, that effective January 2004, the only beverages authorized for sale at the Los Angeles Unified School District before, during and until one half hour after the end of the school day at all sites accessible to students shall be: fruit based drinks that are composed of no less than 50 percent fruit juices and have no added sweeteners; drinking water; milk, including but not limited to, chocolate milk, soy milk, rice milk, and other similar dairy or nondairy milk; and electrolyte replacement bev-

erages and vitamin water that do not contain more than 42 grams of added sweetener per 20 ounce serving.

After the ban had been in place for six months, there would be an audit of sales and a general assessment of the financial impact on the district. I had concerns about promoting the sale of juice—another beverage high in sugar, though without the chemicals. But there was strong support in the coalition for allowing juice, and this resolution was an important step in the right direction, so I capitulated.

The school board held a public hearing on August 27, 2002, to consider the resolution. The hearing was held at the Downtown Business Magnet High School in Los Angeles. When I arrived, the streets in front of the school were packed with reporters from TV and radio. They were interviewing Harold, the coalition leader; Marlene, from the school board; and some of our student support-ers. I could hear reporters speaking in English, Spanish, and even Japanese. If a school district as large as the LAUSD, with over 700,000 students, banned the sale of sodas, it would be big news not only in L.A. and California but throughout the United States and around the world.

A makeshift auditorium had been set up in the school cafeteria. Even with extra rows of folding chairs, there was standing room only. Over a hundred people were packed into the room. Facing them, along a large table, were LAUSD Superintendent Roy Romer, the seven members of the LAUSD school board, and their various assistants. Off to the right was a podium with a microphone for the speakers. A news cameraman stood ready to take pictures. I sat next to colleagues from the Department of Public Health. A few seats away were reporters with big boom microphones. My col-leagues and I didn't dare whisper to each other for fear of being broadcast to the world.

Marlene Canter, author of the resolution, spoke first. She told her fellow board members and the audience that by allowing the sale of sodas in schools, the LAUSD was contributing to obesity and poor health among its students. Therefore, she was proposing a complete ban on sales of all sodas sweetened with sugar or artificial sweeteners; though artificially sweetened sodas might be free of calories, they contained potentially harmful chemicals. A grant funded via the California Department of Education would help schools make the transition. There was wild applause from the audience.

The next speaker was Zev Yaroslavsky, a member of the Los Angeles County Board of Supervisors, the governing body of the county. Supervisor Yaroslavsky had developed type 2 diabetes one year earlier. To control his disease, he'd lost weight through a program of exercise and improved diet. He spoke passionately and eloquently, citing the school board's responsibility to the children of Los Angeles County. He described his own struggles with diabetes. Banning soda, he said, would help people avoid getting diabetes in the first place. The audience responded with a loud clamor of approval.

Then it was my turn. I walked to the podium as if I were going onto a battlefield to wage war. Looking directly at the school board members, I began:

> As a pediatric endocrinologist at Childrens Hospital Los Angeles, my practice has been inundated by children and youth with a new disease: type 2 diabetes, or adult diabetes. This disease is now occurring in children. Diabetes is a killer; diabetes will markedly deteriorate the quality of life of the children it affects and could shorten their lives by twenty or more years. Diabetes is occurring in children and youth because of the epidemic of childhood obesity. Sixteen percent of our children and youth are overweight, 35 percent of our youth of African American and Mexican American descent are overweight. These are the children who are in the Los Angeles Unified School District.
>
> What has made these children obese? It's a combination of genetic and environmental factors. We have no control over the genetic factors, but you, the board members of LAUSD, have control over one of the environmental factors. You have control over what is sold to children in school and you can either decide to contribute to this grave health problem—or today you can be the first to stand up and try to solve it.

The audience applauded, but I'd gotten myself so excited that I could hardly hear them over the throbbing of my own pulse inside my head. I went on to explain that diabetes is a scourge. I described the long-term complications and their costs; I explained the impact that the diabetes epidemic will have on our whole society. Then I finished with this:

> I know we're in a budget crisis now and will likely be in one for years to come. But the fundamental question that you, the members of the LAUSD school board, need to answer today is this: should students be expected to pay for any part of their education by buying things like sodas that are bad for their health? Is this the expectation we have for our students? Is this the legacy we want to leave?

With that, I sat down. And this time I could hear the applause and cheers.

The next speaker was Jacqueline Domac, the head of the health program at Venice High School. Together with a group of students, she'd managed to bring healthier beverage options to her school—but it wasn't easy. A few years earlier, a student in one of Jackie's health classes had asked why the school's beverage vending machines offered soda but not fruit juice. Jackie passed this question to the school's financial manager. The next day she received a reply that stunned her: the school could not sell fruit juice because it would conflict with their exclusive "pouring" contract with the Coca-Cola Beverage Company. According to the contract, all beverages sold in vending machines, other than coffee or milk, must be Coca-Cola products. In return, Coca-Cola paid Venice High School $3,000 per year; the school also received a commission on every can or bottle of soda sold.

Jackie and her students formed a club, called Students for Public Health Advocacy. The group started a petition drive to bring healthier options to the school's vending machines. They also located other vendors willing to match Coke's financial incentives. But the school principal and financial manager refused to consider a change. As a compromise, the students negotiated with Coca-Cola.

The company promised to provide pure apple and orange juice in the vending machines. But out of over 200 vending machine slots, only 4 were devoted to juice; the rest continued to sell soda. Moreover, the juice usually sold out quickly and wasn't restocked promptly.

Jackie described all this to the school board. "Here's what is really sad," she said. "I have freshmen in my health class, and most of them are fairly thin. By the time they're done with high school, they have just ballooned, and I almost don't recognize them. Soda has a lot to do with it."

After all the speeches, the school board members debated the resolution to ban soda in the LAUSD. One board member asked: "Don't students have the right to buy a soda in school if they're thirsty or if they want a pick-me-up?" I was amazed that a school board member would not only sanction soda consumption but justify it as a "pick-me-up." The same argument could sanction drug use. And everyone in the audience knew that student rights was not the real issue. The real issue was money, the projected loss of revenue if students didn't buy sodas.

The debate went on for hours with no break. People became hungry and thirsty; individuals snuck out to grab a bite or use the bathroom, then returned. The meeting had started at 3:00 p.m. At around eight, I realized that I was parched. I looked around the school cafeteria where the meeting was being held. No water fountain. I slipped out of the room and walked through the halls. The only source of fluid I could find was a huge soda machine. There was no way I was going to obtain liquids from that.

Finally, at 10:00, Superintendent Romer took the floor. Until then, he'd said very little. But in a few brief words he ended the debate. He made a personal announcement that surprised many in the audience: like Supervisor Yaroslavsky, he had diabetes. Preventing diabesity was important to him. So he was in favor of banning the sale of sodas in the LAUSD. Since he was also concerned about the fiscal impact of banning soda sales, he suggested a trial period, during which the district would track the impact; if revenues were lost, they would find alternatives to neutralize the effect. Then he called for the vote.

Despite the late hour, the room was still packed with people. Everyone in the audience waited as the individual names of the school board members were called out. The vote was unanimous: sale of soda would be banned in LAUSD schools starting in January 2004. Everyone cheered and applauded. Coalition members hugged each other, delighted by this success. On the way home I stopped at a convenience store, bought the biggest bottle of water I could find, and drank every drop.

The LAUSD decision was reported by the news media worldwide. This was the first soda ban in a major metropolitan school district, the second-largest district in the nation. Over the next few days I was bombarded by phone calls from colleagues all over the country. Pediatric endocrinologists and other doctors wanted to know what we had said and done to achieve such a stunning victory. I was also flooded with e-mails from all over the world—Australia, Mexico, the United Kingdom, Germany, and India. I sent out copies of the resolution and copies of my speech. And I told my colleagues we could do the same thing across the country and around the globe if we persevered.

I'm delighted to report that it's beginning to happen. Individual schools, districts, cities, counties, and states are enacting soda bans or restricting the sale of sodas in schools. New York City, the largest school district in the United States, banned soda in 2003. One of the toughest bans was passed by the Philadelphia public school system in 2004: only water, milk, and 100 percent fruit juice can be sold in the city's public schools, though sports drinks will be available to high school students near sports facilities. The American Academy of Pediatrics and the American Diabetes Association have encouraged their membership to get involved at the local, state, or national level to work toward banning soda and improving the nutritional environment of schools across the country. By the way, Jackie Domac reports that preliminary figures from Venice High School actually show higher profits at the school store and in the vending machines now that they sell only healthy snacks and beverages.

BOOSTING PHYSICAL ACTIVITY

To solve the problem of diabesity, we need to address both sides of the caloric equation: energy expenditure as well as energy intake. To be healthy and fit, children require sixty minutes a day of moderate to vigorous physical activity, on average; teens need even more. Because youngsters spend so much time in school, at least half of that activity should happen during school hours.

Unfortunately, most primary, middle, and secondary schools across the country do not provide thirty minutes of daily physical activity to students. In the Healthy People 2000 report, the United States Surgeon General set a target for 50 percent of schools to require physical education every day. That may sound like a modest goal, but we're far from meeting it. Over the last decade—as school budgets tightened, and as pressure increased to devote more resources to academic subjects—there's been a marked decrease in physical education (PE) in schools. The percentage of students who attended a daily PE class dropped from 42 percent in 1991 to 32 percent in 2001, according to the Centers for Disease Control. What's more, over half the time in PE classes is spent not on physical activity but on changing clothes or sitting on bleachers and listening to instruction. Only 19 percent of high school students taking daily physical education are actually active for at least twenty minutes per class.

One consequence of inactivity in school is lack of fitness. California law requires school districts to administer a physical fitness test to all children in grades five, seven, and nine. In 2003 over 1.3 million students were checked. The test, called the Fitnessgram, was developed by the Cooper Institute for Aerobics Research. It consists of six parts that cover cardiovascular fitness, muscular strength, and flexibility; Body Mass Index is also assessed. To be considered fit, a student must pass all six parts. Having taken the test, which I passed easily at age fifty, I was dismayed to learn that only 23 percent of fifth graders, 27 percent of seventh graders, and 24 percent of ninth graders met all six standards.

Physical activity is not only good for health; it also boosts academic performance. In 2001 California correlated fitness test scores with scores on the standardized academic tests given by the state. The analyses revealed that higher academic achievement was associated with higher levels on fitness tests for all three grade levels. To improve academic test scores in schools throughout the country— and to fight diabesity—physical education should be required, not reduced or eliminated. Experts recommend that elementary school students have 150 minutes of PE per week; middle and secondary school students should have 225 minutes per week. There must be adequate equipment and facilities, as well as a meaningful curriculum. Health-related physical fitness assessments should be performed on students and used as evaluation and goal-setting tools.

Approximately 20 million U.S. children miss the opportunity to exercise and keep off excess weight by walking or bicycling to school. According to a survey by the U.S. Department of Transportation, even among children who live within a mile of their school, only 31 percent of trips to school are made on foot and just 3 percent are made by bike. The most common reason is parental concern about safety.

While dangerous motor vehicle traffic is a real obstacle, schools and communities all around the country are trying to bring back the custom of walking to school. For example, the city of Chicago and its police department created the Walking School Bus program; 175 schools participate. Youngsters who live near each other walk to school together under the supervision of an adult. In addition to encouraging walking and enhancing safety, the Walking School Bus strengthens communities and reduces auto traffic.

MARKETING HEALTHY LIFESTYLES IN SCHOOL

As someone who's a mother as well as a doctor, I know how challenging it is to get kids to give up sweets and soda, eat more fruits and vegetables, and become physically active. Our children live in a toxic media environment. They start to watch television as toddlers, and that's when companies begin marketing junk food to them. But we can appropriate the very same techniques—including advertising, pricing, and packaging—to help kids make better food choices. We can also promote fitness. Students need to be involved in the marketing process, because they know better than we do what will be effective.

Successful school-based promotional efforts are already in place around the country. For example, three California school districts adopted a program to increase fruit and vegetable consumption by middle school children over an eight-week period. Youngsters were taken on supermarket tours; teachers ran intriguing taste tests and cooking demonstrations. The classroom curricula incorporated information about the health value of fruits and vegetables. While all these efforts were taking place in some schools, others made no such changes. After eight weeks, fruit and vegetable consumption was 14 percent higher in schools that had "marketed" healthy eating.

Another success story is the multi-state Fruit and Vegetable Pilot Program, which was part of the federal government's 2002 Farm Act. The program allotted $6 million to twenty-five schools in Iowa, Indiana, Michigan, and Ohio and six schools on one Indian reservation in New Mexico so that children could be offered free fruit and vegetable snacks throughout the school day. Fruits and vegetables were distributed in high schools, middle schools, and elementary schools using a combination of kiosks, vending machines, and in-class methods. Teachers added relevant information to the curriculum, covering such topics as consumer issues, food safety, and techniques of food preparation.

Students and school staff members reported that they enjoyed having a variety of fruits and vegetables available throughout the day. Students liked trying new varieties and picking their favorites. Strawberries and carrots with dip were frequent taste-test winners, with kiwi fruit, apples, pineapple, cucumbers, and celery close behind. Most important, children and faculty appreciated the quality of the fresh fruits and vegetables. To effectively market fruits and vegetables in school, they must be fresh; they must crunch when kids sink their teeth into them. They cannot be items in poor condition that have been rejected for commercial sale.

During the Fruit and Vegetable Pilot Program, NSLP partici-
pation increased in the schools involved. Actual consumption of the
fruits and vegetables in NSLP lunches also increased. One school
reported that 25 percent fewer breakfast doughnuts and 50 percent
fewer lunchtime desserts were purchased. In another school, where
candy bar sales had amounted to $800 per week, candy sales
dropped to $300 per week after the program took hold. School
nurses indicated that fewer kids were visiting their offices, and parents said that children were requesting fruits and vegetables at
home. One unintended positive consequence of the program was
that janitors reported much less candy wrapper litter. Administrators observed other improvements that might have been confirmed
if they'd had more time and funding for research: better behavior,
improved test scores, decreased absenteeism, decreased BMI, and
less vending machine usage.

The success of this pilot program was recognized by Secretary
of Agriculture Ann Veneman during the USDA-sponsored National
Nutrition Connections Conference held in February 2003. She announced that the USDA was committed to stepping up efforts to
support programs such as the Fruit and Vegetable Pilot Program.
Unfortunately, such programs are not yet widespread because
USDA funding is limited.

Schools share with parents the enormous opportunity and responsibility to shape our children. Childhood is when youngsters begin to
develop the habits that will be with them for a lifetime. This is the
time to teach them about the benefits of good nutrition and physical
activity. Health education—which helps students learn the consequences of their lifestyle choices—is critical. And why not incorpo-
rate food labels and meal planning into reading and arithmetic
lessons? But it's not enough to provide formal instruction about
healthy living. The school environment must support what's taught
in the classroom. As Jackie Domac of Venice High School discovered, if health ed. class is teaching students to make wise decisions
about beverages, their education should not be undermined by
school vending machines that promote poor choices.

All this can happen if parents and other concerned citizens become active—find out what is happening at their local schools, familiarize themselves with state laws that deal with health and education, and become advocates. If parents become involved, if they're willing to educate, negotiate, and legislate—and, if necessary, litigate—our schools will become places where healthy lifestyles are taught and modeled every day.

Nine to Five

Children sometimes bring unhealthy snacks—french fries, doughnuts, soda—to their first meeting of KidsNFitness. Usually I take it in stride. After all, these youngsters have joined our program because they need to learn about nutrition and exercise. But I couldn't contain my reaction a year ago when I spotted Alfonso, a fourteen-year-old boy who weighed close to 300 pounds, licking a toy baby bottle filled with blue-colored candy glue. "My God!" I screamed. "Where did you get something so disgusting?"

Alfonso looked hurt. He responded, "I bought it at the gift shop downstairs." Then he added, "If you don't want me to eat it, Dr. Kaufman, then why do you sell it in your hospital?"

He was absolutely right, and I apologized. The minute the KidsNFitness session was over, I ran to the hospital administrator and expressed my outrage. I threw the blue baby bottle on his desk and demanded: "How can I teach children about healthy eating when the hospital—which should be a model—sells junk like this?"

The administrator listened calmly. Then he said something that upset me even more: "Don't worry, Fran. The candy in the gift shop is bought mainly by hospital employees."

"That's even worse!" I said. "Have you looked at our employees? Too many of them are dangerously overweight."

"They have a right to buy and eat what they want," he responded. "People here are under stress, whether they're employees or patients. They need comfort, and sweets are comforting."

"So why did we take away cigarettes?" I retorted, completely exasperated. Then I announced, "I'm going to figure out how to change this hospital." I didn't wait for his answer. I just walked out.

The next morning, when I arrived at the hospital to do teaching rounds, I was still fuming about the gift shop. I sat in the conference room on the fifth floor of the east wing, revising my lecture notes and waiting for the 5 East house staff: two medical students, four interns, and one resident. My topic was infant and childhood nutrition. I planned to talk about parents' responsibility to teach good eating habits, and the culpability of the food and advertising industries. My basic message was that parents were forced to combat these massive industries, which lure their children to consume junk. Parents needed to offer appropriate food in appropriate quantities; they needed to model healthy behaviors. But I also planned to explain that parents couldn't succeed without an environment in which the right choices were accessible and available. I wanted everyone to understand that individuals can't do it alone.

The medical students and interns entered the 5 East conference room at 8:00 on the dot. Since it was customary to eat breakfast during rounds, each person carried a tray from the hospital cafeteria, along with a clipboard and books. As they struggled to hold open the door while balancing their trays, I looked at what they'd brought for breakfast. Most had selected a doughnut, a muffin, or a bagel and cream cheese; only half of them had included a piece of fruit. There were cups of coffee, small cream containers, and sugar packets. One of the interns, Dale, who was at least 20 pounds overweight, had brought an oversized bagel slathered with cream cheese, a big bowl of cereal, a banana, a carton of whole milk, and a container of yogurt. I estimated that his tray held approximately 1,000 calories— close to 40 percent of his recommended daily caloric intake.

Greg, the resident, entered the 5 East conference room last. He was the furthest along in his training—and he was nearly obese. I'd watched Greg over the three years he'd been at Childrens Hospital Los Angeles. He'd been about 15 pounds overweight when he arrived; now, I guessed from looking at him, he was about 40 pounds too heavy. To my astonishment, Greg was carrying a box of Krispy Kreme doughnuts. Apparently he'd brought them to share with his colleagues. He walked over to me and, with a friendly smile, offered me the first doughnut.

I normally try to be polite in a situation like this, but I was still angry about the blue sugar glue sold in the hospital gift shop. So I couldn't conceal my aversion. "No!" I snapped. "I'm not about to eat a Krispy Kreme doughnut while we're discussing appropriate nutrition and how the lack of it has led to the epidemics of obesity and type 2 diabetes!"

Greg looked startled. He put the box, still open, on a table. But he didn't take a doughnut. And neither did anyone else. All through my lecture and our discussion, the Krispy Kremes remained lined up in two neat rows, untouched and glistening in their box.

Looking at the group, I realized that going through medical training was contributing to their weight problems. The two medical students were slender. Dale and the other three interns, who had worked at the hospital longer, all looked flabby or overweight. And Greg, the resident, who'd been here the longest, was obese. Their bodies showed the effects of too many missed meals compensated with junk food, too many on-call nights during which they ate candy to keep going, and too many lunch lectures in which someone, most likely the sponsoring pharmaceutical company representative, brought in pizza or Mexican food. They no longer had—or they had stopped creating—time for exercise. True, they could have made better personal choices about diet and lifestyle. But the hospital didn't provide an environment in which good choices were easy to make. And if we didn't do it, knowing what we know, then who would?

At least 4,000 people work in Childrens Hospital Los Angeles and its surrounding research buildings, day care center, and outpatient towers. This huge workforce consists of doctors and nurses, as well as technical support personnel who draw blood, take X-rays, and help run the clinical and research programs. There's a large cadre of people who keep the hospital clean and free of infectious agents; there are people who make the food, figure out the bills, answer the phones, and sell toys in the gift shop. There are administrators, fund-raisers, students, interns, residents, and fellows. Employees are here around the clock, every day of the year.

To fight diabesity, employers must enable their employees to make healthy choices. You might think that hospitals would be the first employers to do this, but they're not. As I thought about it, I realized that Childrens Hospital, like almost all the hospitals I know, was not a healthy place to work.

Water fountains were scarce—but there was a McDonald's right near the main entrance. There and in the cafeteria, it was easy to buy sweetened soft drinks in 32-ounce cups. Both McDonald's and the cafeteria provided a few healthy options, such as salads, baked pretzels, and soups. But the featured fare was high in salt, fat, sugar, or all three: fried chicken, burgers, fried potatoes, and creamy pastries. And on nearly every floor of the building, vending machines sold sugared sodas, candies, and chips.

Employees had no convenient opportunity for physical activity. The hospital had tried to organize a lunchtime walking program and an end-of-the-day exercise class, but hardly anyone showed up. This wasn't surprising. Lunch breaks barely allow time to sit down and eat. Besides, no one wants to go out in the warm California sun in the middle of the workday and come back all sweaty when there's no place to freshen up. And few employees can stay late at the end of the day: most face long commutes on crowded freeways, and many have second jobs to go to or kids to pick up.

I believed that most people who worked at Childrens Hospital would participate in fitness programs if they were convenient, and that they'd select healthier food if attractive choices were offered. I decided that we needed to create a culture in the hospital that promoted not only the health of our patients but also the health of our employees.

WELLNESS PAYS

Measures that advance employee nutrition and fitness aren't just good for health; they're good for the bottom line. Evidence collected over the past thirty years shows that work site health promotion yields a plethora of positive results: lower healthcare costs, fewer sick days, and healthier, happier employees.

Diabesity is expensive for the nation's employers. In the late 1990s obesity cost American companies $12.7 billion per year because of lost productivity and extra expenses for medical care and insurance. Obesity was associated with 63 million additional doctor visits, 39 million lost workdays, and 239 million restricted activity days, which are days in which a worker can't perform all of his or her normal duties. Indirect costs to employers due to diabetes—including lost workdays, restricted activity days, permanent disabilities, and mortality—totaled $39.8 billion in 2000. High as this number was in 2000, it has undoubtedly climbed higher as the incidence of obesity rises.

Employers, hit by soaring expenses for healthcare benefits, are seeking innovative ways to reduce the drain on their budgets. Wellness programs have proven to be a highly effective solution, almost always saving more money than they cost. They not only reduce medical claims and absenteeism, they also improve productivity and make the workplace more attractive to employees. For example, when Google boasts of its employee benefits, they feature not only stock options but also the fact that people who work at their headquarters enjoy free healthy meals and snacks, as well as an on-site gym and opportunities to hike or ride a bicycle in a neighboring wildlife preserve.

In the fall of 2003 I was invited to Las Vegas, along with U.S. Surgeon General Richard Carmona, to speak to a group of about a hundred people whose work involves health insurance. In the audience were executives and staff members from health plans, insurance companies, Medicare and Medicaid, state government, and employers. My topic was what the diabesity epidemic means for corporations, health care, and our nation's future. I focused on prevention, emphasizing the importance of work site wellness and health promotion.

As soon as I finished, a hand went up in the audience. Gary Earl, vice president of benefits at Caesars Entertainment, introduced himself. I knew that Caesars Entertainment runs some of the largest casinos in Las Vegas, so I pictured smoke-filled rooms with employees hunched over roulette wheels. But Gary was obviously physically fit and didn't match my concept of someone involved with the gaming industry. To my astonishment, he began to describe a weight loss campaign—called the Get Fit Challenge, Weight No More—sponsored by Caesars Entertainment for their employees. Seven thousand of their workers joined teams and competed for prizes. At the end of ninety days, approximately 4,600 workers completed the program. They'd lost a total of about 45,000 pounds, or 22.5 tons. "That's equivalent to four elephants," Gary pointed out.

Their investment in this health promotion and prizes yielded a profit for Caesars Entertainment. Gary explained: "Twelve of our employees with diabetes were able to discontinue diabetes medications. The year prior, we'd spent about $13,000 a year on diabetes medications and treatments for each one of them. In addition, absenteeism went down and productivity went up."

CHANGING ONE STEP AT A TIME

Workplace interventions need not be expensive or complicated. The Centers for Disease Control and Prevention developed a campaign to encourage people to use the stairs at work. They called it the StairWELL to Better Health campaign. Stair climbing is terrific exercise: it gets your heart beating; it works all the major muscles in your lower body. You don't need to change clothes, and stair climbing takes practically no time—instead of standing around waiting for the elevator, you're getting a mini-workout. What's more, the stairs are already in place, because they're required by building codes.

The CDC tested the StairWELL program in an Atlanta office building over a three-and-a-half-year period. Bare walls were painted and decorated with framed artwork, transforming the stairwells into attractive spaces. The steps were carpeted. Speakers were installed and music was piped in. Motivational signs were placed around the building to encourage employees to use the stairs. For instance, a sign at the elevator pointed to the stairwell and read: "No waiting one door over." Other signs delivered health messages such as "Raise your fitness level, one step at a time" and "Your heart needs exercise. Here's your chance." All these measures cost less than $16,000. Yet they produced a significant increase in the number of people who used the stairs, thereby enjoying the benefits of extra exercise.

For years I've taken the stairs at work to help stay fit. When I do teaching rounds on the wards at Childrens Hospital Los Angeles, a group of interns, residents, and fellows traipses behind me. They're spending a month to learn about pediatric diabetes and endocrinology by working with me in my clinics and helping to treat the hospitalized patients under my care. This period is called a rotation, since they'll rotate to a different specialty every month, becoming familiar with all aspects of pediatric medicine. The group follows me wherever I go, from one ward in the hospital to the next, up and down from floor to floor. It's as if we're all glued together. And in my travels, I don't take the elevator. I only take the stairs—and sometimes it's up six flights.

Each year I review my teaching evaluations in the Pediatric Residency Office. For the most part, they're favorable and flattering, laudatory of my skills in teaching pediatrics, particularly diabetes. But until about five years ago, numerous evaluations complained that doing a rotation with me, although intellectually rewarding, was just too physically difficult. Typical comments were: "She makes you take the stairs all day," "No one can walk at her speed," and "She doesn't take any breaks; she just keeps running around." I was astonished. Most of the students and residents were more than twenty years younger than I was.

I decided to announce at the beginning of the next rotation that I would always take the stairs, but anyone who wanted to take the elevator could meet me at our destination. I told them my age—at the time I was approaching forty-eight—and explained that I used the stairs because it was a great way to get some physical activity and stay healthy. From then on, I've made this announcement at the start of every rotation. Ninety percent of my students and residents have taken the stairs with me, and the complaints have ceased.

In 2003, during my ADA presidency, I started wearing a pedometer on my belt. This is a small device, about half the size of a beeper, that counts each step taken. The U.S. Department of Health and Human Services had just announced a Small Steps, Big Rewards campaign to help prevent type 2 diabetes. Secretary Tommy G. Thompson was telling everyone to take 10,000 steps per day. That's the equivalent of about five miles. Sedentary people walk about 2,000 to 3,000 steps in a day, just going about their normal routine. Increasing the total to 10,000 steps is enough to produce impressive health benefits, including weight loss, lower blood pressure, and lower blood glucose. When Secretary Thompson presented me with a pedometer, I decided to make 10,000 steps my personal daily goal.

Most days I log close to 10,000 steps simply by walking my dog in the morning, parking in the most remote part of the parking lot at work, and taking the stairs all the time. But if I've had a less active day than usual, I make sure to walk in the evening after I get home. Even though I've always been strongly committed to exercise, I've found that wearing a pedometer makes me more aware of how well I'm meeting my goals. I recommend it to everyone interested in fitness. You can buy a simple step counter—that's all you need—for $15–$25.

MEETING FOR HEALTH

In 2002, I was invited to chair the Los Angeles County Task Force on Children and Youth Physical Fitness. Our mission was to evaluate the problems of obesity and inactivity among L.A. County youth. We would hold six meetings at Childrens Hospital Los Angeles, then deliver a report to the L.A. County Board of Supervisors. Present at each meeting would be ten task force members, four representatives from the Los Angeles County Department of Health Services, and twenty to thirty people from the general public.

Since we'd be meeting from 3:00 to 5:00 in the afternoon, I wanted to serve refreshments. I wrote up a request for the hospital's catering director, asking for fruits and vegetables, cheese and crackers, water, iced tea, and coffee—nothing more. The next day I received a call from the catering director. "You forgot the cookies and brownies," she said. "Do you want all chocolate chip cookies or an assortment?"

"Thank you, but we don't want any cookies or brownies," I said. "The other refreshments will be plenty."

"Are you sure?" she asked. She wanted to serve food that would impress people coming to Childrens Hospital for a meeting, and clearly her idea of impressive food was something with sugar and fat.

"Yes, I'm sure. This is a meeting about preventing obesity," I explained.

"Well," she said, sounding offended, "people still like a good cookie."

The meeting was held in the Page Conference Hall in the hospital. This wood-paneled room is large and stately. Thanks to modular furnishings, it can be used in multiple ways. With furniture stowed away, this is the room that hosts the physical activity part of our KidsNFitness program. For the task force meeting, the hall was arranged with a long table at the front so all the task force members could sit and face the audience. Before the meeting, I checked the refreshment table and was delighted to see a beautiful display of fresh fruits and vegetables, small cubes of cheese, and crackers. We did have the capability. All that was required was the will.

At 4:00, halfway through the meeting, I announced, "It's time for a Take Ten break." People looked puzzled. Dr. Eloisa Gonzalez and Genaro Sandoval, the director and a staff member from the Health Department's Physical Activity Program, jumped up. Genaro explained: "A Take Ten is a ten-minute break for fitness. We'll stand next to our seats and do a series of exercises."

"You'll invigorate your body and get the blood flowing to your mind!" added Dr. Gonzalez, trying to generate enthusiasm. A few people stood up. But most sat and stared, looking incredulous.

I lectured the audience: "You're sitting in a meeting, and potentially destroying your own health, while you're trying to figure out how to help other people not destroy theirs. That's why we're doing a Take Ten."

Now everyone was standing. For the next ten minutes we marched in place and stretched all the major muscle groups in our arms, legs, and trunk. Right before we started to sweat, we were done. I could feel my heart beating and knew I was breathing faster. I also noticed that I felt energized. Looking around the room, I could see smiles. We decided we would Take Ten at all of our meetings. We would "walk the walk" and show the world we were serious about making a healthier environment for everyone. Even for ourselves.

A HEALTHIER HOSPITAL

Change is beginning at Childrens Hospital Los Angeles. The hospital administrator heard me on that day I barged into his office. Within a month, the gift shop stopped selling the toy baby bottle filled with blue sugar glue—and they also dropped all other candy that was sold with toys. But that minimal victory only whetted my appetite. I began to develop a long-range plan. As one way to find allies to help me, I asked to give grand rounds. All academic medical centers and most community hospitals have grand rounds, a regularly scheduled lecture period designed to inform the medical staff about state-of-the-art medicine. This enables them to meet continuing medical or nursing education requirements.

At my hospital, grand rounds takes place at 8:00 a.m. every Friday. Almost all of the hospital staff attend: doctors, nurses, therapists, and other allied health personnel. In back of the lecture hall are platters of doughnuts, muffins, bagels, and coffee. They're considered part of the attraction of grand rounds. On the way in to hear my lecture—which was titled "Diabesity"—many hospital staff members helped themselves to a breakfast pastry; some took two.

I stood on the podium in front of my colleagues and friends and talked about the epidemics of obesity and diabetes. I explained— passionately—how these epidemics were allowed to flourish in the workplace. I talked about the need for medical facilities to take the lead in improving the workplace environment. And I listed everything that was wrong with the environment at Childrens Hospital Los Angeles, starting with the doughnuts and muffins in back of the room.

"The average nurse in this hospital is in his or her forties. Our full-time medical staff is older than that. Just look around. It's obvious that all of us should be concerned about our health," I said. I could see people putting down their doughnuts. "It's time to make the environment in which we all work conducive to employee wellness," I concluded.

A few days after my lecture, I was invited to appear before the hospital's administrative council. This is the power base of the hospital, comprising all the vice presidents, department heads, and administrators. Bill Noce, the hospital's CEO, told me that I could lead a committee to improve the environment. I decided to call the committee Healthy Hospital and asked Linda Heller, the chief of nutrition services, and Mary Dee Hacker, head of nursing and a key hospital administrator, to co-chair it with me. We added key personnel from communications, building/environmental services, human resources/wellness, and the house staff training program.

Eight months later, I'm thrilled with the progress we've made—though there's still much to be done, and our efforts continue. The gift shop now sells low-fat string cheese, fat-free pretzels, baked chips, and low-fat crackers. Though candy is still available, it's placed high on the display rack, out of the reach of children.

The food services now post charts with the calorie, fat, sugar, and protein content of the food items sold in the cafeteria. There's a daily cooking demonstration, featuring a heart-healthy meal. The cafeteria offers more vegetarian and low-fat options. Near the salad bar one can see model serving sizes for salad dressings and condiments—items that are easily consumed in excess. Gone is the enticing candy rack that used to be right in front of the cafeteria cashier. In its place is a display of fresh fruits and vegetables, to encourage nutritious impulse purchases.

Because many of our employees are overweight, we've arranged for Weight Watchers to give a class at the hospital. That makes it easier for busy people to join and participate in support groups.

They also have the option of joining a Weight Watchers group on-line. To encourage physical activity, we offer discounts for member-ships at nearby gyms. The gyms, eager to enhance their rosters, were more than willing to make these offers. All it required was a few telephone calls from a Healthy Hospital committee member.

The cost of all this positive change is negligible. We're using the hospital newsletter to promote healthy habits at work, to advertise the positive changes in the cafeteria, and to let everyone know about the Weight Watchers group and discounted gym memberships. Each newsletter carries a column with information about nutrition, as well as advice about such risk factors as high BMI, high blood pressure, and high cholesterol.

The Healthy Hospital committee continues to meet monthly. We're gearing up for a health fair in the hospital, which will feature healthy foods and cooking demonstrations. One of our goals for next year is to make all the improvements in the Childrens Hospital stairwells that the CDC recommends—new paint, music, inspira-tional signs—so that more staff members and patients will take the stairs.

We're also planning to promote the use of pedometers, so that people can count the steps they take each day. My center, the Dia-betes and Endocrinology Center, will challenge any other group to see who can walk the most steps. And my group had better win!

I envision that Childrens Hospital Los Angeles will become a place where health is delivered not just to people in operating and exam-ining rooms, but to everyone who walks through its doors. Health will be promoted by what we serve in our cafeteria and vending ma-chines, by how we conduct our meetings, and by a variety of pro-grams and challenges designed to get people moving and fit. In this environment, students, interns, residents, and fellows will learn to practice what they are learning to preach. And I hope that our hos-pital will become a model for other employers.

FIFTEEN

The Healthcare Challenge

I met Consuela on Olvera Street, in a predominantly Latino area of downtown Los Angeles, during the annual American Diabetes Association Health Fair in 2001. She was standing in line to get her blood pressure measured. I was vice president of the ADA at that point, and I spent much of the day walking around the fair talking to people. I wanted to learn more about the men and women who had come to Olvera Street on a Sunday morning for free health screenings.

Consuela caught my eye. She was tall and about 20 pounds overweight. Wearing a traditional Mexican dress, with a brightly colored embroidered belt wrapped tightly around her waist, she stood out in the crowd. Her eyes were big and dark; her beautiful long black hair was streaked with gray. A broad smile lit up her face when she saw me looking at her. I smiled back and approached her. I introduced myself in my broken Spanish, and we began to talk. Since her English was much better than my Spanish, we spoke in English.

Consuela told me she was fifty-three years old. She'd come to the fair to have her blood pressure checked. Her mother had suffered a stroke at age forty-eight, and Consuela wanted to be sure she wasn't destined for the same fate. Her mother's sudden stroke had left her paralyzed and unable to speak. One month to the day after the stroke, she died. "Before her stroke, she not see doctor for almost twenty years. Then she find out about her pressure, but it was too late," Consuela said.

"When was the last time you had your blood pressure checked?" I asked.

"Only with my babies," she told me. And then she added, "My niño is treinta, thirty. When I get green card, five years ago, I want to see doctor. But no time."

Consuela knew she was at risk for hypertension, high blood pressure. But she hadn't had her blood pressure measured for thirty years. As I stood with her, waiting in line for this long-delayed test, I began to worry. She might have serious, potentially devastating hypertension; it might have been damaging her blood vessels for twenty or thirty years. I asked if she was also planning to have a blood test to find out if she had diabetes.

"Sí," she responded. "It is best to know everything."

"Do you have family with diabetes?"

"My abuela, grandmother, in Mexico, many years ago," she said. "She is muerta, dead."

"Do you have a doctor?"

"No," she confessed, her eyes lowered. "Too much money. Dos años, two years before, I was sick con pulmonía," she explained. She expelled a fake cough to show me the symptoms of her illness, which I assumed was pneumonia. "I went to a clínica. I got medicines and radiografía, X-ray." She pointed at her chest with her hands, trying to portray X-ray beams. I nodded again. "Too much money," she said, shaking her head.

As Consuela finished her story, we arrived at the front of the line. A volunteer gave her a paper to fill out. The form asked, in English and Spanish, if she knew what her blood pressure was, if she suffered from any illnesses, and if she was taking any medication. She answered "No" to all of those questions. After she turned in her paper, she was taken to a seat. A nurse approached. I knew her from "the General," the medical center of Los Angeles County, which is associated with the University of Southern California, where I teach. She put a blood pressure cuff around Consuela's arm, cinched it tight, and pressed a button. The cuff inflated. I couldn't see the numbers, but when the nurse deflated the cuff and repeated the procedure, I knew that Consuela had high blood pressure. After the second measurement, a student doctor—another volunteer from the General—came and talked to Consuela in Spanish for about five minutes. When he was finished, he handed her some papers and a small booklet.

As she walked toward me, I could see that the sparkle in her eyes and the smile on her face, which had originally drawn me to her, were gone. "It's too high," she told me.

I asked to see the papers, and she handed them to me. The booklet was a patient information pamphlet in Spanish, from one of the pharmaceutical companies, about the importance of treating hypertension. The paper had her blood pressure numbers written on it: 173/112. This was even worse than I'd feared. Blood pressure under 120/80 is normal; anything over 140/90 is considered significantly elevated. Consuela's blood pressure was high enough to put her at immediate risk for a stroke or even sudden death. In addition to the alarming blood pressure number, the paper provided the telephone numbers of area clinics and of the American Heart Association.

"I will take the diabetes test now," Consuela told me. We headed toward the area where finger-stick blood sugar screenings were being done under the auspices of a pharmaceutical company. This was the first year the local American Diabetes Association had allowed blood tests at the health fair. In the past, the only diabetes screening was a paper-and-pencil test that added up points for diabetes risk factors: family history, age, ethnicity, overweight, history of giving birth to a large baby, and signs of insulin resistance such as high blood pressure and elevated cholesterol levels. Individuals found to be at high risk were offered free blood tests at one of many nearby hospitals or clinic laboratories.

Experts on public health disagree about whether it's desirable to provide finger-stick blood tests at a street fair. The subject has been debated within the American Diabetes Association, the National

Institutes of Health, and the Centers for Disease Control and Prevention. Until 2001 ADA's unofficial policy had been that diabetes blood testing should be done only by a certified laboratory and only in the context of a healthcare visit. Using a certified lab is important because the results are more reliable. A finger-stick blood test is prone to error: sometimes it tells someone they have diabetes when they don't, and sometimes the test misses diabetes and gives false reassurance. Also, if the diagnosis is made during a healthcare visit, it can be properly confirmed and appropriate medical treatment and advice can be given.

Most of the more scientifically oriented people within the ADA were concerned that if blood tests were performed at a street fair, people who tested positive wouldn't follow up with a visit to a healthcare provider. But others in the organization argued that testing would be worthwhile even if it picked up just a few patients who would obtain appropriate care as a result. I could see both sides of this argument. From a purely scientific point of view, I understood the flaws in health fair screening and was concerned about offering tests that were not optimal. But from a personal standpoint, I felt that every person found could potentially benefit from earlier treatment. In 2003, during my presidency, the executive board of the ADA affirmed its position that screening for diabetes should be done in the context of a healthcare visit; this decision was based upon the recommendation of its scientific advisory committee. Finger-stick blood tests are now strongly discouraged at ADA community events.

When we arrived at the diabetes testing booth, a Spanish-speaking volunteer nurse reviewed the obligatory paperwork with Consuela. The nurse swabbed her finger with an alcohol pad, let the alcohol dry, and then pricked Consuela's fingertip with a small needle. As the needle punctured her skin, Consuela winced and pulled back. The nurse pressed out a drop of blood, put the blood onto a special paper strip, then loaded the strip into the glucose meter. Within seconds the number appeared on the screen: 228 mg/dl. That meant diabetes.

"We can't make the diagnosis on the basis of only one test," I told Consuela, "but your sugar level is high and it is very likely that you have diabetes." I tried to be reassuring, but I could tell she felt overwhelmed. She didn't look at me, and she kept wiping her finger-tip where the blood had been drawn. "If you take care of yourself, you'll be all right," I told her. "I can help get you an appointment at the General." I gave her my telephone number and told her to call me the next morning. I asked for her phone number, but she said it would be easier for her to call me.

It was time for me to make a speech to the crowd as vice president of the ADA. I told Consuela how much I had enjoyed meeting her, and once again I urged her to call me first thing in the morning. She said she would. Then I went onto the stage to welcome everyone and announce a dance exhibition. Dancing is an excellent physical activity, so the ADA had arranged for groups to perform traditional Mexican dances to get the crowd active and moving.

When I arrived at my office the next day, I told my secretary, Daisy, that I was expecting a call from a woman named Consuela. At ten o'clock I buzzed Daisy to ask if Consuela had called. She hadn't. At eleven o'clock I buzzed Daisy again, and the answer was still no. By noon I was frantic. I was angry with myself for not insisting that Consuela give me her telephone number, because it was obvious that she was not going to call me. In the afternoon I phoned a colleague at the ADA to ask if there was any way to track down someone who had tested positive at the previous day's diabetes screening. But there wasn't.

I thought about Consuela over the next weeks, trying to think of ways to find her. I asked colleagues at the General if they'd seen her. But no one knew anyone named Consuela who matched her description. After a while I gave up. The following year at the ADA Health Fair on Olvera Street, I looked for Consuela but couldn't find her.

When the time came for the 2003 Olvera Street Health Fair, I was president of the ADA. I spent most of my time on the podium welcoming, announcing, answering questions, and getting my picture taken. It was the third fair with Mexican dancing, and almost everyone in the crowd was participating. I was admiring the dancing when I spotted Consuela—or at least someone I thought was Consuela—at the edge of the crowd. I jumped down from the podium and walked toward her as fast as I could. As I approached, I realized it wasn't Consuela, but someone who looked hauntingly similar. Just to be sure, I said, "Consuela?"

The woman jumped. She asked me how I knew Consuela. I explained. The woman told me that Consuela was her sister.

I felt elated. "How can I reach her?" I asked.

"Not possible," she responded.

"Why not?"

"Ella, she is dead," she whispered.

I gasped. "What happened?" I cried.

"She had stroke, and with diabetes, she died," she explained, as if it made sense.

"Did she go to the doctor two years ago?" I asked. I needed to find out.

"She went to clinic, but wait so long. She miss too much work and almost lose her job. She heard about medicine, but medicine too much money. She got sick and sicker. She went to the clinic again. Then the clinic was closed. She found another clinic. Sometimes she get medicine and sometimes she cannot pay for everything. It was too hard for Consuela."

"Why didn't she call me?" I asked, feeling anguished and frustrated. "I could have helped."

"She not take charity," Consuela's sister informed me. "Consuela proud. She try to do for herself. But she could not."

"It wasn't her fault," I said. "Consuela didn't fail," I whispered under my breath. "The system failed Consuela." She was the victim of a fragmented, disconnected healthcare system that denies people adequate access, that's difficult to navigate, and that withholds sufficient funding. I might have been able to help her, but she didn't accept my offer. Pride got in her way, or maybe she didn't think I would really help. And if it was hard for her, it was equally difficult for all the other people who must find their way through the system on their own.

According to our best estimates today, 5 to 6 million people have type 2 diabetes and don't know it. Tens of millions more are at risk because of their weight and may even have pre-diabetes. We will reach more of these people thanks to increased public concern about the disease, as well as increased education efforts by the

American Diabetes Association, the federal government, and others. But once we find them, we must provide them with affordable, coordinated medical care. Until we can meet that challenge, people like Consuela will continue to die too young from this treatable—and preventable—disease.

THE UNINSURED—AND THE UNDERINSURED

Each year when I attend the ADA's annual conference, I visit the displays set up by the pharmaceutical companies and marvel at the latest advances. I learn about a host of new medications that promise to improve insulin sensitivity. I see gadgets that make it easier for people with diabetes to control their blood sugar, improved glucose meters for home use, insulin pumps that can be worn to deliver a constant infusion of insulin throughout the day, pen-like syringes that make injections simple and painless. But even as I rejoice at the progress we're making, I wonder how many people will be able to afford these medications and devices, let alone the consistent, personalized health care that makes them truly effective. More than 43.6 million people in the United States have no health insurance coverage, and at least another 29 million are underinsured. Many of these people have medical conditions, such as diabetes, that require expensive treatments and medications they can't afford. The dilemmas they face are heartbreaking.

Bill and Nancy are a hard-working couple in their late twenties; I know them because Nancy's mother is a secretary at the hospital. Shortly after they paid off their college loans, Bill and Nancy bought a modest condo and took on additional debt to purchase a copy shop franchise. Though their business did well, money was tight. Because they no longer had employers to contribute to their health insurance premiums, the cost jumped by more than 50 percent. So they made a decision that many of their friends had made: they dropped their insurance and decided to gamble on their health. They did this even though they knew that Bill was at risk for diabetes—he was obese, and his father had died of diabetes complications two years earlier. Because Bill's father had been diagnosed at age forty-three, they assumed they had plenty of time. Sadly, they did not.

About a year and a half after Bill and Nancy joined the ranks of the uninsured, Bill developed the classic symptoms of diabetes: he was urinating frequently and felt constantly thirsty. He put off going for a checkup. He was too busy, he told Nancy, and it would be too expensive; besides, maybe it was just the hot weather making him drink too much. But when his vision became blurry, Nancy insisted he see a doctor immediately. His blood sugar was over 250 mg/dl; together with his symptoms, that meant he had diabetes.

Bill was referred to an ophthalmologist, who examined his eyes. The ophthalmologist told them that Bill was lucky, because there was no sign of retinopathy or retinal damage; his vision was very likely to clear up when he brought his blood sugar under control. Though Bill tested negative for kidney damage, his blood pressure and cholesterol were elevated, putting him at high risk for heart disease.

When his doctor reviewed all the test results with Bill and Nancy, she emphasized that he could achieve excellent control of his disease, and also improve his blood pressure and cholesterol, with a combination of pills, diet, exercise, and weight loss. She offered a referral to a nutritionist and exercise physiologist, but Bill and Nancy refused—they were too alarmed by their mounting medical bills, including the cost for medication.

Both of them mined the Internet to learn all they could about diabetes. Following a suggestion from an online patient support forum, they arranged to swap copying services for membership in a gym near their store; Nancy designed a brochure for a nutritionist in exchange for a consultation. Now strongly motivated to lose weight, Bill made significant changes in his eating habits. He and Nancy worked out at the gym four times a week. Within three months, Bill had lost 21 pounds. Now his blood sugar levels were almost always within the normal range, and his vision was no longer blurry. He was able to stop taking medication, but he still required medical checkups and lab tests, as well as equipment to monitor his blood sugar every day.

Because of Bill's diagnosis, affordable health insurance was now even more out of reach. The couple consulted a health advocate, who offered devastating choices: give up their home or lose their budding new business. When they balked at these options, the consultant suggested divorce—Nancy could keep the house and the business in her name, and Bill could become a medically indigent adult. This was even more unacceptable. As a temporary measure, they negotiated reduced payments with Bill's doctors and borrowed money from their parents to pay their medical bills. Though both of them had hoped to work full time building their business, Bill found employment elsewhere simply to gain access to insurance.

Even those fortunate enough to have health insurance may struggle if they develop diabetes. People who are underinsured may face huge deductibles and gaps in coverage. Or they may be financially strained by co-payments that can amount to hundreds of dollars per month—for doctor visits, medication, strips to measure blood sugar, syringes, and other essential supplies. Yet another problem may be the limitations of managed care.

Managed care organizations or health maintenance organizations (HMOs) were designed to help keep people healthy, thereby saving money for the patient, the HMO, and the entire medical system. In the 1970s my father-in-law, who had been a private medical practitioner for decades, helped set up HMOs in the Midwest. He believed they would allow all Americans access to affordable, high-quality health care. Many HMOs, including Kaiser Permanente and others, continue to reflect that dream. They ensure that patients with diabetes receive the services and support they need; they perform essential tests and checkups according to medical guidelines. But, sadly, some HMOs have changed so that their primary goals are to contain medical costs or to make a profit for the HMO's shareholders.

In the original HMO concept, the primary care physician was supposed to oversee the patient's medical care, ensuring that everything was coordinated. That can be an extremely valuable function, especially with a complex illness such as diabetes, where a patient might be under the care of half a dozen specialists, each ordering tests and prescribing medications. But some HMOs have turned the primary care physician into a gatekeeper rather than a coordinator, with too much emphasis on cost containment and too little on providing needed services. This can be very frustrating for a specialist like me.

My hospital clinic sees patients referred by doctors, other clinics, and emergency rooms from all over Los Angeles County and beyond. Some of these patients are uninsured; the rest have a wide variety of medical coverage: private insurance of many kinds, Medicaid, California entitlement programs for the needy or those with chronic illnesses (such as California Children's Services), or an HMO. Most insurers permit me to treat patients as I deem necessary, with minimal oversight. But others require that all tests and treatments I recommend be approved ahead of time and be done in particular laboratories. I can understand their motives: they want to ensure that the care they provide is truly necessary and reasonably priced. But unfortunately, this can make it very difficult for me to get a timely turnaround on labs and tests—and to make sure the results don't get lost in the shuffle. When the person acting as gatekeeper is not familiar with appropriate care for youngsters with diabetes, the approval process can involve unnecessary delays and inappropriate denials, and may even lead to worsening health or a poor outcome for my patients.

Two years ago, one of my patients, a seventeen-year-old named Alissa, entered a managed care program. I'd seen her for two years before that under a private insurance plan. Alissa had type 2 diabetes. But that was not all she had. Alissa also suffered from polycystic ovarian syndrome (PCOS), and her cholesterol was high—both conditions related to her diabetes. Alissa was overweight, but her arms and legs were skinny; she carried all of her excess weight in her abdomen. Her round face was covered with terrible acne, a consequence of her PCOS. She'd grown her blond hair long and wore bangs to hide her pimples and acne scars. But that only made things worse, because her hair irritated her skin.

When I first saw Alissa at age fifteen, right after her diabetes diagnosis, her multiple, interlocking problems made her a challenging case. But after two years she was doing well with a combination of measures. Thanks to insulin and metformin, a diabetes pill that reduces insulin resistance, as well as exercise and dietary change, Alissa's blood sugar was under good control, and she had lost weight; other medication had brought her cholesterol down into the normal range. Acne treatments with a dermatologist had improved her skin. This made her more self-confident. She no longer tried to hide her face. At that point her father changed jobs, and the only available health insurance involved managed care. Now the real challenge of caring for her began.

I could no longer simply order the lab tests I needed to manage Alissa's many conditions; I could no longer refer her to the dermatologist. First I had to write a letter or call her primary care physician and explain the obvious: Alissa needed lab tests because she had diabetes and a host of other problems related to her insulin resistance; visits to the dermatologist would maintain the improvement in her skin. Sometimes the primary care physician would ask, "Are you sure?" I would become frustrated.

The tests were always approved eventually. Alissa's blood would be drawn and her urine collected at a lab of the managed care organization's choosing. It would take weeks to get the results back. When a test had to be repeated, results could take another few weeks. For example, Alissa needed a test once a year to screen her urine for protein. The appearance of protein in the urine is the first sign that diabetes is affecting the kidneys. I called her primary care physician to request authorization. "Why does she need this test?" he asked.

"Because she has type 2 diabetes," I responded. "She's at risk for kidney damage, and this test can detect it early, before symptoms develop. If we find it early, we can stop ongoing damage by giving her appropriate medication. That means she can avoid or delay kidney failure."

The annual test would cost $35; the medication, if she needed it, would cost hundreds of dollars per year. If we didn't perform the test and simply waited for problems to appear, her kidneys might be irreversibly damaged. In that case, she'd require dialysis, which costs over $50,000 per year, or a kidney transplant, which would cost over $100,000, plus several thousand dollars annually for the special drugs she'd need to take for the rest of her life to prevent rejection of the transplanted kidney. By ordering the test, not only was I protecting Alissa's kidneys, but I also could be saving her insurance company many thousands of dollars.

The doctor persisted: "Are you sure this needs to be done?"

"Yes!" I barked, completely exasperated. Six weeks later, the results came back, and they were abnormal: Alissa had too much protein in her urine. Once again, I called the primary care provider. I told him the urine test result was abnormal, so it needed to be repeated. We never make a diagnosis based on a single test, because we can get false positive results if a patient is menstruating, has a urine infection, or has recently engaged in vigorous physical activity. The ADA Standards of Care call for three tests over at least a month to confirm the persistence of protein in the urine.

Once again Alissa's primary care doctor asked if I was sure. It was a good thing I wasn't in the same room with him, because I was ready to explode. Instead I just shouted a loud, emphatic "Yes!" Vanquished, he authorized the repeat urine test. This showed that Alissa was still spilling protein into her urine. One more test a few weeks later confirmed that diabetes had begun to affect her kidneys. I immediately prescribed medication. Six months later I tested Alissa again, and the protein value had returned to the normal range. This meant that treatment was working, and I was greatly relieved.

Meanwhile, her acne had returned, so I called the primary physician to get authorization for the referral. "Her acne doesn't look all that bad," the doctor said.

"Not that bad to whom?" I snapped. "My patient thinks it's bad; her parents think it's bad; I think it's bad. When she was under the care of a dermatologist, it was markedly improved. Now my patient hides her face behind her hair again, and that's making matters worse. If we wait too much longer, all the benefit from her previous treatments will be gone."

He sighed. "Okay. She can see the dermatologist on our list. But this is for one time only."

HEALTH CARE, NOT DISEASE CARE

Diabesity is a health problem that desperately calls for education and other preventive services. We know that lifestyle changes can prevent diabetes. We've proven that if people eat right, lose weight, and become physically active, they can halt the progression to full-blown diabetes. But currently, health insurance plans, HMOs, and the entitlement programs of Medicare and Medicaid focus on disease management. Health insurance pays for doctor visits, medications, surgeries, and hospitalizations. Prevention—all the measures that people can take to ward off diseases and improve their ability to live not only a long life but a healthy one—is another story. Less than 1 percent of the billions spent annually on health care in the United States is spent on prevention. This is a profound flaw in our healthcare system, and it must be addressed if we are to fight diabesity.

For example, most insurers will not pay for measures to treat obesity—unless the obese person has already suffered a health problem as a result. The mother of one of my patients tried to get her insurance company to pay for a consultation with a nutritionist. Although this woman did not have heart disease or diabetes, she was at extremely high risk for both because she weighed 280 pounds. Her doctor appealed to the insurance company repeatedly. But every time, the appeal was denied with the explanation that "health insurance does not cover obesity treatment." They would not pay a few hundred dollars to help this markedly obese woman lose weight. Instead, the insurance company wound up forking over more than $100,000 when she had a heart attack at age forty-eight, followed by a mild stroke that required months of rehabilitative care.

In 2004, Health and Human Services Secretary Thompson announced a promising change in Medicare policy: obesity treatment would be eligible for coverage even for otherwise healthy individuals. I was delighted by this change because I've spent my career as a physician "eating the cost" so that my multidisciplinary team of nurses, nutritionists, and psychologists can teach my patients how to adopt healthy lifestyles to prevent type 2 diabetes. Insurance companies usually won't pay for the services of these team members, even though they're meeting with patients, educating them, counseling them, and talking to them on the phone to avert catastrophes. So I must find other ways to pay their salaries. Sometimes the money comes from research grants or clinical trials; sometimes I raise funds from foundations or private philanthropists.

Another great obstacle to preventive health care is time. On average, I have only fifteen to twenty minutes for each patient visit; primary care providers typically have even less. That brief period is overloaded with essential tasks that must be accomplished, from taking a history to examining the patient and explaining what's required for treatment. It's incredibly frustrating for me, and for every physician I know, not to have time to talk about lifestyle changes and other preventive measures. Our patients benefit from the educational efforts of public health workers, government agencies (particularly agencies within Health and Human Services), schools, and voluntary health associations such as the ADA. But health promotion must be built into the healthcare system.

Who should pay to promote healthy living? There must be multiple payers, including individuals, the insurance industry, employers, unions, and the private sector via philanthropy. But the predominant payer must remain the government. As an ever-increasing portion of the gross national product is consumed by healthcare costs—with a large proportion of those dollars coming from government coffers—the government stands to gain the most. That's because preventing disease is much more cost-effective than treating it.

PUSHING PREVENTION IN THE RESEARCH AGENDA

I've been pleased to see increasing government efforts aimed at preventing diabesity. Secretary of Health and Human Services Tommy G. Thompson has been a vocal force in focusing our nation on prevention—and he's set an inspiring personal example. Concerned about curbing the obesity and diabetes epidemics, he lost 15 pounds and began an exercise program. To ensure that he took 10,000 steps every day—the equivalent of walking nearly five miles—he started wearing a pedometer. He challenged the staff of his agency to do the same. Every time he climbs up on a podium to speak, he tells his audience about the benefits of taking 10,000 steps a day.

Secretary Thompson has talked about prevention, and he's funded preventive efforts through the Centers for Disease Control and Prevention and the National Institutes of Health. But much more is needed to combat diabesity. For example, in 2001 the CDC spent approximately $16 million on the promotion of healthy lifestyles and obesity prevention combined. In contrast, $100 million was spent on tobacco control. Yet the physical harm done by obesity is comparable to that associated with smoking.

Research on preventive measures also is critically needed. I've spent my career as a clinical researcher, and two years ago I started the project of my life, becoming the chair of STOPP-T2D—Studies to Treat or Prevent Pediatric Type 2 Diabetes. These NIH-funded studies, under the auspices of the National Institute of Diabetes and Digestive and Kidney Diseases (NIDDK), involve investigators from sixteen university medical centers around the country and will last for five years. When Dr. Judith Fradkin, head of the diabetes branch of the NIH, asked if I wanted to chair these trials, I was beyond flattered—I was speechless. NIH is spending nearly $10 million per year on STOPP-T2D, attesting to concern about the diabesity epidemic in children.

The study groups are made up of pediatric endocrinologists, psychologists, nurses, nutritionists, and research coordinators from the participating medical centers. Before we began to write our research protocols, Dr. Fradkin, Dr. Barbara Linder, the project coordinator from the NIDDK, and I convened a planning meeting in Washington, D.C. Together with the investigators, we discussed goals and possible projects. At the meeting, and during the numerous follow-up conference calls, there was a huge debate about whether it was possible to devise programs that could help children and their parents change their lifestyle habits.

Many members of the study group argued that it wasn't possible to accomplish such a monumental task. They said that families were set in their ways. If they hadn't exercised or eaten fresh fruits and vegetables in years, was there any reason to think we could persuade them to behave differently? These investigators felt that most people weren't prepared to make changes because they didn't see the necessity; they didn't understand that they were compromising their health by being sedentary or weighing too much. Furthermore, even if they wanted to change, there were simply too many environmental barriers in the way.

On the other side of the argument were group members who insisted that people could get past the obstacles if only they were given the tools. If they could have a place to exercise, a nutrition plan to follow, and plenty of support and encouragement, they'd be able to adopt healthy lifestyle habits. I share this view and was delighted when it prevailed. STOPP-T2D will fund research to see whether weekly meetings with a lifestyle coach can help children with diabetes eat better and exercise more. We will know that these meetings are successful if the youngsters lose weight and improve their diabetes management. We will also test whether middle school children can be persuaded to select healthy food options at school and to exercise strenuously enough during physical education classes to elevate their heart rates. And we will figure out if creating a buzz about health in school helps kids form good habits.

I believe our research will show that children are capable of improving their lifestyles. The techniques we develop may not be "rocket science," the high-tech solutions that most people associate with NIH-funded research. But our interventions will be even more important if they show us simple, practical ways to combat diabesity.

CONNECTING WITH COMMUNITIES

We in the healthcare profession can't fight diabesity without community support. A myriad of commercial and nonprofit community organizations deliver health-related programs and services. Community resources—including service centers, churches, synagogues, mosques, shopping malls, parks, libraries, and local newspapers—are our natural allies in preventing obesity and diabetes. All of them can serve as platforms to improve nutrition and physical activity levels and to help people become motivated to change.

I've been encouraged by a national trend for hospitals, including mine, to forge links with the communities they serve. In the past, I wasn't aware of the resources available near where my patients live, resources that could help them become healthier. There was no mechanism by which I could bridge the gap between advice like "I suggest you swim or walk together as a family" and all the practical steps necessary for them to do that. I didn't know if they had access to a beach or swimming pool; I had no idea whether there was a park or safe place to walk nearby.

Now, however, communities around the country are creating Internet-based ways to locate health resources. My own hospital recently launched an initiative with several local partners to develop an online asset map of Los Angeles. This map lists family programs, parks and recreation facilities, social service agencies, and health-care facilities. I can use it to locate resources for my patients and their families.

For example, one of my patients—a fourteen-year-old boy named Todd—was interested in tennis lessons. I was delighted. Todd was inactive and obese; he had diabetes. He'd never held a tennis racket or hit a tennis ball. But after watching an exciting match on TV, he wanted to play this game. I thought it was a great idea. But Todd knew of no place in his neighborhood to learn tennis. So I went to the asset map Web site and typed in his zip code and "tennis lessons." Within seconds, I discovered that a boys' club not far from his house offers tennis lessons in the spring. The mother of another patient wanted to find fresh vegetables that she could afford. Her neighborhood had no health food stores and no supermarkets, only convenience stores. I entered her zip code, typed in "fresh produce," and learned about a Friday farmers' market just one bus stop away from her home.

REACHING OUT TO THE BARRIOS

In the spring of 2003, I was asked to speak about diabesity at a Catholic church in one of the barrios, a center of L.A.'s Latino community. I jumped at the opportunity. I know that if I am to have an

impact in the war against diabesity, I must spread the message beyond the hospital. So I was eager to speak with people from a community that has been hit particularly hard by this epidemic.

As I prepared my presentation, I tried to decide which of my
PowerPoint slides to show at the church. I wanted them to understand that Latino youth and young adults were increasingly affected.
But I also was eager to show slides explaining how over-consumption
of calories, sedentary behavior, and thrifty genes caused insulin resistance, and how insulin resistance led to obesity and diabetes. I
planned to emphasize how important it was to identify people at risk
and to diagnose diabetes as early as possible in order to manage it effectively and to avoid complications such as cardiovascular disease.
To lighten my presentation, I added a few PowerPoint pictures from
my trips to Ecuador and India. I clicked through the images,
arranged them carefully, and I was set.

At the church I was greeted by a vigorous man of about fifty who
was in charge of maintenance. He brought me into the community
hall and immediately made me feel welcome. As we walked, he told
me about his family—a wife and five children ages four to nineteen.
He said that he and his wife would do anything for their children.
When I told him about the subject of my talk, he expressed pride in
his own good health and that of his family. But he said that he was
concerned about the health of many of his friends, the members of
the church.

The streets outside the church had been dark and quiet, but inside were bright lights, a cacophony of voices, and the aroma of tortillas and fried meat. At least a hundred people were waiting to hear
me speak: old men and women, young couples with babies, multi-
generational families, and singles. I found Katie, the community
worker who had invited me. She was clearly Anglo, with blond hair
and a pleasant face. I asked her where I could plug in my computer
and connect to their projector. "Projector?" Katie responded in astonishment. "I'm not sure we have a working projector. I didn't
know you needed one."

"I put together a PowerPoint presentation about obesity and diabetes," I said. Katie looked dismayed. I felt embarrassed. Obviously, I'd totally misread my audience. The people who'd gathered

to hear me needed a friendly question-and-answer period, not a lecture on the diabetes disease process illustrated with PowerPoint slides filled with arrows and equations. They wanted my interest and attention, evidence that the healthcare system is concerned about them.

"I can just talk, Katie. That will be better," I said.

Katie looked relieved. "First you'll have some food, and then we can start," she said, leading me to the back of the hall, in the direction of the incredible smell. As we walked, Katie greeted people. Unlike me, she spoke perfect Spanish, and I was grateful that she could translate.

Two older women approached us. One handed me a full plate with a corn tortilla, beans, and salad; the other gave me a tall glass of lemonade. The woman who'd given me the plate said, "Eat, es bueno, good." Then she said something to Katie. Katie laughed, then turned to me and translated: "She thinks you're too thin. She says she guesses that's why you're here, to tell us how to be too thin, too." I thanked the women and asked Katie to tell them that the food smelled fantastic. I ate the salad and the beans; after I picked out the fried meat, I ate the tortilla, too. The food was home-cooked, and it really was fantastic.

Katie moved to the front of the room, gesturing for me to follow. As I did, everyone picked up chairs and created four big concentric semicircles with me in the middle. The older people sat in the front rows. In the outer row were the young mothers, positioned so they could watch their children, who were either jumping around or asleep in strollers. The man who had greeted me brought two chairs to the front for Katie and me.

"This is Doctora Francine Kaufman," Katie began. She spoke first in English, then repeated what she said in Spanish. "She is a very famous doctor for children who have diabetes. And she is president of the American Diabetes Association, the group that helps to run our health fair. Doctora Kaufman will say a few words, and then she will answer your questions."

By now it was after eight. I hoped the session wouldn't run past nine, since I was tired and I had an early meeting at the hospital the following morning. I thanked Katie for giving me the opportunity to speak, and I thanked everyone for a wonderful dinner. As Katie translated, I looked at the two women who had served me. They smiled and nodded. Then I asked how many people in the audience had been told that they or someone in their family had diabetes. Almost all of the hands went up. This wasn't surprising; usually people who attend community diabetes talks are connected to the disease directly or through a loved one. I told them diabetes was common, particularly among Latinos. And then I told them diabetes was very serious, that people with diabetes were at risk for a lot of problems, including heart attacks and stroke. I paused for a minute while Katie translated. As she did, heads nodded again.

I asked how many with diabetes were checking their blood sugar levels at home. Very few hands went up. I went through the ABCs of diabetes. A: Know your glucose level by taking the A1c blood test at least every six to twelve months, more often if you are on insulin or other medications. B: Know your blood pressure. C: Know your cholesterol level. I asked how many knew their blood pressure, and a few more hands went up. Then I asked about cholesterol. Hands went down again.

I already knew from research reports that many patients with diabetes are unaware of their blood sugar, blood pressure, and cholesterol levels. But even though I was prepared, I was still disheartened. There I was, in a room filled with people with diabetes or at risk for the disease, and only a few of them had essential information about their own health status. I emphasized how important it was that they learn these numbers. I told them I would leave brochures in Spanish from the American Diabetes Association to explain more about glucose testing, blood pressure, and cholesterol. And then I invited questions.

A woman in the first row struggled to her feet. She looked about fifty years old and at least 70 pounds overweight. Speaking in Spanish, she asked, "Why is it bad to weigh too much? And why is it bad to fry food?" I understood her questions, but I waited for Katie to translate because I needed more time to think about what to say. I needed simple answers, but there are no simple answers to these questions, which are so complicated that they will be studied and restudied until the end of time.

"Weighing too much is a strain on the body and on all the organs inside the body. Fried foods make you weigh too much," I responded. Not a bad start, but I wanted to say so much more. I wanted to explain about thrifty genes; I wanted to talk about adipocytes, the fat cells, and to tell her about insulin resistance. But as Katie translated, the woman sat down. Clearly, I'd told her enough.

A young mother asked from the back of the room, "What does it mean when su baby es too fat when borned?" She was rocking a stroller, and she was at least 30 pounds overweight. I knew I needed to be careful. She might have had gestational diabetes, and it might have persisted. Her baby might have a medical problem. Katie translated the question into Spanish.

I measured every word. "Sometimes a baby's weight indicates that the mother had sugar problems during pregnancy—we call that diabetes of pregnancy. But women without diabetes can have large babies, too. Usually a woman is checked for diabetes, particularly if it looks like she's carrying a big baby. She is checked during pregnancy—sometimes more than once—and again after birth, if needed. A baby who is born large is observed right after birth. That is the critical time, because the baby's blood sugar can drop too low. Also, the baby needs to be checked for problems."

The woman leaned forward, listening intently. When I was finished, she asked, "Should the woman do something, like examinar her blood after she have birth? And her child? If no problems right away, no worry later?"

"She should talk to her doctor about herself and to the baby's doctor about the baby," I told her. How could I offer medical advice concerning a baby and a woman that I hadn't examined? But I didn't know if this young woman actually had a doctor she could talk to. My head was filled with thoughts I wasn't saying aloud: that I hoped she'd had a glucose test during pregnancy and that the results were normal. That I hoped her baby had been born normal, without evidence of exposure to diabetes in utero and without low blood sugar problems after birth. I didn't want to imagine that she'd had inadequate medical care during her pregnancy and that gestational diabetes was missed, or that the baby had suffered undiagnosed sugar problems during the immediate neonatal period, something that could result in brain damage. I added, "It would be important for that woman to lose weight and to start an exercise program. And it would be important for her to be physically fit and at a normal weight before she considered having another baby."

Katie translated, then put in her own contribution: "Women like that can come to the church's Walk on Sunday Program and the American Diabetes Association Health Fair." She told them about the Women, Infants, and Children (WIC) program of the U.S. Department of Agriculture, which encourages breast-feeding and also provides nutrition information and supplemental food to those in need. As she spoke, I felt relieved. I was sitting in a church inside a community that had resources to help. I could be a catalyst to make them aware of programs within their reach.

I continued to answer questions. "Why did my doctor tell me I had a little stroke?" "Why did my husband lose his leg?" "What is a kidney machine?" "Why does insulin have to come only in a needle?" "What does diabetes do to the eyes?" "Why do my medicines cost so much?" The questions were as good as those I get from the college students who do community service with us at Childrens Hospital Los Angeles, and the questioners were just as interested. When I glanced at my watch at the end of the meeting, I was astonished to see that it was nearly ten, an hour later than I had hoped to leave. But I was the one who had to be torn away. I was having too good a time talking with people from a community that cared.

On the way home, I envisioned all the roadblocks that kept people from good, affordable medical care. I thought about the power of a concerned healthcare team—doctors, nurses, and nutritionists—when they approach patients in a nonjudgmental, supportive way. And I thought about Consuela. I remembered the bright colored band wrapped around her waist on that day I met her. I remembered how the sunlight made the few gray strands of her hair dance against the black background. And I remembered how devastated I was when the words "She died" spilled out of her sister's mouth.

Until we resolve as a nation to make fundamental changes in the healthcare system, people will die unnecessarily, and doctors, no matter how caring, will not be able to treat everyone who needs their help. In the meantime, I was comforted to know that the young mother at the church has support from her community as she struggles to find her way through the healthcare maze. And I liked to think that my words had empowered her to take personal steps toward a healthier life for herself and her baby.

A Choice of Futures

In the year 2020, I will be sixty-nine years old. I hope to still be working as a professor and a doctor in academic medicine, teaching, seeing patients, and conducting research. I hope to continue giving talks about diabetes prevention and treatment. But as I stand on a podium in the year 2020, what will I see? What national and international landscapes will stretch out before me? How will my audience look? I see two possibilities, depending on whether or not we commit ourselves to a comprehensive approach to diabesity prevention.

If we choose to conduct business as usual; if we fail to work together to hold back the diabetes epidemic; if individuals, families, neighborhoods, schools, community programs, corporations, the healthcare system, and the government deny that each of them is part of the fabric of an interwoven solution—then I will be on a podium describing a world in which 300 million people have diabetes.

I will talk about the 72 percent increase in diabetes worldwide since 2005. I will reveal that in North America there are now 36 million people with diabetes, in South America 26 million, in Europe 58 million, and in India and Asia 120 million. I will describe how the economies of whole nations have collapsed trying to care for this horrid disease. I will explain that in the developed world and in emerging nations a large percentage of the workforce is on permanent disability because of a wide array of obesity-related orthopedic disabilities and cardiovascular catastrophes.

Three-quarters of the people in my audience will be overweight or obese. In the back of the room will be platters of doughnuts and cans of soda. Many of the people in front of me will be asleep in their seats due to obesity-related apnea. As a result, my words will fall on deaf ears. No one will care that I'm still talking about preventing diabetes and obesity, because no one will think it can be done. Many will have tried "magic bullets" manufactured by the pharmaceutical industry to curb their appetites, increase their energy expenditure, and interfere with their nutrient absorption. Some will have submitted to bariatric surgery that permanently alters their digestive tract.

They will have tried a bucket of pills and a host of surgical procedures, but none of these interventions can work for long in an environment where food is served in supersize portions, where fat is freely added for taste, where sugar and corn syrup are universal ingredients, where sweetened soda is gulped by the gallon, where advertisements and inducements for junk food are on every TV and on every billboard, and where few engage in physical activity. The hope of a bailout by fancy drugs and high-tech procedures will not have been realized, and we will be in the midst of an epidemic the likes of which the world has never seen.

Most people over age forty will be on pills to control high blood pressure, to counteract insulin resistance, to lower cholesterol and triglycerides, to treat erectile dysfunction, or to combat depression. Obesity will be common in toddlers; third graders will have type 2 diabetes; thirty-year-olds will experience their first heart attack. The disabilities we now associate with old age will be common in midlife. Life expectancy will decline. Our overburdened healthcare system will be struggling unsuccessfully to relieve widespread suffering.

Or I could be standing on another podium in the year 2020. I imagine an auditorium where every chair has exercise resistance bands and exercise cycle pedals attached to it. As I speak, half of my audience will be strengthening their muscles and lowering their insulin resistance, while the other half will be pedaling at a moderate rate to improve cardiovascular fitness. In the back of the room will be platters of fresh fruits and vegetables, along with pitchers of water.

My audience will be living in a city in which urban sprawl has been conquered. People will use public transportation and routinely walk part of the way to work. This city will have safe parks and playgrounds located near homes, schools, libraries, and community centers. Employers will encourage physical activity. Children will be tested on physical performance in school and the results will be given equal weight with academic testing. Just about all youngsters will pass these exercise tests.

Schools will serve wholesome meals and snacks. Soda vending machines will be as unthinkable in schools and hospitals as cigarette vending machines were in 2005. Fast food restaurants will still sprinkle the landscape, but their menus will have changed markedly. Beverages will be unsweetened. They'll offer salads, crunchy vegetable sticks, and fresh fruit. Meat, fish, and poultry will be lean, with greatly reduced saturated fat. In school, in restaurants, and at home, portion sizes will be appropriate.

From my vantage point atop this podium, I can see that most people in my audience are of normal weight. Few need pharmaceutical agents to be healthy. High blood pressure and high cholesterol have become uncommon. Thanks to comprehensive healthcare reform, everyone has health insurance. The system has been funded in part by cost savings realized by turning to a preventive rather than a treatment model; taxes on junk food and sweetened beverages provide supplemental funding. People look forward to living well into their eighties, nineties, and even past a hundred in good health, able to accomplish their personal goals and dreams.

Which scenario will we see in 2020? I don't know. But the future is up to us. We must determine what legacy we will leave to our children and to all the children yet to come. I only hope we make the right decisions.

APPENDIX

Resources

Peonle diagnosed with diabetes must learn to navigate in a new
world, the world of living with diabetes. Managing this complicated disease involves new knowledge and new routines. Typically,
the whole family is involved. Adjustments continue over the years.
This isn't easy, and no one should try to go it alone. Just as it takes a
village to raise a child, it takes a team of professionals to help a person and family coping with diabetes—physicians, nurses, nutritionists, social workers, psychologists, community health workers,
exercise physiologists, pharmacists, and other healthcare providers.
This team can be assembled in a doctor's office, health maintenance
organization, community hospital, or academic medical center.

I suggest the following survival steps for anyone who has just
been diagnosed: assemble a team and then find the American Diabetes Association. The ADA has a Web site filled with information for
people with diabetes (www.diabetes.org); it has a call center for those
who need to talk with a live person (1–800-DIABETES). The ADA's
bookstore offers a wide selection of books that inform, motivate, and
inspire, including books on general self-care, nutrition, fitness, and
parenting. Cookbooks abound. The ADA publishes a monthly magazine and even sells pedometers as part of the Small Steps Big Rewards

program. It runs seminars, camps, walks, and programs—including programs designed especially for children, for the elderly, and for members of particular racial or ethnic groups. The ADA helps protect people with diabetes through its advocacy activities. It trains professionals, funds research, and forms partnerships with the pharmaceutical companies and other diabetes-related businesses. The American Diabetes Association is like glue for people with diabetes. After they receive their diagnosis, they may feel that they're falling apart. The ADA is there to help put them back together.

The following resources provide additional information and assistance:

OTHER ORGANIZATIONS AND AGENCIES

The Juvenile Diabetes Research Foundation International (JDRFI) supports research aimed at finding a cure for type 1 diabetes. They are strong advocates for research funding, and they let people know how they can help move the research agenda forward. Their Web site has a special section for children that provides help for dealing with diabetes day-to-day. (1-800-533-CURE; www.jdrf.org)

The International Diabetes Federation (IDF), based in Brussels, Belgium, works worldwide to promote diabetes awareness and access to diabetes prevention and care. Their magazine, *Diabetes Voice*, and other information are available online (www.idf.org).

The National Diabetes Education Program (NDEP) is a partnership of the National Institutes of Health, the Centers for Disease Control and Prevention, and more than 200 public and private organizations, including the American Diabetes Association. NDEP focuses on three major campaigns: Control Your Diabetes for Life; Be Smart About Your Heart—Control the ABCs of Diabetes; and Small Steps Big Rewards—Preventing Type 2 Diabetes. The NDEP offers a directory of diabetes organizations, fact sheets, and information on prevention and treatment—all in multiple languages. (1-800-438-5383; www.ndep.nih.gov)

The Centers for Disease Control and Prevention (CDC) has a diabetes division that translates diabetes research into daily practice. Their goals are to help people understand the impact of the disease, influence health outcomes, and improve access to quality health care. The CDC publishes fact sheets and other helpful information about diabetes, and offers suggestions about healthy eating and physical activity (1-877-CDC-DIAB; www.cdc.gov/diabetes). A page on the CDC Web site calculates your BMI if you enter your height and weight, and it displays normal growth curves for children (www.cdc.gov/nccdphp/dnpa/bmi).

The National Institute of Diabetes and Digestive and Kidney Diseases (NIDDK) offers the National Diabetes Information Clearinghouse, which provides extensive information in English and Spanish for people with diabetes—including a list of clinical trials (1-800-860-8747; www.diabetes.niddk.nih.gov).

OTHER ONLINE RESOURCES

MedlinePlus (www.medlineplus.gov), part of the National Library of Medicine, has extensive information from the National Institutes of Health and other trusted sources about over 650 diseases and conditions—including diabetes and obesity. The site also provides lists of hospitals and physicians, a medical encyclopedia and a medical dictionary, extensive information on prescription and nonprescription drugs, and links to thousands of clinical trials. There is no advertising on this site, nor does MedlinePlus endorse any company or product. Information is offered in English and Spanish.

Children with Diabetes (www.childrenwithdiabetes.com) was established by a concerned and talented father, Jeff Hitchcock. The site serves as an online community for youngsters with diabetes and their families. It provides updates on the latest diabetes research, discussions of school issues, practical information, and a chat room. Members have the opportunity to meet in person during the summer for a family seminar (locations alternate between the East and West coast), where

fun activities are coupled with educational and motivational
sessions.

BOOKS

For a comprehensive book about living with diabetes, see *The
American Diabetes Association Complete Guide to Diabetes, Third Edition* (Bantam, 2003)

Other self-help books include:

Healing Our Village: A Self-Care Guide to Diabetes Control by Lenore
    T. Coleman and James R. Gavin (Healing Our Village Publish-
    ing, 2004)

*Dr. Gavin's Health Guide for African Americans: How to Keep Yourself
    and Children Well* by James R. Gavin (American Diabetes Asso-
    ciation, 2004)

The Way to Eat: A Six-Step Path to Lifelong Weight Control by David
    L. Katz and Harrigan Gonzales (Sourcebooks, 2004)

Many books have covered the obesity epidemic. These include:

Fat Land: How Americans Became the Fattest People in the World by
    Greg Critser (Mariner Books, 2004)

*Food Fight: The Inside Story of the Food Industry, America's Obesity Cri-
    sis, and What We Can Do About It* by Kelly D. Brownell and
    Katherine Battle Horgen (McGraw-Hill, 2003)

Food Politics: How the Food Industry Influences Nutrition and Health by
    Marion Nestle (University of California Press, 2003)

Fat: Fighting the Obesity Epidemic by Robert Pool (Oxford University
    Press, 2001)

Fast Food Nation: The Dark Side of the All-American Meal by Eric
    Schlosser (Perennial, 2002)

Notes

1. A Tale of Two Children

7   *Ninety percent of people with diabetes:* World Health Organization. Fact sheet no. 138. April 2002. Available at www.diabetes.org.

8   *In fact, the symptoms are so subtle:* Dallo FJ, Weller SC. Effectiveness of diabetes mellitus screening recommendations. Proceedings of the National Academy of Sciences of the United States of America 2003;100(18). Available at http://www.pnas.org/cgi/content/full/100/18/10574. Harris MI, Flegal KM, Cowie CC, Eberhardt MS, Goldstein DE, Little RR, Wiedmeyer HM, Byrd-Holt DD. Prevalence of diabetes, impaired fasting glucose, and impaired glucose tolerance in U.S. adults. The Third National Health and Nutrition Examination Survey, 1988–1994. Diabetes Care 1998;21:518–524. American Diabetes Association. All About Diabetes. Available at http://www.diabetes.org/about-diabetes.jsp.

13   *In 1990, 4.9 percent of the American adult population:* Mokdad AH, Ford ES, Bowman BA, Nelson DE, Engelgau MM, Vinicor F, Marks JS. Diabetes trends in the U.S.: 1990–1998. Diabetes Care 2000;23(9):1278–1283.
     ...and by 2002, it had soared to 8.7 percent in adults: American Diabetes Association Web site. Available at http://www.diabetes.org/diabetes-statistics/national-diabetes-fact-sheet.jsp.
     Ninety percent of them have type 2: American Diabetes Association Web site. Available at www.diabetes.org. National Institute of Diabetes and Digestive and Kidney Diseases. National diabetes statistics fact sheet: general information and national estimates on diabetes in the United States, 2003. Bethesda, MD: U.S. Department of Health and Human

Services, National Institutes of Health, 2003. 1999–2001 National
Health Interview Survey (NHIS), National Center for Health Statistics,
Centers for Disease Control and Prevention. U.S. Bureau of the Census,
2002 population estimates. Fagot-Campagna A, Pettitt DJ, Engelgau
MM, Burrows NR, Geiss LS, Valdez R, Beckles GL, Saadine J, Gregg
EW, Williamson DF, Narayan KM. Type 2 diabetes among North
American children and adolescents: an epidemiologic review and a pub-
lic health perspective. Journal of Pediatrics 2000;136:664–672. Ludwig
DS, Ebbeling CB. Type 2 diabetes mellitus in children: primary care and
public health considerations. Journal of the American Medical Association 2001;286:1427–1430.

That is almost 30 percent of the adult population: U.S. Department of Health
and Human Services, National Center for Health Statistics. Obesity still
on the rise, new data show. Available at http://www.cdc.gov/nchs/
releases/02news/obesityonrise.htm. U.S. Department of Health and
Human Services, National Center for Health Statistics. Healthy weight,
overweight, and obesity among persons 20 years of age and over, according to sex, age, race, and Hispanic origin: United States, 1960–62, 1971–
74, 1976–80, 1988–94, and 1999–2000. Available at http://www.cdc.gov/
nchs/data/hus/tables/2002/02hus070.pdf. Flegal KM, Carroll MD,
Ogden CL, Johnson CL. Prevalence and trends in obesity among U.S.
adults, 1999–2000. Journal of the American Medical Association
2002;288:1723–1727.

14   *Shape Up America, an organization founded in 1994:* The contributions of
diet and inactivity to diabesity in America: an agenda for action. Available at http://www.shapeup.org/profcenter/diabesity/. Accessed March
8, 2004. Dunstan D, Zimmet P, Welborn T, Sicree R, Armstrong T,
Atkins R, Cameron A, Shaw J, Chadban S, on behalf of the Australian
Diabetes Steering Committee. Diabesity and associated disorders in
Australia 2000: the accelerating epidemic. Melbourne: International Diabetes Institute, 2001. Mokdad A, Bowman B, Ford E, Vinicor F,
Marks J, Kaplan J. The continuing epidemic of obesity and diabesity
in the United States. Journal of the American Medical Association
2001;286:1195–2000.

Over the past three decades: U.S. Department of Health and Human Services, National Center for Health Statistics. Overweight children and
adolescents 6–19 years of age, according to sex, age, race, and Hispanic
origin: United States, selected years 1963–65 through 1999–2000. Available at http://www.cdc.gov/nchs/data/hus/tables/2002/02hus071.pdf.

An estimated 18.2 million Americans: American Diabetes Association.
National Diabetes Fact Sheet. Available at http://www.diabetes.org/
diabetes-statistics/national-diabetes-fact-sheet.jsp. National Institute of
Diabetes and Digestive and Kidney Diseases. National diabetes statistics
fact sheet: general information and national estimates on diabetes in the
United States, 2003. Bethesda, MD: U.S. Department of Health and
Human Services, National Institutes of Health, 2003. 1999–2001 Na-
tional Health Interview Survey (NHIS), National Center for Health Sta-
tistics, Centers for Disease Control and Prevention. U.S. Bureau of the
Census, 2002 population estimates. Cowie CC, Rust KF, Byrd-Holt D,
Eberhardt MS, Saydah S, Geiss LS, Engelgau MM, Ford ES, Gregg
EW. Prevalence of diabetes and impaired fasting glucose in adults—

United States, 1999–2000. Morbidity and Mortality Weekly Review 2003;52(35):833–837.

Even more ominous: more than twice as many people: American Diabetes Association. Diagnosis and classification of diabetes. Diabetes Care 2004;27(suppl 1):S5–S10. American Diabetes Association. What is prediabetes? Available at http://www.diabetes.org/pre-diabetes.jsp. Accessed July 8, 2004.

15   *Diabetes is the sixth leading cause of death:* American Diabetes Association. Economic costs of diabetes in the U.S. in 2002. Diabetes Care 2003;26:917–932. National Institute of Diabetes and Digestive and Kidney Diseases. National diabetes statistics fact sheet: general information and national estimates on diabetes in the United States, 2003. Bethesda, MD: U.S. Department of Health and Human Services, National Institutes of Health, 2003. Geiss LS, Herman WH, Smith PJ. Mortality in non-insulin-dependent diabetes. In: National Diabetes Data Group, eds. Diabetes in America. 2nd ed. NIH publication no. 95-1468. Washington, DC: U.S. Department of Health and Human Services, National Institutes of Health, National Institute of Diabetes and Digestive and Kidney Diseases, 1995. pp. 233–257. Kuller LH. Stroke and diabetes. In: National Diabetes Data Group, eds. Diabetes in America. 2nd ed. NIH publication no. 95-1468. Washington, DC: U.S. Department of Health and Human Services, National Institutes of Health, National Institute of Diabetes and Digestive and Kidney Diseases, 1995. pp. 449–456.

Every year in the United States, 24,000 people: American Diabetes Association. Diabetes and retinopathy. Available at http://www.diabetes. org/diabetes-statistics/eye-complications.jsp. Fong DS, Aiello L, Gardner TW, King GL, Blankenship G, Cavallerano JD, Ferris FL III, Klein R, for the American Diabetes Association. Retinopathy in diabetes. Diabetes Care 2004;27(suppl 1):S84–S87. Klein R, Klein BEK. Vision disorders in diabetes. In: National Diabetes Data Group, eds. Diabetes in America. 2nd ed. NIH publication no. 95-1468. Washington, DC: U.S. Department of Health and Human Services, National Institutes of Health, National Institute of Diabetes and Digestive and Kidney Diseases, 1995. pp. 293–336. Will JC, Geiss LS, Wetterhall SF. Diabetic retinopathy [letter]. New England Journal of Medicine 1990;323:613.

Twenty-eight thousand people end up in kidney failure: American Diabetes Association. Diabetes and nephropathy. Available at http://www.diabetes. org/diabetes-statistics/kidney-disease.jsp. U.S. Renal Data System. USRDS 2003 annual data report: atlas of end-stage renal disease in the United States. Bethesda, MD: National Institutes of Health, National Institute of Diabetes and Digestive and Kidney Diseases, 2003. American Diabetes Association. Diabetes and cardiovascular disease. Available at http://www.diabetes.org/diabetes-statistics/heart-disease.jsp.

Eighty-two thousand people with diabetes will have an amputation: Unpublished data from the 2000–2001 National Hospital Discharge Survey, National Center for Health Statistics, Centers for Disease Control and Prevention.

African Americans are 1.6 times more likely to develop diabetes: American Diabetes Association. Diabetes statistics for African Americans. Available at http://www.diabetes.org/diabetes-statistics/african-americans.jsp.

On average, the risk is 1.5 times higher for Hispanic Americans: American

Diabetes Association. Diabetes statistics for Latinos. Available at http://www.diabetes.org/diabetes-statistics/latinos.jsp.

16   *In the U.S. in 2002, the tab for diabetes-related doctor visits:* Hogan P, Dall T, Nikolov P, for the American Diabetes Association. Economic costs of diabetes mellitus in the U.S. in 2002. Diabetes Care 2003;26:917–932. *The bottom line comes to $137.7 billion:* Ibid.

18   *We don't have to watch 300 million people worldwide develop diabetes:* King H, Aubert R, Herman W. Global burden of diabetes, 1995–2025: prevalence, numerical estimates, and projections. Diabetes Care 1998;21(9). Zimmet P. Diabetes epidemiology as a trigger to diabetes research. Diabetologia 1999;42:499–518. World Health Organization. Fact sheet no. 138. April 2002.

2. Diabetes Descends on My Grandma Sadie

24   *Diabetes is a terrible affliction, not very frequent among men:* Bliss M. The discovery of insulin. Chicago: University of Chicago Press, 1984. (Earliest known record of diabetes mentioned on 3rd dynasty Egyptian papyrus by physician Hesy-Ra; mentions polyuria [frequent urination] as a symptom.) von Engelhardt D, ed. Diabetes: its medical and cultural history. Berlin: Springer-Verlag, 1989. p. 3.

25   *In 1869 Paul Langerhans—a German doctor who studied anatomy—identified special cells:* Saudek CD. 2002 presidential address: a tide in the affairs of medicine. 62nd annual American Diabetes Association meeting, June 14–18, 2002. Diabetes Care 2003;26. Bliss M. The discovery of insulin. Chicago: University of Chicago Press, 1984. Bliss M. William Osler: a life in medicine. New York: Oxford University Press, 1999. Bliss M. Rewriting medical history: Charles Best and the Banting and Best myth. Journal of the History of Medical Allied Science 1993;48:253–274. Bliss M: Banting: a biography. 2nd ed. Toronto: University of Toronto Press, 1992.

This verified that the pancreas was responsible for maintaining normal sugar metabolism: Houssay BA. The discovery of pancreatic diabetes: the role of Oskar Minkowski. In: von Engelhardt D, ed. Diabetes: its medical and cultural history. Berlin: Springer-Verlag, 1989. Saudek CD. 2002 presidential address: a tide in the affairs of medicine. 62nd annual American Diabetes Association meeting, June 14–18, 2002. Diabetes Care 2003;26. Joseph, Baron von Mering. Encyclopædia Britannica. 2004. Canadian Diabetes Association. The history of diabetes. Available at http://www.diabetes.ca/Section_About/timeline.asp. Adams F, ed. and trans. The extant works of Aretaeus, the Capadocian. London: The Sydenham Society, 1856. pp. 38–40. Quoted in Sanders LJ. The philatelic history of diabetes: in search of a cure. Alexandria, VA: American Diabetes Association, 2001. Macleod JJR. History of the researches leading to the discovery of insulin (1922), letter of Macleod to Col. Albert Gooderham. Bulletin of the History of Medicine 1978;52:295–312. Saudek CD. 2002 presidential address: a tide in the affairs of medicine. 62nd annual American Diabetes Association meeting, June 14–18, 2002. Diabetes Care 2003;26.

26   *In 1923, Frederick Banting and one of his associates shared a Nobel prize:* Canadian Diabetes Association. The history of diabetes. Available at http://www.diabetes.ca/Section_About/timeline.asp.
        Leonard Thompson—who had not been expected to live for more than a few months: Ibid.
30   *Approximately 4 percent of pregnancies—about 135,000 per year—are complicated by gestational diabetes:* American Diabetes Association. Diabetes statistics for women. Available at http://www.diabetes.org/diabetes-statistics/women.jsp.
        Finding and treating gestational diabetes is important for both baby and mother: Coustan D, Reece AE. Diabetes mellitus in pregnancy. 2nd ed. New York: Churchill Livingstone, 1995. Jovanovic-Peterson L, Biermann J, Toohey B. The diabetic woman. 2nd ed. New York: Putnam, 1996. American Diabetes Association. Gestational diabetes. Available at http://www.diabetes.org/gestational-diabetes.jsp.

3. The March to Type 2 Diabetes

36   *According to a study published in the* New England Journal of Medicine: Klein S, Fontana L, Young VL, Coggan AR, Kilo C, Patterson BW, Mohammed BS. Absence of an effect of liposuction on insulin action and risk factors for coronary heart disease. New England Journal of Medicine 2004;350:2549–2557.
38   *Overnight, when no food is consumed, blood sugar drops to its lowest point:* Blood sugar levels: what's normal? Mayo Foundation for Medical Education and Research (MFMER) Web site. Available at www.mayoclinic.com.
        Pre-diabetes is diagnosed when fasting blood sugar is elevated but not high enough to be considered diabetic: American Diabetes Association. Frequently asked questions about pre-diabetes. Available at http://www.diabetes.org/pre-diabetes/faq.jsp. Meigs JB, Nathan DM, D'Agostino RB Sr, Wilson PW, for the Framingham Offspring Study. Fasting and postchallenge glycemia and cardiovascular disease risk: the Framingham Offspring Study. Diabetes Care 2002;10:1845–1850. Smith NL, Barzilay JI, Shaffer D, Savage PJ, Heckbert SR, Kuller LH, Kronmal RA, Resnick HE, Psaty BM. Fasting and 2-hour postchallenge serum glucose measures and risk of incident cardiovascular events in the elderly: the Cardiovascular Health Study. Archives of Internal Medicine 2002;162:209–216.
38–39   *Though many of them don't know it, more than 41 million Americans have pre-diabetes:* American Diabetes Association. What is pre-diabetes? Available at http://www.diabetes.org/pre-diabetes.jsp. Accessed July 8, 2004. Third National Health and Nutrition Examination Survey (NHANES III), National Center for Health Statistics, Centers for Disease Control and Prevention. U.S. Bureau of the Census, 2000 population estimates. Methods: The prevalence of IGT, IFG, and pre-diabetes were estimated from NHANES III. Persons previously diagnosed with diabetes and persons with undiagnosed diabetes (i.e., persons without a history of diabetes but with a fasting plasma glucose of 126 or more) were excluded from the prevalence counts of IGT, IFG, and pre-diabetes. Persons were classified as having IGT if they had a 2-hour plasma glucose value of 140

to 199 mg/dL after an oral glucose tolerance test. Persons were classified as having IFG if they had a fasting plasma glucose of 100 to 125 mg/dl (regardless of their 2-hour plasma glucose value). Persons were classified as having pre-diabetes if they had IGT or IFG or both. To estimate the number of people in 2000 with these conditions, these prevalence estimates were applied to 2000 population estimates.

39   *Studies have shown that each year about 10 percent of people with pre-diabetes will develop diabetes:* American Diabetes Association. Frequently asked questions about pre-diabetes. Available at http://www.diabetes.org/pre-diabetes/faq.jsp.

This investigation, which began in the mid-1990s, was the single most important study ever conducted in diabetes prevention: National Institute of Diabetes and Digestive and Kidney Diseases (NIDDK), National Institutes of Health. Diabetes Prevention Program questions and answers. Available at http://www.niddk.nih.gov/patient/dpp/dpp-q&a.htm. Delahanty LM, Meigs JB, Hayden D, Williamson DA, Nathan DM. Psychological and behavioral correlates of baseline BMI in the Diabetes Prevention Program (DPP). Diabetes Care 2002;25:1992–1998. Diabetes Prevention Program Research Group. Reduction in the evidence of type 2 diabetes with life-style intervention or metformin. New England Journal of Medicine 2002;346:393–403. The Diabetes Prevention Program: design and methods for a clinical trial in the prevention of type 2 diabetes. Diabetes Care 1999;22:623–634. Diabetes Prevention Program Research Group. The Diabetes Prevention Program: baseline characteristics of the randomized cohort. Diabetes Care 2000;23:1619–1629.

Twenty-seven medical centers across the United States participated: Diabetes Prevention Program Research Group. The Diabetes Prevention Program: baseline characteristics of the randomized cohort. Diabetes Care 2000;23:1619–1629.

41   *Metabolic syndrome is defined as a cluster of risk factors for diabetes and cardiovascular disease:* Reaven GM. Banting lecture 1988: role of insulin resistance in human disease. Diabetes 1988;37:1595–1607. Meigs JB. Invited commentary: insulin resistance syndrome? Syndrome X? Multiple metabolic syndrome? A syndrome at all? Factor analysis reveals patterns in the fabric of correlated metabolic risk factors [review]. American Journal of Epidemiology 2000;152:908–911. Trevisan M, Liu J, Bahsas FB, Menotti A. Syndrome X and mortality: a population-based study: Risk Factor and Life Expectancy Research Group. American Journal of Epidemiology 1998;148:958–966. American Diabetes Association. The metabolic syndrome. Available at http://www.diabetes.org/weightloss-and-exercise/weightloss/metabolicsyndrome.jsp.

42   *In 2002, a landmark study in the* New England Journal of Medicine *reported that CRP level predicted cardiovascular events:* Ridker PM, Rifai N, Rose L, Buring JE, Cook NR. Comparison of C-reactive protein and low-density lipoprotein cholesterol levels in the prediction of first cardiovascular events. New England Journal of Medicine 2002;347:1557–1565.

4. The Blood Sugar Balancing Act

54–56   *[History, background, results, and outcomes of the Diabetes Control and Complications Trial]:* DCCT Research Group. The Diabetes Control and Complications Trial (DCCT): design and methodologic considerations for the feasibility phase. Diabetes 1986;35:530–545. DCCT Research Group. Feasibility of centralized measurements of glycated hemoglobin in the Diabetes Control and Complications Trial: a multicenter study. Clinical Chemistry 1987;33:2267–2271. DCCT Research Group. The effect of intensive treatment of diabetes on the development and progression of long-term complications in insulin-dependent diabetes mellitus. New England Journal of Medicine 1993;329:977–986. DCCT Research Group. Resource utilization and costs of care in the Diabetes Control and Complications Trial. Diabetes Care 1995;18:1468–1478. DCCT Research Group. The relationship of glycemic exposure (HbA1c) to the risk of development and progression of retinopathy in the Diabetes Control and Complications Trial. Diabetes 1995;44:968–983. DCCT Research Group, Klein R, Moss S. A comparison of the study populations in the Diabetes Control and Complications Trial and the Wisconsin Epidemiologic Study of Diabetic Retinopathy. Archives of Internal Medicine 1995;155:745–754. DCCT Research Group. The effect of intensive treatment of diabetes on the development and progression of long-term complications in insulin-dependent diabetes mellitus. New England Journal of Medicine 1993;329:977–986. DCCT Research Group. Lifetime benefits and costs of intensive therapy as practiced in the Diabetes Control and Complications Trial. Journal of the American Medical Association 1996;276:1409–1415. DCCT Research Group. The absence of a glycemic threshold for the development of long-term complications: the perspective of the Diabetes Control and Complications Trial. Diabetes 1996;45:1289–1298. DCCT Research Group. Implications of the Diabetes Control and Complications Trial. Diabetes Care 2002;25:25S–27S. DCCT Research Group. Diabetes Control and Complications Trial (DCCT): update. Diabetes Care 2002;13:427–433.

57   *With type 1 diabetes, the body makes no insulin:* American Diabetes Association. Type 1 diabetes. Available at http://www.diabetes.org/type-1-diabetes.jsp.

58   *About a fifth of people with type 2 diabetes require insulin injections:* American Diabetes Association. About insulin. Available at http://www.diabetes.org/type-2-diabetes/insulin.jsp.

60   *But starting in the early 1980s, when home glucose monitors became available, guidelines became more liberal:* American Diabetes Association. Clinical practice recommendations 1996. Diabetes Care 1996;19(suppl 1):S1–S118.

         Clinical research showed that improved testing allowed patients to balance food: Böhme P, Floriot M, Sirveaux M-A, Durain D, Ziegler O, Drouin P, Guerci B. Evolution of analytical performance in portable glucose meters in the last decade. Diabetes Care 2003;26:1170–1175. Brunner GA, Ellmerer M, Sendlhofer G, Wutte A, Trajanoski Z, Schaupp L, Quehenberger F, Wach P, Krejs GJ, Pieber TR. Validation of home blood glucose meters with respect to clinical and analytical approaches. Diabetes

Care 1998;21:585–590. Poirier JY, Le Prieur N, Campion L, Guilhem I, Allannic H, Maugendre D. Clinical and statistical evaluation of self-monitoring blood glucose meters. Diabetes Care 1998;21:1919–1924.

62   *The page—called "Helping the Student with Diabetes Succeed"—explains the rights of children with diabetes:* National Diabetes Education Program. Helping the student with diabetes succeed. Available at http://www.ndep.nih.gov/resources/school.htm.

5. A Life-Altering Diagnosis

74   *Employers are not supposed to discriminate against people with any kind of disability who are qualified for a job and can carry out the work:* American Diabetes Association. Hypoglycemia and employment/licensure [position statement]. Diabetes Care 2003;26(suppl 1):S141. The role of healthcare professionals in diabetes discrimination issues at work and school. Clinical Diabetes 2003;fall.

        In 2003, a man named Jeff Kapche won an important victory: Kapche v. San Antonio, 304 F.3d 493 (5th Cir. 2002); 176 F.3d 840(5th Cir. 1999). McCarren M. Lone star. Diabetes Forecast 2003;56:56–61. Arent S, Greene M. The age of legal advocacy for diabetes. Diabetes Spectrum 1999;12:214–221.

6. Running on Empty

77   *Hypoglycemia is not a complication of diabetes itself:* American Diabetes Association. Hypoglycemia. Available at http://www.diabetes.org/type-1-diabetes/hypoglycemia.jsp.

78   *Associated with this, he or she may experience symptoms:* Ibid.

        The problem occurs in only about a quarter of people with type 2 diabetes: Cryer PE, Davis SN, Shamoon H. Hypoglycemia in diabetes. Diabetes Care 203;26:1902–1912.

86   *In the Diabetes Control and Complications Trial:* Steffes MW, Sibley S, Jackson M, Thomas W. ß-cell function and the development of diabetes-related complications in the Diabetes Control and Complications Trial. Diabetes Care 2003;26:832–836.

90   *Sixty-five teens enrolled in our study:* Kaufman FR, Halvorson M, Kaufman ND. A randomized, blinded trial of uncooked cornstarch to diminish nocturnal hypoglycemia at Diabetes Camp. Diabetes Research and Clinical Practice 1995;30(3):205–209.

91   *[Background on the creation of ExtendBars]:* Kaufman FR, Halvorson M, Kaufman ND. Evaluation of a snack bar containing uncooked cornstarch in subjects with diabetes. Diabetes Research and Clinical Practice 1997;35:25–33. Kaufman FR, Devgan S. Use of uncooked cornstarch to avert nocturnal hypoglycemia in children and adolescents with type I diabetes. Journal of Diabetes Complications 1996;10:84–87.

7. The Long Haul

95   *Dr. Heather Dean of Children's Hospital of Winnipeg:* Dean HJ. Dancing
         with many different ghosts: treatment of youth with type 2 diabetes. Di-
         abetes Care 2002;25:237–238. Sellers EA, Dean HJ. Diabetic ketoacido-
         sis: a complication of type 2 diabetes in Canadian aboriginal youth.
         Diabetes Care 2000;23:1202–1204. Sellers EAC, Triggs-Raine B,
         Rockman-Greenberg C, Dean HJ. The prevalence of the HNF-1α
         G319S mutation in Canadian aboriginal youth with type 2 diabetes. Di-
         abetes Care 2002;25: 2202–2206.

96   *The most serious complication of diabetes is cardiovascular disease:* Geiss LS,
         Herman WH, Smith PJ. Mortality in non-insulin-dependent diabetes.
         In: National Diabetes Data Group, eds. Diabetes in America. 2nd ed.
         NIH publication no. 95-1468. Washington, DC: U.S. Department of
         Health and Human Services, National Institutes of Health, National In-
         stitute of Diabetes and Digestive and Kidney Diseases, 1995. pp. 233–
         257. Kuller LH. Stroke and diabetes. In: National Diabetes Data Group,
         eds. Diabetes in America. 2nd ed. NIH publication no. 95-1468. Wash-
         ington, DC: U.S. Department of Health and Human Services, National
         Institutes of Health, National Institute of Diabetes and Digestive and
         Kidney Diseases, 1995. pp. 449–456. Geiss LS, Rolka DB, Engelgau
         MM. Elevated blood pressure among U.S. adults with diabetes, 1988–
         1994. American Journal of Preventive Medicine 2002;22:43–49. Na-
         tional Institute of Diabetes and Digestive and Kidney Diseases. National
         diabetes statistics fact sheet: general information and national estimates
         on diabetes in the United States, 2003. Bethesda, MD: U.S. Department
         of Health and Human Services, National Institutes of Health, 2003.
         Diabetes elevates heart risk even more for women than for men: Franklin K,
         Goldberg RJ, Spencer F, Klein W, Budaj A, Brieger D, Marre M, Steg PG,
         Gowda N, Gore JM, for the GRACE investigators. Implications of dia-
         betes in patients with acute coronary syndromes: the Global Registry of
         Acute Coronary Events. Archives of Internal Medicine 2004;164:1457–
         1463.

97   *This program emphasizes the importance of knowing your A1c:* Gottlieb SH.
         Know your ABC's: "A" is for A1C. Diabetes Forecast 2002.
         *In a 2003 survey of more than a thousand women, sponsored by the American
         Heart Association:* American Diabetes Association. Heart disease is great-
         est threat to women: survey shows growing awareness. Available at
         http://www.diabetes.org/diabetes-cholesterol/news-women.jsp.

101   *People with diabetes are 60 percent more likely to develop cataracts:* Klein R,
         Klein BEK. Vision disorders in diabetes. In: National Diabetes Data
         Group, eds. Diabetes in America. 2nd ed. NIH publication no. 95-1468.
         Washington, DC: U.S. Department of Health and Human Services, Na-
         tional Institutes of Health, National Institute of Diabetes and Digestive
         and Kidney Diseases, 1995. pp. 293–336. Will JC, Geiss LS, Wetterhall
         SF. Diabetic retinopathy [letter]. New England Journal of Medicine
         1990;323:613. Lang-Muritano M, La Roche GR, Stevens JL, Gloor BR,
         Schoenle EJ. Acute cataracts in newly diagnosed IDDM in five chil-
         dren and adolescents. Diabetes Care 1995;18:1395–1396. Ehrlich RM,
         Kirsch S, Daneman D. Cataracts in children with diabetes mellitus. Dia-
         betes Care 1987;10:798–799.

Glaucoma—dangerously elevated pressure inside the eye: Mapstone R, Clark CV. Prevalence of diabetes in glaucoma. British Medical Journal 1985;291:93–95. Becker B. Diabetes mellitus and primary open-angle glaucoma: the XXVII Edward Jackson memorial lecture. American Journal of Ophthalmology 1971;71:1–16. Sugar HS. Modern ophthalmology. 4th ed. London: Butterworths, 1964. chap. 6:554. Safir A, Poulsen E, Klayman J. Elevated intraocular pressure in diabetic children. Diabetes 1964;13:161. Armstrong JR, Dailv RK, Dobson HL, et al. The incidence of glaucoma in diabetes mellitus: a comparison with the incidence of glaucoma in the general population. American Journal of Ophthalmology 1960;50:55–63.

108   *Between 10 and 21 percent of people with diabetes suffer from kidney disease:* National Institute of Diabetes and Digestive and Kidney Diseases. National diabetes statistics fact sheet: general information and national estimates on diabetes in the United States, 2003. Bethesda, MD: U.S. Department of Health and Human Services, National Institutes of Health, 2003. Lewis EJ, Hunsicker LG, Clarke WR, Berl T, Pohl MA, Lewis JB, Ritz E, Atkins RC, Rohde R, Raz I, for the Collaborative Study Group. Renoprotective effect of the angiotensin-receptor antagonist irbesartan in patients with nephropathy due to type 2 diabetes. New England Journal of Medicine 2001;345:851–860. Brenner BM, Cooper ME, de Zeeuw D, Keane WF, Mitch WE, Parving HH, Remuzzi G, Snapinn SM, Zhang Z, Shahinfar S, for the RENAAL Study Investigators. Effects of losartan on renal and cardiovascular outcomes in patients with type 2 diabetes and nephropathy. New England Journal of Medicine 2001:345:861–869. Parving HH, Lehnert H, Brochner-Mortensen J, Gomis R, Andersen S, Arner P; Irbesartan in Patients with Type 2 Diabetes and Microalbuminuria Study Group. The effect of irbesartan on the development of diabetic nephropathy in patients with type 2 diabetes. New England Journal of Medicine 2001;345:870–878. Hostetter TH. Prevention of end-stage renal disease due to type 2 diabetes. New England Journal of Medicine 2001;345:910–912. Lewis EJ, Hunsicker LG, Bain RP, Rohde RD. The effect of angiotensin-converting-enzyme inhibition on diabetic nephropathy. New England Journal of Medicine 1993;329:1456–1462. U.S. Renal Data System. USRDS 2003 annual data report: atlas of end-stage renal disease in the United States. Bethesda, MD: National Institutes of Health, National Institute of Diabetes and Digestive and Kidney Diseases, 2003.
       Approximately 43 percent of new ESRD cases are attributed to diabetes: American Diabetes Association. Diabetes and nephropathy (kidney complications). Available at http://www.diabetes.org/diabetes-statistics/kidney-disease.jsp.

111   *In addition, we have novel and experimental wound treatments:* Hirn M. Hyperbaric oxygen in the treatment of gas gangrene and perineal necrotizing fasciitis. A clinical and experimental study. European Journal of Surgery (Supplement) 1993;570:1–36. Hirn M, Niinikoski J, Lehtonen OP. Effect of hyperbaric oxygen and surgery on experimental gas gangrene. European Surgical Research 1992;24(6):356–362. Bakker DJ. Hyperbaric oxygen therapy and the diabetic foot. Diabetes Metabolism Research and Review 2000;16(suppl 1):S55–S58. Baroni G, Porro T, Fuglia E et al. Hyperbaric oxygen in diabetic gangrene treatment.

Diabetes Care 1987;10:81–86. Brakora MJ, Sheffield PJ. Hyperbaric oxygen therapy for diabetic wounds. Clinic in Podiatric Medicine and Surgery 1995;12(1):105–117. Cavanagh PR, Buse JB, Frykberg RG, et al. Consensus development conference on diabetic foot wound care. Diabetes Care 1999;22(8):1354–1360. Cianci P, Hunt TK. Adjunctive hyperbaric oxygen therapy in treatment of diabetic foot wounds. In: Levin ME, O'Neal LW, Bowker JE, eds. The Diabetic Foot. 5th ed. St. Louis: Mosby Year Book, 1992. chap. 14:306–319.

Each year, approximately 82,000 people with diabetes lose one or more toes, a foot, or even a leg: Unpublished data from the 2000–2001 National Hospital Discharge Survey, National Center for Health Statistics, Centers for Disease Control and Prevention. American Diabetes Association Web site. National Diabetes Fact Sheet. Available at http://www.diabetes.org/diabetes-statistics/national-diabetes-fact-sheet.jsp. Faglia E, Favales F, Aldeghi A, et al. Change in major amputation rate in a center dedicated to diabetic foot care during the 1980s: prognostic determinants for major amputation. Journal of Diabetic Complications 1998;12:96–102. Bild DE, Selby JV, Sinnock P, Browner WS, Braveman P, Showstack JA. Lower extremity amputation in people with diabetes. Epidemiology and prevention. Diabetes Care 1989;12:24–31. Litzelman DK, Slemenda CW, Langefeld CD, Hays LM, Welch MA, Bild DE, Ford ES, Vinicor F. Reduction of lower extremity clinical abnormalities in patients with non-insulin-dependent diabetes mellitus. A randomized, controlled trial. Annals of Internal Medicine 1993;119:36–41.

115   *By age sixty, more than half of all men with diabetes experience erectile dysfunction:* De Berardis G, Franciosi M, Belfiglio M, Di Nardo B, Greenfield S, Kaplan SH, Pellegrini F, Sacco M, Tognoni G, Valentini M, Nicolucci A. Erectile dysfunction and quality of life in type 2 diabetic patients: a serious problem too often overlooked. Diabetes Care 2002;25:284–291. McCulloch DK, Campbell IW, Wu FC, Prescott RJ, Clarke BF. The prevalence of diabetic impotence. Diabetologia 1980;18:279–283. Rubin A, Babbott D. Impotence in diabetes mellitus. Journal of the American Medical Association 1958;168:498–500. Zemel P. Sexual dysfunction in the diabetic patient with hypertension. Amercian Journal of Cardiology 1988;61:27H–33H. Fedele D, Bortolotti A, Coscelli C, Santeusanio F, Chatenoud L, Colli E, Lavezzari M, Landoni M, Parazzini F, on behalf of Gruppo Italiano Studio Deficit Erettile nei Diabetici. Erectile dysfunction in type 1 and type 2 diabetics in Italy. International Journal of Epidemiology 2000;29:524–531. Fedele D, Coscelli C, Santeusanio F, Bortolotti A, Chatenoud L, Colli E, Landoni M, Parazzini F, on behalf of Gruppo Italiano Studio Deficit Erettile nei Diabetici. Erectile dysfunction in diabetic subjects in Italy. Diabetes Care 1998;21:1973–1977. Hekim LS, Goldstein I. Diabetic sexual dysfunction. Endocrinology and Metabolic Clinic North America 1996;23:379–400. Chew KK, Earle CM, Stuckey BGA, Jamrozik K, Keogh EJ. Erectile dysfunction in general medicine practice: prevalence and clinical correlates. International Journal of Impotence Research 2000;12:41–45. Klein R, Klein BEK, Lee KE, Moss SE, Cruickshanks KJ. Prevalence of self-reported erectile dysfunction in people with long-term IDDM. Diabetes Care 1996;19:135–141. Braunstein GD. Impotence in diabetic men. Mt. Sinai Journal of Medicine 1987;54:236–240.

8. Designed for Feast or Famine

125   *About 40,000 years ago, on some savanna, a Paleolithic man and woman emerged to become the great, great, great... grandparents of us all:* Eaton SB, Eaton SB III, Konner MJ, et al. An evolutionary perspective enhances understanding of human nutritional requirements. Journal of Nutrition 1996;126:1732–1740. Harman D. Aging: prospects for further increases in the functional life span. Age 1994;17:119–146. Eaton SB, Shostak M, Konner M. The Paleolithic prescription: a program of diet and exercise and a design for living. New York: Harper & Row, 1988. p. 39. Eaton SB, Konner M. Paleolithic nutrition: a consideration of its nature and current implications. New England Journal of Medicine 1983;312:283–289.

127   *In an influential article published in 1962, the late geneticist James Neel called them "thrifty" genes:* Neel JV. Diabetes mellitus: a "thrifty" genotype rendered detrimental by progress? American Journal of Human Genetics 1962;14:353–362.

128   *His theory helps explain why diabesity is more common in some parts of the world than in others:* Gutersohn A, Naber C, Muller N, Erbel R, Siffert W. G protein beta3 subunit 825TT genotype and post-pregnancy weight retention. Lancet 2000;355:1240–1241.

129   *Their thrifty genes remained important—and became all the more so when these peoples were conquered:* Neel JV. The thrifty genotype revisited. In: Konnerling J, Tattersall R, eds. The genetics of diabetes mellitus. New York: Academic Press, 1982. pp. 283–293. Rittenbaugh C, Goodby CS. Beyond the thrifty gene: metabolic implications of prehistoric migrations into the New World. Medical Anthropology 1989;11:227–237. Hales CN, Barker DJP. Type 2 (non-insulin-dependent) diabetes mellitus: the thrifty phenotype hypothesis. Diabetologia 1992;35:595–601.

Their traditional diet had been low in fat and high in starch and fiber: Smith CJ, Schakel SF, Nelson RG. Selected traditional and contemporary foods currently used by the Pima Indians. Journal of the American Dietetic Association 1991;91:338–341. Smith CJ, Manahan EM, Pablo SG. Food habit and cultural changes among the Pima Indians. In: Joe JR, Young RS, eds. Diabetes as a disease of civilization. Berlin, New York: Mouton de Gruyter, 1993. Brand JC, Snow BJ, Nabhan GP, Truswell AS. Plasma glucose and insulin responses to traditional Pima Indian meals. American Journal of Clinical Nutrition 1990;51:416–420. Jenkins DJ, Wolever TM, Jenkins AL, Thorne MJ, Lee R, Almusky J, Reichert R, Wong GS. The glycaemic index of foods tested in diabetic patients: a new basis for carbohydrate exchange favoring the use of legumes. Diabetologia 1983;24:257–264. O'Dea K. Marked improvement in carbohydrate and lipid metabolism in diabetic Australian Aborigines after temporary reversion to traditional lifestyle. Diabetes 1984;33:596–603.

...now their fat consumption increased significantly: Swinburn BA, Boyce VL, Bergman RN, Howard BV, Bogardus C. Deterioration in carbohydrate metabolism and lipoprotein changes induced by modern, high fat diet in Pima Indians and Caucasians. Journal of Clinical Endocrinology and Metabolism 1991;73:156–165. McMurry MP, Cerqueira MT, Connor SL, Connor WE. Changes in lipid and lipoprotein levels and body

weight in Tarahumara Indians after consumption of an affluent diet. New England Journal of Medicine 1991;325:1704–1708.

130   *As they examined members of the tribe:* Reid JM, Fullmer SD, Pettigrew KD, Burch TA, Bennett PH, Miller M, Whedon GD. Nutrient intake of Pima Indian women: relationships to diabetes mellitus and gallbladder disease. American Journal of Clinical Nutrition 1971;24:1281–1289.

Over 50 percent of Pimas over the age of thirty: Knowler WC, Pettitt DJ, Saad MF, Charles MA, Nelson RG, Howard BV, Bogardus C, Bennett PH. Obesity in the Pima Indians: its magnitude and relationship with diabetes. American Journal of Clinical Nutrition 1991;53:1543S–1551S.

This discovery inspired an extraordinary collaboration: Smith CJ, Nelson RG, Hardy SA, Manahan EM, Bennett PH, Knowler WC. Survey of the diet of Pima Indians using quantitative food frequency assessment and 24-hour recall: the Diabetic Renal Disease Study. Journal of the American Dietetic Association 1996;96:778–784. Shulz LO, Harper IT, Smith CJ, Kriska AM, Ravussin E. Energy intake and physical activity in Pima Indians: comparison with energy expenditure measured by doubly labeled water. Obesity Research 1994;2:541–548.

And we've also learned that increased physical activity: Kriska AM, Bennett PH. An epidemiological perspective of the relationship between physical activity and NIDDM: from activity assessment to intervention. Diabetes and Metabolism Review 1992;8:355–372. Kriska AM, LaPorte RE, Pettitt DJ, Charles MA, Nelson RG, Kuller LH, Bennett PH, Knowler WC. The association of physical activity with obesity, fat distribution, and glucose intolerance in Pima Indians. Diabetologia 1993;36:863–869.

135   *The concept that nutrition in the womb and the cradle helps determine risk:* Barker DJP. The fetal origins of disease. European Journal of Clinical Investigation 1995;25:457–463. Barker DJ, Hales CN, Fall CH, Osmond C, Phipps K, Clark PM. Type 2 (non-insulin-dependent) diabetes mellitus, hypertension and hyperlipidaemia (syndrome X): relation to reduced fetal growth. Diabetologia 1993;36:62–67.

136   *But their growth may have been limited by their mother's malnutrition:* Godfrey KM, Barker DJP. Fetal malnutrition and adult disease. American Journal of Clinical Nutrition 2000;71:1344S–1352S. Godfrey KM, Barker DJP, Robinson S, Osmond C. Mother's birthweight and diet in pregnancy in relation to the baby's thinness at birth. British Journal of Obstetrics and Gynaecology 1997;104:663–667. Seghieri G, Anichini R, De Bellis A, Alviggi L, Franconi F, Breschi MC. Relationship between gestational diabetes mellitus and low maternal birth weight. Diabetes Care 2002;25:1761–1765. Saldana TM, Siega-Riz AM, Adair LS, Savitz DA, Thorp JM Jr. The association between impaired glucose tolerance and birth weight among black and white women in central North Carolina. Diabetes Care 2003;26:656–661.

137   *How can it matter fifty or more years later that a person was born small:* Hales CN, Barker DJP, Clark PMS, Cox LJ, Fall C, Osmond C, Winter PD. Fetal and infant growth and impaired glucose tolerance at age 64. British Medical Journal 1991;303:1019–1022.

9. The Land of Plenty

141   *These changes would increase our average daily caloric consumption:* Trends in
       intake of energy and macronutrients—United States, 1971–2000. Mor-
       bidity and Mortality Weekly Review 2004;53(04);80–82.

142   *The Body Mass Index is sometimes called the Quetelet Index:* Stigler SM.
       Adolphe Quetelet. Encyclopedia of Statistical Sciences. New York: John
       Wiley & Sons, 1986. Hankins FH. Quetelet as a statistician. New York:
       1908. Lécuyer B-P. Probability in vital and social statistics: Quetelet,
       Farr, and the Bertillons. In: Krüger L, Daston LJ, Heidelberger M, eds.
       The probabilistic revolution, vol. 1: ideas in history (Cambridge, MA:
       MIT Press, 1987). pp. 317–335. Lazarsfeld PF. Notes on the history of
       quantification in sociology—trends, sources and problems. In: Kendall
       MG, Plackett RL, eds. Studies in the history of statistics and probability
       II (London: 1977). pp. 213–270. Porter TM. The mathematics of soci-
       ety: variation and error in Quetelet's statistics. British Journal for the
       History of Science 1985;18(58)(1):51–69. Sheynin BA. Quetelet as a stat-
       istician. Archives of the History of Exact Sciences 1986;36(4):281–325.
       Stigler SM. The history of statistics: the measurement of uncertainty be-
       fore 1900 (Cambridge, MA: MIT Press, 1986).

143   *The 1999–2000 National Health and Nutrition Examination Survey found:*
       Finkelstein EA, Fiebelkorn IC, Wang G. National medical spending at-
       tributable to overweight and obesity: how much, and who's paying?
       Health Affairs 2003;W3;219–226. Finkelstein EA, Fiebelkorn IC,
       Wang G. State-level estimates of annual medical expenditures attributa-
       ble to obesity. Obesity Research 2004;12(1):18–24. U.S. Department of
       Health and Human Services. The surgeon general's call to action to pre-
       vent and decrease overweight and obesity. [Rockville, MD]: U.S. De-
       partment of Health and Human Services, Public Health Service, Office
       of the Surgeon General, [2001]. Wolf AM, Colditz GA. Current esti-
       mates of the economic cost of obesity in the United States. Obesity Re-
       search 1998;6(2):97–106. Wolf A. What is the economic case for treating
       obesity? Obesity Research 1998;6(suppl):2S–7S.
       Rates of overweight in American children have increased similarly: U.S. De-
       partment of Health and Human Services, National Center for Health
       Statistics. Overweight children and adolescents 6–19 years of age, ac-
       cording to sex, age, race, and Hispanic origin: United States, selected
       years 1963–65 through 1999–2000. Available at http://www.cdc.gov/
       nchs/data/hus/tables/2002/02hus071.pdf. Ogden CL, Flegal KM, Car-
       roll MD, Johnson CL. Prevalence and trends in overweight among U.S.
       children and adolescents, 1999–2000. Journal of the American Medical
       Association 2002;288:1728–32.
       For African American and Hispanic children: Centers for Disease Control
       and Prevention, National Center for Health Statistics, National Health
       and Nutrition Examination Survey, Hispanic Health and Nutrition Ex-
       amination Survey (1982–84), and National Health Examination Survey
       (1963–65 and 1966–70).

150   *In 2002, the most recent year for which numbers are available:* NPDFood-
       world. 17th annual eating patterns in America. 2002.

152–153 *From 1971 to 2000, average consumption by men:* Trends in intake of energy and macronutrients—United States, 1971–2000. Morbidity and Mortality Weekly Review 2004;53(04);80–82.

153   *In current surveys, 40 percent of American adults report that they are completely sedentary:* Dong L, Block G, Mandel S. Activities contributing to total energy expenditure in the United States: results from the NHAPS study. International Journal of Behavioral Nutrition and Physical Activity 2004;Feb. 12:4. Centers for Disease Control and Prevention. Physical activity and health: a report of the surgeon general. Atlanta: U.S. Department of Health and Human Services, 1996. Barnes PM, Schoenborn CA. Physical activity among adults: United States, 2000. Advance data from vital and health statistics, no. 333. Hyattsville, MD: National Center for Health Statistics, 2003.

154   *According to government transportation surveys:* A report to the president from the secretary of health and human services and the secretary of education. Promoting better health for young people through physical activity and sports. Washington, DC: 2000.

       Physical education, which was once a required part of the school curriculum: Centers for Disease Control and Prevention. Physical activity and health: a report of the surgeon general. Atlanta: U.S. Department of Health and Human Services, 1996. American Council on Exercise, Adams PF, et al. Health risk behaviors among our nation's youth: United States, 1992. National Center for Health Statistics, 1995. Vital Health Statistics 10(192). DHHS publication no. PHS 95-1520.

       But by 1990, kids spent an average of three hours daily: Children and watching TV. American Academy of Child and Adolescent Psychiatry 2003;54.

       These days, when kids are asked about their physical activity: U.S. Department of Health and Human Services. Physical activity and health, 1996; call to action to prevent and decrease overweight and obesity, 2001.

10. Diabesity Around the World

157   *In 2000, 151 million adults worldwide:* McCarty D, Zimmet P. Diabetes 1994 to 2010: global estimates and projections. Melbourne: International Diabetes Institute, 1994. Amos AF, McCarty DJ, Zimmet P. The rising global burden of diabetes and its complications: estimates and projections to the year 2010. Diabetic Medicine 1997;14(suppl 5):S1–S85. King H, Rewers M. Global estimates for prevalence of diabetes mellitus and impaired glucose tolerance in adults. Diabetes Care 1993;16:157–177. Zimmet P, Alberti KGMM, Shaw J. Global and societal implications of the diabetes epidemic. Nature 2001;414: 782–787. King H, Aubert RE, Herman WH. Global burden of diabetes, 1995–2025: prevalence, numerical estimates, and projections. Diabetes Care 1998;21:1414–1431.

158   *In Latin America, diabetes is expected to increase by 44 percent:* World Health Organization Web site. Available at http://www.who.int/en/.

       According to the International Obesity Task Force: Diabetes Atlas. 2nd ed. International Diabetes Federation, 2003. Cost-effective approaches to diabetes care and prevention. International Diabetes Federation, 2003. World Health Organization. Prevention of diabetes mellitus. Technical Report Series no. 844. Geneva, 1994.

Each year 34 million people die from obesity-related causes: World Health Organization. The global strategy on diet, physical activity and health. Available at http://www.who.int/dietphysicalactivity/media/en/gsfs_general.pdf. World Health Organization. The world health report 2002: reducing risks, promoting healthy life. Geneva, 2002.

Obesity has doubled in Japan since 1982: Diabetes around the world. International Diabetes Federation, 1998. Kanazawa M, Yoshiike N, Osaka T, Numba Y, Zimmet P, Inoue S. Criteria and classification of obesity in Japan and Asia-Oceania. Asia Pacific Journal of Clinical Nutrition 2002;11(suppl 8):S732–S737.

The prevalence of obesity has increased by 10 to 40 percent: Ibid.

According to the International Obesity Task Force, 0.7 percent of children in Africa: World Health Organization. Prevention of diabetes mellitus. Technical Report Series no. 844. Geneva, 1994. Diabetes Atlas. 2nd ed. International Diabetes Federation, 2003. Available at http://www.idf.org/e-atlas/home/index.cfm?node=195. Diabetes and kidney disease: time to act. International Diabetes Federation, 2003.

159   *In the U.S., where 43.6 million people are without health insurance:* U.S. Census Bureau. Current population survey, 2002 and 2003 annual social and economic supplements. U.S. Census Bureau. Health insurance coverage in the United States: 2002. September 2003.

With increased prosperity and adoption of Western ways: Diabetes Atlas. 2nd ed. International Diabetes Federation, 2003. Diabetes and cardiovascular disease: time to act. International Diabetes Federation, 2001. World Health Organization Web site. Available at http://www.who.int/en/. Diabetes around the world. International Diabetes Federation, 1998. Cost-effective approaches to diabetes care and prevention. International Diabetes Federation, 2003. Popkin BM, Horton S, Kim S. The nutritional transition and diet-related chronic diseases in Asia: implications for prevention. Discussion paper 105. Food Consumption and Nutrition Division of the International Food Policy Research Institute. Haddad L. What can food policy do to redirect the diet transition? Discussion paper 165. Food Consumption and Nutrition Division of the International Food Policy Research Institute. Bell AC, Keyou GE, Popkin BM. The road to obesity or the path to prevention: motorized transportation and obesity in China. Obesity Research 2002;10:277–283. Popkin BM. The nutrition transition and its health implications in lower income countries. Public Health Nutrition 1998;1:5–21.

160   *Both of us knew that the Mexican healthcare system:* Aguilar-Salinas C. Prevalence and characteristics of early-onset type 2 diabetes in Mexico. American Journal of Medicine 2002;113(7):569–574.

Almost 6 percent of the Indian population between ages twenty and seventy-nine: International Association for the Study of Obesity Web site. Available at http://www.iotf.org/. Diabetes Atlas. 2nd ed. International Diabetes Federation, 2003. Diabetes and cardiovascular disease: time to act. International Diabetes Federation, 2001. World Health Organization Web site. Available at http://www.who.int/en/. Diabetes around the world. International Diabetes Federation, 1998. Wild S, Roglic G, Green A, Sicree R, King H. Global prevalence of diabetes: estimates for the year 2000 and projections for 2030. Diabetes Care 2004;27(5):1047–1053.

173   *They founded an international nonprofit organization called AYUDA, which*
       stands for American Youth Understanding Diabetes Abroad: American Youth
       Understanding Diabetes Abroad (AYUDA) Web site. Available at http://
       www.ayudainc.net/.

176   *According to the International Obesity Task Force, obesity is on the rise in*
       Ecuador: International Association for the Study of Obesity Web site.
       Available at http://www.iotf.org/.
       A 1999 study found that 19 percent of schoolchildren in Quito: Pan American
       Health Organization, 2002.

11. The New Normal

183   *...growth charts developed by the Centers for Disease Control and Preven-*
       tion (CDC): CDC growth charts. Available at http://www.cdc.gov/
       growthcharts/.

191   *The glycemic index was invented by Dr. David Jenkins and his colleagues at the*
       University of Toronto: Wolever TMS, Jenkins DJA, Josse RG, Wong GS,
       Lee R. The glycemic index: similarity of values derived in insulin-
       dependent and non-insulin-dependent diabetic patients. Journal of the
       American College of Nutrition 1987;6:295–305. Jenkins DJ, Wolever
       TM, Jenkins AL. Starchy foods and glycemic index. Diabetes Care
       1988;11:149–159. Wolever TM, Jenkins DJ, Vuksan V, Jenkins AL,
       Wong GS, Josse RG. Beneficial effect of low-glycemic index diet in
       overweight NIDDM subjects. Diabetes Care 1992;15:562–564.

192   *In one such study, reported in the* New England Journal of Medicine: Foster
       GD, Wyatt HR, Hill JO, McGuckin BG, Brill C, Mohammed BS, Sza-
       pary PO, Rader DJ, Edman JS, Klein S. A randomized trial of a low-
       carbohydrate diet for obesity. New England Journal of Medicine
       2003;348:2082–2090.
       However, research suggests that this is not the case: Bravata DM, Sanders L,
       Huang J, Krumholz HM, Olkin I, Gardner CD. Efficacy and safety of
       low-carbohydrate diets: a systematic review. Journal of the American Med-
       ical Association 2003;289:1837–1850. Brehm BJ, Seely RJ, Daniels SR, et
       al. A randomized trial comparing a very low carbohydrate diet and a
       calorie-restricted low fat diet on body weight and cardiovascular risk fac-
       tors in healthy women. Journal of Clinical Endocrinology and Metabolism
       2003;88(4):1617–1623. Bonow RO, Eckel RH. Diet, obesity, and cardio-
       vascular risk. New England Journal of Medicine 2003;348:2057–2058.

193   *This database includes more than 4,000 people who have maintained a weight*
       loss of at least 30 pounds for at least one year: National Weight Control Reg-
       istry Web site. Available at http://www.lifespan.org/services/bmed/wt_
       loss/nwcr/.
       A study of their participants: Klem ML, Wing RR, McGuire MT, Seagle
       HM, Hill JO. A descriptive study of individuals successful at long-term
       maintenance of substantial weight loss. American Journal of Clinical
       Nutrition 1997;66:239–246.

194   *For example, in 1994 scientists were excited by the discovery of a hormone:*
       Zhang Y, Proenca R, Maffei M, Barone M, Leopold L, Friedman JM.
       Positional cloning of the mouse obese gene and its human homologue.
       Nature 1994;372(6505):425–432.

195   *An estimated 10 to 20 percent of those who undergo bariatric surgery subsequently require additional surgery:* National Institute of Diabetes and Digestive and Kidney Diseases. Gastrointestinal surgery for severe obesity. NIH Publication No. 01-4006. 2001. Steinbrook R. Surgery for severe obesity. New England Journal of Medicine 2004;350:1075–1079.

196   *In 1991 the National Institutes of Health issued a consensus statement:* Gastrointestinal surgery for severe obesity. Consensus statement, NIH Consensus Development Conference, March 25–27, 1991. Public Health Service, National Institutes of Health, Office of Medical Applications of Research.
        In 2003 there were 103,000: Data from American Society for Bariatric Surgery. Steinbrook R. Surgery for severe obesity. New England Journal of Medicine 2004;350:1075–1079.
        Bariatric surgery costs approximately $20,000 to $50,000: Ibid.
        The National Institutes of Health has established a study group to answer key questions about the risks and benefits: National Institutes of Health Web site. Available at http://grants2.nih.gov/grants/guide/rfa-files/RFA-DK-03-006.html.

200   *Blue Cross/Blue Shield of Massachusetts came up with a super-simple message that I repeat constantly:* Blue Cross Blue Shield of Massachusetts Web site. Available at http://www.bcbsma.com. Jump up and go! [brochure]. Available at http://www.bcbsma.com/common/en_US/pdfs/JumpUpAndGoBrochure.pdf. Jump Up and Go! Web site. Available at http://www.jumpupandgo.com.

204   *In 2000, at the annual American Diabetes Association meeting in San Antonio, Texas, we presented our initial analysis of KidsNFitness:* Mackenzie M, Halvorson M, Kaufman FR, Braun S, Conrad BP. Effect of a KidsNFitness weight management program on obesity and other pediatric health factors. Diabetes 2001;50:A22.
        In 2004 we reported at the annual ADA meeting in Orlando, Florida, that the first group of thirty-five youths who attended our new twelve-week KidsNFitness program: Monzavi R, Dreimane D, Geffner ME, Braun S, Conrad B, Klier M, Kaufman FR. Improvement in metabolic syndrome and insulin resistance in obese youth treated with lifestyle intervention. Diabetes 2004;53:A7.

12. Who's Responsible?

212   *A Los Angeles County Health Survey conducted in 1999:* 1999–2000 Los Angeles County Health Survey. Los Angeles County Department of Health Services, Public Health.
        Americans are ambivalent about the role society and government should play in fighting obesity: The Harvard Forums on Health, a project of Harvard University's Interfaculty Program for Health Systems Improvement, commissioned Lake Snell Perry & Associates to conduct a national poll to explore the public's knowledge about obesity as a public health issue and their opinions about various policy options to fight obesity in adults and children. This national survey of 1,002 Americans age 18 and older was conducted May 28 through June 1, 2003. Available at http://www.phsi.harvard.edu/health_reform/poll_results.pdf.

213   *In 2003 the National Cancer Institute's 5-a-Day program, which encourages Americans to eat five fruits and vegetables every day:* National Cancer Institute's 5 a Day for Better Health Program Web site. Available at http://www.5aday.gov.

Meanwhile, the food industry spends approximately $25 billion a year on advertising to deliver their messages: Elitzak H. Food marketing costs at a glance. Food Marketing 2001;24(3):47–48. Available at http://www.ers.usda.gov/publications/FoodReview/septdec01/FRv24i3g.pdf.

According to Marion Nestle, author of Food Politics: Nestle M. Food politics: how the food industry influences nutrition and health. Berkeley: University of California Press, 2002. Nestle M, Wootan M, as quoted in Spending on marketing to kids up $5 billion in last decade. Food Institute Report 2002;April 15.

214   *Moreover, industry experts believe brand loyalty begins as early as age two:* Brand aware. Children's Business 2000;June.

Four out of five food ads aimed at children are for sugary cereals, snack foods: Center for Science in the Public Interest. Available at http://www.cspinet.org/nutritionpolicy/food_advertising.html.

217   *Currently Arkansas, Missouri, Rhode Island, Tennessee:* Jacobson and Brownell. Small taxes on soft drinks and snack foods to promote health. American Journal of Public Health 2000;90:854–857.

218   *Today, veterans of the tobacco wars are retooling their weapons to go into battle against "big food":* Cohan A. Editorial observer; the mcnugget of truth in the lawsuits against fast-food restaurants. New York Times 2003;February 3. Available at http://www.pinniped.net/mcfrankenstein.html. Wald J. McDonald's obesity suit tossed. CNN Online, February 17, 2003. Available at http://money.cnn.com/2003/01/22/news/companies/mcdonalds.

220   *The bill, H.R. 339, bars consumers from bringing obesity-related lawsuits against restaurants and food manufacturers:* H.R. 339. Personal Responsibility in Food Consumption Act. Available at http://www.congress.gov/cgi-bin/bdquery/z?d108:H.R.339:.

13. Reading, Writing, and Diabesity

223   *"Competitive foods"—so called because they compete with USDA meals:* Child nutrition policy brief: competitive foods in schools. Food Research & Action Center, Washington, DC. Available at http://www.frac.org/pdf/cncompfoods.pdf. Foods sold in competition with USDA school meal programs. U.S. House Appropriations Committee Report, House Report 106-619. Available at http://www.gao.gov/new.items/d04673.pdf. National School Lunch Program/School Breakfast Program: foods of minimal nutritional value. USDA School and Community Nutrition Program Policy memorandum. January 16, 2001. Available at http://www.fns.usda.gov/cnd/Lunch/CompetitiveFoods/fmnv.pdf. School Health Policies and Programs Study (SHPPS). Journal of School Health 2001;71(7).

But not all schools comply with this rule: State of the states: a profile of food and nutrition programs across the nation. Food Research and Action Center. February 2003. Available at http://www.frac.org/pdf/021903SOS.pdf.

224   *In the School Health Policies and Programs Study 2000, conducted by the*

Centers for Disease Control and Prevention: School Health Policies and Program Study (2000). Centers for Disease Control and Prevention (CDC), National Center for Chronic Disease Prevention and Health Promotion, Division of Adolescent and School Health. Available at http://www.cdc.gov/HealthyYouth/shpps/index.htm.

After the war, in 1946, President Truman started the NSLP: Child nutrition fact sheet: National School Lunch Program. Food Research and Action Center. Available at http://www.frac.org/pdf/cnnslp.pdf. National School Lunch Program: frequently asked questions. Food Research and Action Center. School Lunch Program—efforts needed to improve nutrition and encourage healthy eating. GAO report GAO-03-506.

During the 2002–2003 school year more than 27.8 million children received meals: Child nutrition fact sheet: National School Lunch Program. Food Research and Action Center. Available at http://www.frac.org/pdf/cnnslp.pdf.

Caloric requirements for lunch are: National School Lunch Program regulations.

225   *Over the years, the NSLP expanded to add breakfast:* Nutrition insights (15): eating breakfast greatly improves schoolchildren's diet quality. USDA Center for Nutrition Policy and Promotion. December 1999. Available at http://www.usda.gov/cnpp/Insights/insight15.pdf. School breakfast scorecard: 2003. Thirteenth annual status report on the School Breakfast Program. Food Research and Action Center. Available at http://www.frac.org/pdf/2003Breakfast.pdf. Universal School Breakfast Program. Food Research & Action Center. Available at http://www.frac.org/pdf/universal_sbp.pdf.

But on a typical day during the 2002–2003 school year: School Breakfast Program: frequently asked questions. Food Research and Action Center. Available at http://www.frac.org/pdf/cnsbp.pdf.

Of these children, 79 percent received: Ibid.

According to the CDC's School Health Policies and Program Study 2000: School Health Policies and Program Study (2000). Centers for Disease Control and Prevention (CDC), National Center for Chronic Disease Prevention and Health Promotion, Division of Adolescent and School Health. Available at http://www.cdc.gov/HealthyYouth/shpps/index.htm.

Candy and sodas aren't supposed to be sold during meals: Centers for Disease Control and Prevention. Guidelines for school health programs to promote lifelong healthy eating. Morbidity and Mortality Weekly Report 1996;45(RR-9):1–33. American Dietetic Association. Local support for nutrition integrity in schools—position of ADA. Journal of the American Dietetic Association 2000;100:108–111.

225–226 *Schools share in vending machine profits:* Nestle M. Soft drink pouring right. Public Health Reports 2000;115:308–317. Harnack L, Stang J, Story M. Soft drink consumption among U.S. children and adolescents: nutrition consequences. Journal of the American Dietetic Association 1999;99(4):436–441. Jacobson MF. Liquid candy: how soft drinks are harming Americans' health. Center for Science in the Public Interest. 1998.

226   *In one telling study, investigators from Baylor College of Medicine in Houston:* Cullen KW, Zakeri I. Fruits, vegetables, milk, and sweetened beverages

consumption and access to à la carte/snack bar meals at school. American Journal of Public Health 2004;94:463–467.

Many states are trying to regain control by instituting standards for the sale of competitive foods: School Health Policies and Programs Study (SHPPS). Journal of School Health 2001;71(7).

227 *The problem of competitive foods is one of quantity as well as quality:* Foods sold in competition with USDA school meal programs. U.S. House Appropriations Committee Report, House Report 106-619.

231 *Another problem is that schools often serve lunch at inappropriate times:* Sanchez A, Hoover L, Sanchez N, Miller J. Measurement and evaluation of school lunch time elements in elementary, junior high and high school levels. Journal of Child Nutritional Management 1999;1:16–21. Bergman EA, Buergel NS, Joseph E, Sanchez A. Time spent by schoolchildren to eat lunch. Journal of the American Dietetic Association 2000;100(6):696–698.

232 *In an influential report titled* Liquid Candy, *the Center for Science in the Public Interest (CSPI) documented:* Jacobson MF. Liquid candy: how soft drinks are harming Americans' health. Center for Science in the Public Interest. 1998.

From 1977 to 1996, soda consumption by teens jumped: Soda consumption puts kids at risk for obesity, bone fractures, osteoporosis, and cavities fact sheet. California Center for Public Health Advocacy. Continuing Survey of Food Intake by Individuals, 1977–1996. Available at http://www.publichealthadvocacy.org/resources/Soda%20Fact%20Sheet.pdf.

Sixty-five percent of adolescent girls and 74 percent of adolescent boys consume sodas daily: Ludwig OS, Peterson KE, Gortmaker SL. Relation between consumption of sugar-sweetened drinks and childhood obesity: a prospective, observational analysis. Lancet 2001;357:505–508.

Teenage girls consume an average of 36.2 grams: Ibid.

Teenage boys consume 57.7 grams on average: Ibid.

A 2001 study of sixth and seventh grade children in Boston, published in The Lancet: Ibid.

In a 2004 report in the British Medical Journal, *another team of investigators documented the benefits:* James J, Thomas P, Cavan D, Kerr D. Preventing childhood obesity by reducing consumption of carbonated drinks: cluster randomised controlled trial. British Medical Journal 2004;328:1237.

233 *But here's just one example, from an article in Beverage World, a trade publication for the U.S. beverage industry:* Beverage World Web site. Available at http://www.beverageworld.com/beverageworld/index.jsp.

In a 2001 survey by the National Association of Secondary School Principals: National Soft Drink Association Web site. School principals overwhelmingly support business partnerships that provide revenue for education programs. Available at http://www.nsda.org/About/news/2001%20Releases/principals.html.

234 *Marlene crafted the Healthy Beverage Resolution and enlisted the support of two other school board members as co-sponsors:* Canter M, Hayes G, Korenstein J. Motion to promote healthy beverage sales in the LAUSD. Available at http://www.publichealthadvocacy.org/legislation/Healthy%20Beverage%20Resolution.pdf.

239 *Individual schools, districts, cities, counties, and states are enacting soda bans or*

restricting the sale of sodas in schools: Snyder P. Advocates push for more healthy foods in schools. Philadelphia Inquirer 2003;July 10. Available at http://www.philly.com/mld/inquirer/news/local/6268825.htm?1c. Joy K. Junk food is facing school expulsion. Boston Globe 2004;March 4. Available at http://www.boston.com/news/education/k_12/articles/2004/03/04/junk_food_is_facing_school_expulsion/.

240   *In the Healthy People 2000 report, the United States Surgeon General set a target for 50 percent of schools to require physical education every day:* Healthy People 2000. Available at http://odphp.osophs.dhhs.gov/pubs/hp2000/. Healthy People 2000 Review. Available at http://www.cdc.gov/nchs/products/pubs/pubd/hp2k/review/review.htm.

The percentage of students who attended a daily PE class: Kann L, et al. Youth risk behavior surveillance—United States, 2001. Morbidity and Mortality Weekly Report 2002;57(SS-4):1–64. Youth Risk Behaviors Surveillance Survey fact sheet. Centers for Disease Control and Prevention, National Center for Chronic Disease Prevention and Health Promotion. Available at http://www.cdc.gov/od/oc/media/pressrel/fs020627.htm.

Only 19 percent of high school students taking daily physical education are actually active for at least twenty minutes per class: Centers for Disease Control and Prevention, National Center for Chronic Disease Prevention and Health Promotion, Division of Nutrition and Physical Activity. A report of the surgeon general: physical activity and health—adolescents and young adults. Available at http://www.cdc.gov/nccdphp/sgr/pdf/adoles.pdf.

The test, called the Fitnessgram, was developed by the Cooper Institute for Aerobics Research: The Fitness Gram Assessment. Cooper Institute Web site. Available at http://www.cooperinst.org/ftgmain.asp.

241   *According to a survey by the U.S. Department of Transportation:* Barriers to children walking and biking to school—United States, 1999. Morbidity and Mortality Weekly Report 2002;51:701–703. Promoting better health for young people through physical activity and sports. A report to the president from the secretary of health and human services and the secretary of education. 2000. Available at http://www.cdc.gov/HealthyYouth/physicalactivity/promoting_health/.

For example, the city of Chicago and its police department created the Walking School Bus program: The Walking School Bus. Available at http://www.cityofchicago.org/cp/Alerts/SafetyTips/ChildSafety/WalkingSchoolbus.html.

242   *Another success story is the multi-state Fruit and Vegetable Pilot Program, which was part of the federal government's 2002 Farm Act:* Farm Security and Rural Investment Act of 2002. United States Department of Agriculture, Economic Research Service Web site. Available at http://www.ers.usda.gov/features/farmbill/.

243   *During the Fruit and Vegetable Pilot Program:* Evaluation of the USDA Fruit and Vegetable Pilot Program: report to Congress. Economic Research Service/USDA. Available at http://www.fns.usda.gov/cnd/Research/FV030063.pdf.

14. Nine to Five

249   *Evidence collected over the past thirty years shows that work site health promotion:* Pelletier K. A review and analysis of the health and cost-effective outcome studies of comprehensive health promotion and disease prevention programs at the worksite: 1991–1993 update. American Journal of Health Promotion 1993;8(1):50–62. Holzbach RL, Piserchia PV, McFadden DW, Hartwell TD, Herrmann A, Fielding JE. Effect of a comprehensive health promotion program on employee attitudes. Journal of Occupational Medicine 1990;32(10):973–978. Bertera R. Behavioral risk factors and illness day changes with workplace health promotion. American Journal of Health Promotion 1993;7(5):365–373.

       Diabesity is expensive for the nation's employers. In the late 1990s obesity cost American companies $12.7 billion per year: Thompson D, Edelsberg J, Kinsey KL, Oster G. Estimated economic costs of obesity to U.S. business. American Journal of Health Promotion 1998;13(2):120–127.

       Obesity was associated with 63 million additional doctor visits: Wellman NS, Friedberg B. Causes and consequences of adult obesity: health, social and economic impacts in the United States. Asia Pacific Journal of Clinical Nutrition 2002;11(8):S705.

       Indirect costs to employers due to diabetes: Hogan P, Dall T, Nikolov P, American Diabetes Association. Economic costs of diabetes in the U.S. in 2002. Diabetes Care 2003;26:917–932.

250   *The Centers for Disease Control and Prevention developed a campaign:* CDC's Division of Nutrition and Physical Activity. StairWELL to better health: a worksite intervention. Kerr NA, Yore MM, Ham SA, Dietz, WH. Increasing stair use in a worksite through environmental changes. American Journal of Health Promotion 2004;18(4):312–315.

252   *The U.S. Department of Health and Human Services had just announced a Small Steps, Big Rewards campaign:* National Diabetes Education Program Web site. Available at http://www.ndep.nih.gov/campaigns/SmallSteps/SmallSteps_index.htm.

       In 2002, I was invited to chair the Los Angeles County Task Force on Children and Youth Physical Fitness: Los Angeles Task Force on Fitness Web site. Available at http://www.lapublichealth.org/mch/reports/Board%20ReportFinal.pdf.

15. The Healthcare Challenge

259   *Experts on public health disagree about whether it's desirable to provide fingerstick blood tests at a street fair:* American Diabetes Association. Screening for type 2 diabetes. Diabetes Care 2004;27:11S–14S.

262   *According to our best estimates today, 5 million to 6 million people have type 2 diabetes and don't know it:* American Diabetes Association Web site. Available at www.diabetes.org.

263   *More than 43.6 million people in the United States have no health insurance coverage:* U.S. Census Bureau. Health insurance coverage: 2002.

276   *I went through the ABCs of diabetes:* Gottlieb SH. Know your ABC's: "A" is for A1C. Diabetes Forecast 2002;55(10):34–36.

Epilogue: A Choice of Futures

280   *I will reveal that in North America there are now 36 million people with dia-*
        betes: McCarty D, Zimmet P. Diabetes 1994 to 2010: global estimates
        and projections. Melbourne: International Diabetes Institute, 1994.
        Amos AF, McCarty DJ, Zimmet P. The rising global burden of diabetes
        and its complications: estimates and projections to the year 2010. Dia-
        betic Medicine 1997;14(suppl 5):S1–S85. King H, Rewers M. Global es-
        timates for prevalence of diabetes mellitus and impaired glucose
        tolerance in adults. Diabetes Care 1993;16:157–177. Zimmet P, Alberti
        KGMM, Shaw J. Global and societal implications of the diabetes epi-
        demic. Nature 2001;414:782–787. King H, Aubert RE, Herman WH.
        Global burden of diabetes, 1995–2025: prevalence, numerical estimates,
        and projections. Diabetes Care 1998;21:1414–1431.

Acknowledgments

This book stems from memories of my Grandma Sadie and her struggle with diabetes. Every time I inform a child that he or she has developed diabetes, I picture my grandmother's first insulin injection and how she winced. And when I talk to the child's parents, I remember the look of anguish on my father's face as he pushed the needle into his mother's skin. I wanted to tell stories about diabesity that would convey the pain and triumph of those afflicted. I wrote this book to help people understand the roots of the epidemic and compel them to demand change—in our society and within ourselves.

Throughout my career I've been inspired by my many patients and their families. Children diagnosed with this devastating disease react with fear and dignity. Parents eventually replace shock with acceptance and unending determination to one day see the end of diabetes. I'm privileged to have participated in their lives. To respect my patients' privacy—something I am required to do by law as well as by personal conviction—I have changed names and disguised personal details so that individual patients cannot be identified by themselves or by anyone else.

Over the years I have been inspired and motivated by many

mentors. Drs. Maury Kogut, George Donnell, and Barbara Korsch filled the early days of my pediatric career with knowledge and passion. They were shining examples of how to practice medicine. Dr. Thomas Roe was my boss and my friend for the first twenty years I was at Childrens Hospital. He practiced medicine with dignity and dedication. I would like to thank my incredible colleagues at Childrens Hospital Los Angeles Center for Diabetes, Endocrinology and Metabolism: Drs. Gertrude Costin (also a most valued mentor, who taught me by example how to be not only a physician but also a mother), Daina Dreimane, Lynda Fisher, Mitchell Geffner, Debra Jeandron, Kevin Kaiserman (who gave me valuable critical comments on *Diabesity*), and Pisit Pitukcheewanont. Mary Halvorson has been my collaborator on almost all important projects. There is no finer example of brilliance and dedication. The doctors in training at the Center—Maria Karantza, Roschi Monzavi, Steve Mittelman, Tariq Ahmad, Lily Chao, Joshua May, and Andriette Ward—teach us all by making us be our best.

The individuals who make up the staff of the Center for Diabetes, Endocrinology and Metabolism at Childrens Hospital Los Angeles—nurses, nutritionists, social workers, psychologists, research assistants, clerks, secretaries, and support personnel—are my inspiration. They are led by Sue Carpenter, whose gentle demeanor and unending patience enable her to extract the best from staff and patients alike, and Ryan Keefer, who has tremendous organizational and leadership skills. I am grateful to the entire staff for working overtime to enable me to be president of the American Diabetes Association, for caring about and for our patients and their families, and for working to triumph over diabetes. These people are among the most compassionate, capable, and caring individuals I know. I am honored to work with them every day. I am particularly indebted to Daisy Mondaca, my administrative secretary, for always getting me to the right place at the right time and for going beyond what is expected.

Dr. Roberta Williams, chair of the Department of Pediatrics; Paul King, vice president; and William Noce, CEO of Childrens Hospital Los Angeles, gave me their blessings and enough leeway to write this book. The staff of the Foundation Office of Childrens

Hospital Los Angeles—Terry Green, Bethany Taylor, Martha St. Romain, Claudia Looney, Ken Wildes, and Alissa Spargo—enables us to succeed in our work by finding continuing support for our clinical and research efforts. I am indebted to Dr. Richard MacKenzie for organizing many of the international medical missions and for making them valuable experiences for all who participated. The entire medical and surgical staff and the residents of Childrens Hospital Los Angeles make the hospital environment conducive to academic endeavor and a premier place to care for children and families.

I am indebted to my many collaborators in the United States and around the globe in the field of diabetes. I will mention only a few who have been extraordinary friends and collaborators: Drs. Paul Zimmet, Bernie Zinman, Stephanie Amiel, George Alberti, Philippe Halban, Paolo Pozzilli, Pesach Segal, Itamar Raz, Pierre Lefèbvre, and Martin Silink. My close friends in endocrinology in the United States have enlightened and improved the lives of so many: Drs. Irl Hirsch, Jay Skyler, Bruce Buckingham, Richard Rubin, Lois Jovanovic, Janet Silverstein, Jim Gavin, and Des Schatz.

My colleagues at the University of Southern California are devoted academics who have improved the lives of people with diabesity through their research, teaching, and advocacy: Drs. Michael Goran, Richard Bergman, Tom Buchanan, Glen Melnick, Peter Clarke, Susan Evans, and Geoff Cowan. I work particularly closely with Dr. Anne Peters Harmel, to whom I refer most of my patients when they grow beyond my pediatric practice. I partner with her on the Keck Diabetes Prevention Initiative, and I am led by her strength and spirit.

The National Institute of Diabetes and Digestive and Kidney Diseases (NIDDK) is fortunate to have Drs. Barbara Linder, Judy Fradkin, and Alan Spiegel at the helm of the diabetes effort. The investigators of the STOPP-T2, DPT-1, and TrialNet study groups are inspiring examples of dedicated physicians and scientists who have devoted themselves to advancing diabetes research and clinical care.

Gifted researchers at the Centers for Disease Control and Prevention, including Bill Dietz and Frank Vinicor, deserve thanks for bringing diabetes into greater focus. Those who work tirelessly for the National Diabetes Education Project (NDEP) should be lauded for helping to get the information about diabetes and obesity out to the public.

Because they shun recognition, I have changed the names of some of the physicians and scientists mentioned in the book. But to all of them: knowing and working with you has been an honor and a privilege.

One of the most rewarding aspects of my career has been my involvement with the American Diabetes Association. The incredible staff and volunteers of the American Diabetes Association have earned my respect over and over. My years with John Graham, Marti Funnell, Mike Weiss, Richard Kahn, Mike Mawby, Caroline Stevens, Jerry Franz, Nathaniel Clark, Shereen Arent, Bronwyn Reynolds, Lisa Murdock, Mike Clinkenbeard, Linda Gledhill, and the boards of directors have been challenging and inspiring. These people, plus thousands of others, have been instrumental in moving the mission of the association forward.

Unending appreciation and accolades go to U.S. Secretary of Health and Human Services Tommy G. Thompson. I have worked by his side, listened to him speak, and been thankful for his visionary leadership. He has made a difference by thoughtfully waging a war against diabesity. The hard-working legions within his department deserve much credit. Surgeon General Richard Carmona has instilled in all of us the desire to help people help themselves. Ann Albright, who is currently working within HHS, has a firm grasp on the issues and enviable abilities—as a result she is able to effect positive change. In addition, I have been particularly inspired by Tracy Self, HHS assistant secretary for public affairs, and her ability to get the word out.

The Department of Health Services in the County of Los Angeles is filled with people dedicated to improving health and combating disease. Under the incredible leadership of Tom Garthwaite, there are places for people to receive compassionate care in the immense county in which I live. Jonathan Fielding has dazzled me with his brilliance, Cindy Harding with her dedication, and Eloisa Gonzales with her humanity.

Zev Yaroslavsky, one of the members of the Los Angeles County Board of Supervisors, exemplifies that diabesity can be triumphed over. Supervisor Yaroslavsky was the push behind the L.A. County Task Force on Youth Fitness, which evaluated the problems of obesity and inactivity among youth in the county. He deserves unending gratitude for putting the citizens of Los Angeles County first at all times. Marlene Canter of the Los Angeles Unified School District School Board has devoted herself to improving the school environment for 700,000 children. She serves as an example for us all. Other elected officials—particularly Henry Waxman, Hilda Solis, Loretta and Linda Sanchez, Alex Padilla, Marta Escutia, Paul Koretz, Debra Ortiz, and Tom Torlakson from California and Valerie Weiner from Nevada—have worked hard to formulate legislation to improve the landscape of our lives.

The hard-working staff at Camp Chinnock made each summer an experience to remember. Neal Halfon, Robert Gottleib, and Robert Ross have devoted themselves to advancing the public's health. The writings of Adam Drewnowski, David Ludwig, Kelly Brownell, Jared Diamond, Eric Schlosser, and Marion Nestle serve as road maps for what needs to be accomplished.

Valerie Ruelas, who is currently the Program Director of the Keck Diabetes Prevention Initiative, worked with me on the L.A. County Task Force and many other L.A. County Department of Health Services programs. She is one of the most capable people I know and someone who can do almost any job. I thank her for her help in reviewing *Diabesity* to assure that I captured the flavor of our joint efforts. Ruth Hirsch, a dedicated diabetes educator, gave me invaluable comments on this manuscript. Ruth and her family are truly immersed in helping people with diabetes. Cynthia Landes helped in the early versions of *Diabesity*. Her guidance and encouragement were critical in helping me feel I could go on with my writing. Rosa Soto of the Center for Public Health Advocacy willingly reviewed scenes and facts and served as inspiration, and Harold Goldstein, at the same center, showed me time and time again that dedicated people can make a difference.

The day I met Greg Critser, author of *Fat Land*, I started feeling that I had a torrent of stories inside me about diabesity. I am grateful to him for encouraging me to let that torrent out—and for standing by to ensure I did not drown in the process.

Dena Chwan and Joyce Ho were the most dedicated and industrious research assistants I could have hoped for in mining data for *Diabesity*. They endured my many e-mails, reading segment after segment to check on details. Their careful work made a difficult process much easier.

Debbie Birns, a cherished friend, helped me with my first trial at writing. Thanks to her encouragement, I did not stop writing. I also want to thank Chuck Hurewitz for advice and guidance.

I am grateful to Adam Chromy, my literary agent. He found me one day in Minnesota and told me this book needed to be written. He never lost faith in me even during the times when I was ready to give up. My editor, Toni Burbank, helped form the vision of what *Diabesity* was to be and extracted the best from me. My thanks to her are effusive. Toni's brilliance was obvious in every suggestion she made about *Diabesity*. I want to express appreciation for the extraordinary support and enthusiasm I received from my publisher, Bantam. I always presumed there was an army of people behind each book published, but the army at Bantam was even more impressive than I had imagined. My book benefited greatly from the critical input of three insightful writers: Anita Bartholomew, Sally Wendkos Olds, and Barbara Sofer. I am also thankful for the careful, intelligent review by Willie Lockeretz. But my deepest thanks goes to Sarah Wernick. Sarah dedicated her time and effort—and her brilliance—to transforming *Diabesity* into something that non-medical people could understand and appreciate. She was meticulous, tenacious, and my guide. She was a virtual zen master.

From the time I was four years old, I never wavered in my commitment to my father to become a physician. I treasure my memories of the days I sat by his side, listening to his medical lectures and stories. However, it was really my mother who enabled me to succeed as a doctor. For twelve years—from the time my children entered middle school until they finished college—she helped run my household. She put dinner on the table and she had an answer for every problem. Though she tried to protect me from myself when she thought I was taking on too much, I know my accomplishments filled her with pride. I miss her commitment to giving my family fresh food and love every day.

Delmi (Lupe) Pena, whom I met the day she was diagnosed with diabetes at age eight, has brightened my home while she has gone to college and now graduate school. She showed me how someone with diabetes can succeed and enjoy life. She is my inspiration.

Lance Kinkead earned my respect and love the day he entered my life. He taught me more about diabetes than anyone or anything else. My heart is filled with thanks for the honor of being first his doctor and then his family. With his wife Sussie and his children Saige and Bryce, he has filled my house with laughter.

Barry Behrstock (who brilliantly helped edit every word of *Diabesity*), Gwen Behrstock, Tobi Inlender, Nachum Inlender, Nan Zaitlen, Richard Zaitlen, and Benita Sakin are the best friends anyone could ever have. For decades, they have filled my life with good times and warmth. They each gave me invaluable advice and were by my side late at night while I was picking away at my computer.

My sons Adam and Jonah have participated in every aspect of my career, learning all the diabetes jargon and intricacies. When they were growing up, they joined me on medical missions and at diabetes camp—and they hardly ever complained. Now they are young adults and I'm proud that they've chosen to work on diabetes solutions at this early point in their careers. I thank them for enthusiastically reading my manuscript and for providing valuable suggestions. Most of all, I thank them for making being a mom the most rewarding aspect of my life.

I can't do justice to my husband Neal in print. No matter what I have tried to do in my life, he has stood by my side, with advice, support, and love. He has helped me rewrite and realign *Diabesity*—he's read numerous drafts of every chapter and has gone over everything in detail, with endless patience and good humor. He encouraged me, brought me sustenance, and let me know how proud he was of my accomplishment. I have built a professional and personal life with him that has brought me honor. Simply, he has been the most supportive and loving husband any woman physician, or any woman at all, could ever hope to have.

Index

ABOUT THE AUTHOR

FRANCINE RATNER KAUFMAN, M.D., is a past president of the American Diabetes Association; head, Center for Diabetes, Endocrinology and Metabolism at Childrens Hospital Los Angeles; and professor of pediatrics, Keck School of Medicine of the University of Southern California. The author of more than 150 articles, she is also a tireless public advocate who was instrumental in banning the sale of soda in the L.A. Unified School District. She lives in Los Angeles with her husband and is the mother of two sons.